AF323681

The Scientific Basis of Tissue Transplantation

Advances in Tissue Banking Vol. 5

The Scientific Basis of Tissue Transplantation

Editor-in-Chief

G O Phillips

Research Transfer Ltd, Cardiff, Wales, UK

Volume Editor

A Nather

National University Hospital Tissue Bank, Singapore

Regional Editors

D M Strong

Puget Sound Blood Center, USA

R von Versen (Europe)

German Institute for Cell and Tissue Replacement, Germany

World Scientific
New Jersey • London • Singapore • Hong Kong

Published by

World Scientific Publishing Co. Pte. Ltd.

P O Box 128, Farrer Road, Singapore 912805

USA office: Suite 1B, 1060 Main Street, River Edge, NJ 07661

UK office: 57 Shelton Street, Covent Garden, London WC2H 9HE

British Library Cataloguing-in-Publication Data
A catalogue record for this book is available from the British Library.

ISBN 981-02-4583-1

Printed in Singapore by FuIsland Offset Printing

ADVANCES IN TISSUE BANKING

International Advisory Board

LIST OF CONTRIBUTORS

JIRI ADLER
Tissue Bank University Hospital
Brno, Czech Republic

KENNETH M.C. CHEUNG
Department of Orthopaedic Surgery
The University of Hong Kong
The Duchess of Kent Children's Hospital
12 Sandy Bay Road, Hong Kong

JOHN CHIA
Department of Orthopaedic Surgery
National University Hospital
Lower Kent Ridge Road, Singapore 119074

LOUIS T.C. CHOW
Department of Anatomical & Cellular Pathology
The Chinese University of Hong Kong
Prince of Wales Hospital, Shatin, NT, Hong Kong, SAR

KHAIRUL ZAMAN HAJI MOHD DAHLAN
Radiation Processing Technology Division
Malaysian Institute for Nuclear Technology Research (MINT)
Bangi, 43000 Kajang, Selangor, Malaysia

MALCOLM DAVIES
Institute of Nephrology
University of Wales College of Medicine
Heath Park, Cardiff CF14 4XN, Wales, UK

MOHMOOD FARAZDAGHI
International Federation of Eye Banks
Tissue Banks International, 815 Park Avenue
Baltimore, MD 21201, USA

SAMEERA M. FARAZDAGHI
Johns Hopkins University
Johns Hopkins School of Hygiene and Public Health
615 N Wolfe Street, Baltimore, MD 21205, USA

LINDA L.-K. FU
Musculoskeletal Tissue Bank
at Sir Y.K. Pao Centre for Cancer
The Chinese University of Hong Kong
Prince of Wales Hospital, Shatin, NT, Hong Kong, SAR

JAMES GRIFFITH
Department of Diagnostic Radiology & Organ Imaging
The Chinese University of Hong Kong
Prince of Wales Hospital, Shatin, NT, Hong Kong, SAR

HO KEE HAI
Department of Oral and Maxillofacial Surgery
National University Hospital
Lower Kent Ridge Road, Singapore 119074

N. HILMY
Batan Research Tissue Bank
Centre for Research and Development of Isotopes
and Radiation Technology
National Nuclear Energy Agency of Indonesia
Jalan Cinere Ps. Jumat
P.O. Box 7002, Jakarta 12070 JKSKL
Indonesia

CHARANJIT KAUR
Department of Anatomy, Faculty of Medicine
National University of Singapore
4 Medical Drive, MD10, Singapore 117597

JAN KOLLER
Ruzinov General Hospital
Centre for Burns and Reconstructive Surgery
Central Tissue Bank, Ruzinovka 6, 82606 Bratislava
Slovak Republic

GAMINI KUMARASINGHE
Division of Microbiology
Department of Laboratory Medicine
National University Hospital
5 Lower Kent Ridge Road, Singapore 119074

SHEKHAR M. KUMTA
Department of Orthopaedics & Traumatology
The Chinese University of Hong Kong
Prince of Wales Hospital, Shatin, NT, Hong Kong, SAR

P.C. LEUNG
Department of Orthopaedics & Traumatology
The Chinese University of Hong Kong
Prince of Wales Hospital, Shatin, NT, Hong Kong, SAR

M. LINA
Batan Research Tissue Bank
Centre for Research and Development of Isotopes and
Radiation Technology
National Nuclear Energy Agency of Indonesia
Jalan Cinere Ps. Jumat
P.O. Box 7002, Jakarta 12070 JKSKL
Indonesia

KEITH D.K. LUK
Department of Orthopaedic Surgery
The University of Hong Kong
The Duchess of Kent Children's Hospital
12 Sandy Bay Road, Hong Kong

HASIM MOHAMAD
Department of Surgery, Hospital Kota Bharu
155867 Kota Bharu, Kelantan, Malaysia
and
National Tissue Bank
Hospital University Sains Malaysia
Kubang Kerian, 16150 Kota Bharu, Kelantan, Malaysia

KEITH MOORE
Clinical Research Laboratory
Wound Management Division
Smith & Nephew Medical Limited
Imperial House, Imperial Way
Newport, South Wales NP10 8UH, UK

S.Z. MORDIFFI
Major Operating Theatre Suite
Nursing Department, National University Hospital
5 Lower Kent Ridge Road, Singapore 119074

AZIZ NATHER
NUH Tissue Bank
National University Hospital
5 Lower Kent Ridge Road, Singapore 119074

KAREN A. NELSON
Puget Sound Blood Center
921 Terry Avenue, Seattle, WA 98104
USA

BARRY P. PEREIRA
Department of Orthopaedic Surgery
National University Hospital
Lower Kent Ridge Road, Singapore 119074

GLYN O. PHILLIPS
Research Transfer Ltd
2 Plymouth Drive
Radyr, Cardiff CF15 8BL, UK

JOSEPH THAMBIAH
Department of Orthopaedic Surgery
National University Hospital
Lower Kent Ridge Road, Singapore 119074

P. THIAGARAJAN
Division of Adult Reconstructive Surgery
Department of Orthopaedic Surgery
National University Hospital
Lower Kent Ridge Road, Singapore 119074

GARETH J. THOMAS
Institute of Nephrology
University of Wales College of Medicine
Heath Park, Cardiff CF14 4XN, Wales, UK

M. YEGAPPAN
Division of Adult Reconstructive Surgery
Department of Orthopaedic Surgery
National University Hospital
Lower Kent Ridge Road, Singapore 119074

CHANG JOON YIM
Dankook University School of Dentistry
Infirmary Dental Hospital and Dankook University Hospital
Department of Oral & Maxillofacial Surgery
7-1 Sinbudong, Cheonan, 330-716, Republic of Korea

NORIMAH YUSOF
Tissue Bank
Malaysian Institute for Nuclear Technology Research (MINT)
Bangi, 43000 Kajang, Selangor, Malaysia

PREFACE

This Preface need only be short, since the rationale and basis for the volume is given below in the Introduction. My objective now is to acknowledge the central role of Professor Aziz Nather in editing and planning this volume. As the Director of the International Atomic Energy Agency Training Courses in tissue banking at the Regional Centre at the National University Hospital in Singapore, he recognised the need for the tissue banker, not only to be well versed in the production techniques, but also in the scientific principles which underpin the entire subject. With such an inter-disciplinary subject, access to the various scientific and medically-related materials is often difficult for the student. In the one-year National University of Singapore University Diploma Course which he initiated, Prof. Nather, therefore, introduced lectures by specialists which covered these associated subjects. It then became even clearer that the student did not have access to appropriate texts to study the subject in more depth. Consequently, this volume was conceived. It now provides another building unit to give the tissue banker and tissue user a foundation to the subject. He is uniquely qualified to pilot this volume, for he himself is both a tissue banker and user, and additionally a pioneering educationalist in the subject. The product in this volume will prove valuable to all involved in tissue banking and provide a ready reference to the various scientific basic parts of the field. We must all thank him and congratulate him and his colleagues on the outcome.

Glyn O. Phillips
Editor-in-Chief

CONTENTS

List of Contributors   vii

Preface   xiii

Introduction   xix

Section I: Anatomy

Chapter 1   Anatomy of the Upper Limb   3

Chapter 2   Anatomy of the Lower Limb   25

Chapter 3   Anatomy of the Spine   42

Chapter 4   Anatomy of the Pelvis   51

Chapter 5   Anatomy of the Oral Maxillofacial Region   58

Section II: Matrix Biology and Physiology of Tissues

Chapter 6   The Organisation of the Extracellular Matrix   73

Chapter 7   Histology of Bone   97

Chapter 8   Histology of Cartilage   115

Chapter 9   Basic Anatomy and Physiology of Human Skin   123

Chapter 10   Anatomy and Embryology of Human Placenta, Amnion and Chorion   139

Chapter 11   Electron Microscopy of Human Amniotic Membrane   149

Section III: Microbiology

Chapter 12 Introduction to Medical Microbiology   175

Chapter 13 Bioburden Estimation in Relation to
Sterilisation   200

Chapter 14 Transmissible Diseases of Particular
Importance in the Immunocompromised
and Transplant Recipients   212

Section IV: Sterile Techniques

Chapter 15 Principles of Sterile Technique   235

Chapter 16 Sterile Procurement of Bones and Ligaments   265

Chapter 17 Sterile Preparation of Tissue Grafts During
Transplantation   291

Section V: Radiation Sciences

Chapter 18 Radiation Sciences   309

Chapter 19 Effect of Radiation on Microorganisms —
Mechanism of Radiation Sterilisation   342

Chapter 20 Effects of Ionising Radiation on Viruses,
Proteins and Prions   358

Section VI: Biology of Healing of Allografts

Chapter 21 The Scientific Basis of Wound Healing   379

Chapter 22 Skin and Amnion Grafts   398

Chapter 23 The Role of BMP in Bone Incorporation   419

Chapter 24 Biology of Healing of Large Deep-Frozen
Cortical Bone Allografts   434

Chapter 25 The Biology of Massive Bone Allografts:
Understanding Allograft Biology
and Adapting it Towards Successful
Clinical Application   455

Chapter 26 Effect of Growth Factors on Healing and the
Clinical Applications of Autogenous Platelet
Rich Plasma Gel to Enhance Bone Formation   473

Chapter 27 Biology and Biomechanics of Anterior
Cruciate Ligament Allograft Reconstruction   491

Section VII: Biomechanics of Allografts

Chapter 28 Some Principles of Biomechanics —
Structural and Material Properties   507

Chapter 29 Biomechanics of Bone Allograft
Transplantation   534

Section VIII: Immunology

Chapter 30 Basic Principles of Transplantation
Immunology   553

Subject Index   567

INTRODUCTION

AZIZ NATHER and GLYN O. PHILLIPS

1. Background

The International Atomic Energy Agency (IAEA) through its programme "Radiation Sterilisation of Tissue Grafts", produced a distance learning package on the procedures involved in tissue banking, particularly in the application of radiation to sterilise tissues (Nather, 1999a; 1999b; Phillips and Strong, 1999; Nather, 2000a; 2000b; Phillips, 2000). The individual modules are: 0 — Historical Background; 1 — Rules and Regulations; 2 — Organisation; 3 — Quality Assurance; 4 — Procurement; 5 — Processing; 6 — Distribution & Utilisation; 7 — Future Developments in Tissue Banking. This curriculum has been used extensively throughout the Asia Pacific region itself, and in other regions such as Latin America, Africa and parts of Europe.

The IAEA draft curriculum was first piloted in Singapore during the IAEA/RCA Workshop on Tissue Banking in September 1995. Consequently, IAEA established a Regional Training Centre in the National University Hospital, Singapore to train tissue bank operators in the Asia Pacific region using the curriculum. Since then, the training centre has conducted several distance learning programmes for tissue-bank operators in the region.

To enable this development to proceed effectively, the Singapore Government (Ministry of Environment) provided a grant to the NUH Tissue Bank through the National Science and Technology Board to develop the centre to be equipped with facilities for hands-on training. This grant also provided for sufficient funds to convert the draft curriculum into a multimedia curriculum. The National

University Hospital provided the space in which the NUH Tissue Bank was constructed. Both NUH and NUS contributed renovation funds for the building of a purpose-built tissue bank with a reception area, documentation room, wet processing and dry processing laboratories as well as a library for resource materials in tissue procurement and processing, and in tissue transplantation.

Simultaneously, the National University of Singapore (NUS) approved the development of a one-year distance learning Diploma Course in Tissue Banking to be conducted by the NUH Tissue Bank at the NUS Training Centre. The syllabus for the Diploma Course basically consisted of three components: the multimedia curriculum on tissue banking, a basic sciences component and a recommended textbook — the book selected being the series *Advances in Tissue Banking*. With these three components together, a comprehensive training could be provided.

With funds from the Singapore Government in April 1998, a multimedia element could be introduced. This required further editing of text from draft to module and the editing of illustrative materials into video demonstrations of not more than 30 minutes each. Special box containers were designed to house each module to include a booklet, accompanying videotapes and illustrative case slides from the region and available reference texts. With the first module, an audiocassette was introduced with instructions on how to use the distance learning package. The complete package — seven box containers in all, was distributed to all tissue banks in the Asia Pacific member states. In April 1998, a "Train the Trainers" workshop was held in Singapore to instruct the national trainers on the use of multimedia curriculum. Since then, this multimedia curriculum has replaced the draft curriculum as the first component of the syllabus for the Diploma Course.

The University Diploma Course is conducted over a period of one-year. First, the trainees attend a face-to-face two-week intensive training course in Singapore. Over the subsequent year, they are given progressive study of the curriculum, guided by National Coordinators. Over this period, they pursue a number of practical and written assignments which are then remitted to the University for assessment. Finally, at the end of the year, they return to Singapore for the final examination. The overall diploma is awarded by continuous assessment over the entire one-year course.

Development has continued regularly. The seven videotapes have now been converted into two compact discs contained in a jewel case. The curriculum has been in great demand. The initial 100 sets produced were quickly exhausted. Therefore, another 250 sets were produced in April 2000. The multimedia curriculum package has been further redesigned to have all the seven module booklets conveniently housed in one specially printed box container, which contains the seven modules, two compact discs, an audiocassette and a new updated textbook as a companion volume to the multimedia curriculum. This new compact design makes the distribution of the curriculum more convenient. The updated volume *Radiation and Tissue Banking* (2000) was written by experts contracted by IAEA and printed with funds from the Singapore Government. It is an appropriate companion volume to the IAEA multimedia curriculum. It was released in July 2000 and provided free of charge to tissue banks in the member states throughout the world.

2. The Present Development

The basic sciences component of the syllabus for the Diploma Course, which is presented in the training course, includes subjects such as Anatomy, Matrix Biology and Physiology of Tissues, Microbiology, Sterile Techniques, Radiation Sciences, Biology of Healing of Allografts, Biomechanics of Allografts and Immunology. It was quickly realised that students found difficulty in obtaining basic text for this part of the Diploma Course curriculum. Available specialist textbooks on the diverse subjects addressed, such as Anatomy, Microbiology, Immunology etc., were too detailed to meet the needs of the Diploma students. It was therefore decided to produce a specifically-designed specialist textbook incorporating the various topics and to be directed at the appropriate level so as to address the specific needs of the Diploma Course students and generally that of the tissue banker, tissue procurer, tissue processer and tissue transplanter. This textbook is written with this objective in mind. Authors were selected to write the various chapters, with specific instructions to address the needs of tissue-bank operators.

Section I: Anatomy

Tissue bankers need to have a basic knowledge of anatomy of the various regions ranging from the upper limb, lower limb, spine, pelvis to the maxillo-facial region. Several tissue-bank operators without a medical background will find this section especially useful when carrying out their daily work. Personnel with a medical background will also find this section a joy to read, rather than having to access detailed texts from anatomy textbooks since no textbook of anatomy for tissue-bank operators exists. Technologists too can now understand better the anatomy of the tissues they have been procuring or processing, and also the types of tissues that could be used for different anatomical regions.

Section II: Matrix Biology & Physiology of Tissues

The microscopic structure of tissues are detailed in this section, starting with the extracellular matrix, bone, cartilage, skin and amnion. Again, the major attractive feature is its descriptive nature with excellent illustrations. Worthy of mention is a special chapter on electron microscopy of the amnion, a tissue widely used in the Asia Pacific region.

Section III: Microbiology

Microbiology is a very important subject for tissue bankers and tissue transplant surgeons alike. The basic concepts in medical microbiology are carefully explained. Bioburden estimation itself merits one whole chapter. Equally important is the knowledge of the various transmissible diseases. Tissue bankers seek to maintain a high quality control standard to ensure safe tissue transplantation practice. No efforts must be spared to prevent possible disease transmission during tissue transplantation. It is therefore important that tissue-bank operators have a good knowledge of the seriousness of these diseases, including AIDS, Hepatitis B and C, and syphilis.

Section IV: Sterile Techniques

To achieve high quality control standards, tissue procurement should be performed as far as possible under sterile conditions. One whole chapter is devoted to the principles of aseptic technique from scrubbing techniques, monitoring of sterility in the operating room to methods of sterilisation of equipment and materials. Another chapter is devoted to procuring tissues under sterile conditions and a third chapter to ensuring that the tissues transplanted are prepared in the correct aseptic manner so as to avoid the much dreaded complication of infection. Again, excellent illustrations have been used to make the text more readable and easier to understand.

Section V: Radiation Sciences

This section contains chapters written by three radiation scientists. The basic principles of radiation sciences are presented in the first chapter with good illustrations, so that technologists with medical background and no training in the radiation sciences can better appreciate the principles of ionising radiations. The second chapter deals with the effect of radiation on microorganisms and the third the effect of radiation on viruses, proteins and prions.

Section VI: Biology of Healing of Allografts

The biology of the healing of tissues is described, starting from the scientific basis of wound healing to the healing of the skin and amnion, and the healing of bones and ligaments. The role of various growth factors, including bone morphogenetic proteins and platelet-derived growth factor to promote bone healing, is also described and discussed in greater detail.

This section is important to surgeons who use allografts and who need to understand how the transplanted tissues heal so that they can choose more wisely the right type of graft for the various clinical conditions they encounter. In this way, better results can be obtained and complications minimised. Similarly, tissue bankers who prepare the tissue grafts will also better understand the functions of the various types of tissues they process.

Section VII: Biomechanics of Allografts

The first chapter is written by a mechanical engineer to introduce the basic concepts of biomechanics, and which could be readily understood by the tissue-bank technologists. Ample illustrations have been used to make this section user-friendly. In another chapter, the structural requirements of bone allografts for the various reconstructions performed are described by an orthopaedic surgeon, covering deep-frozen cortical bone allografts for massive allograft reconstruction of lower limbs requiring weight-bearing functions, the adequacy of lyophilised cortical allografts for massive spine reconstruction and the adequacy of lyophilised morsellised bone allografts for packing cavities in bones.

Section VIII: Immunology

This last section, written by an immunologist, outlines the basic principles of the immunology of tissue transplantation. This is vital both for the end-users (surgeons), using the bone allografts to avoid the dreaded complication of immune rejection and resulting infection and for the tissue-bank operators who need to process the tissue grafts to eliminate as much as possible any immunogenic properties of the tissue graft products.

3. References

NATHER, A. (1999a). Tissue banking in Asia Pacific region — The Asia Pacific Association of Surgical Tissue Banking. In: *Advances in Tissue Banking*, Vol. 3, G.O. Phillips, R. von Versen, M. Strong and A. Nather, eds., World Scientific, Singapore, pp. 419–425.

NATHER, A. (1999b). Tissue Banking in the Asia Pacific region: current status and future developments, *J. Orthop. Surg.* **7**(2), 89–93.

NATHER, A. (2000a). Diploma training for technologists in tissue banking, *Cell And Tissue Banking* **1**(1), 41–44.

NATHER, A. (2000b). Tissue banking in Asia Pacific region — Ethical, legal, religious, cultural and other regulatory aspects, *J. ASEAN Orthop. Assoc.* **13**(1), 60–63.

PHILLIPS, G.O. (2000). The future role of the International Atomic Energy Agency (IAEA), *Cell and Tissue Banking* **1**, 27–40.

PHILLIPS G.O. and STRONG D.M. (1999). The contribution of the International Atomic Energy Agency (IAEA) to tissue banking. In: *Advances in Tissue Banking*, Vol. 3, G.O. Phillips, R. von Versen, M. Strong and A. Nather, eds., World Scientific, Singapore, pp. 403–417.

SECTION I:

ANATOMY

Advances in Tissue Banking Vol. 5
© 2001 by World Scientific Publishing Co. Pte. Ltd.

1 ANATOMY OF THE UPPER LIMB

JOHN CHIA

Department of Orthopaedic Surgery
National University Hospital
Lower Kent Ridge Road, Singapore 119074

1. Introduction

The upper limb of man is built for prehension. The hand is a grasping mechanism, with four fingers flexing against an opposed thumb. The hand is a major tactile organ. It is provided with a rich nerve supply for this function. In order to be able to grasp in any position, the forearm is provided with a range of 180 degrees of pronation and supination, and at the elbow, has a range of flexion and extension of similar amount. In addition, free mobility is provided at the shoulder joint, and this mobility is further increased by the mobility of the pectoral girdle through which the upper limb articulates with the axial skeleton.

All vertebrates possess four limbs. The limbs are connected to the axial skeleton by means of bones known as the pectoral and pelvic girdles. The pectoral girdle does not articulate with the vertebral column. In many vertebrates, it does not articulate with the axial skeleton at all; in these, it consists only of a shoulder blade slung in muscle, the clavicle being absent or so rudimentary as to be functionless. The muscles act as shock absorbers, the weight of the bounding body being received on a fore limb that articulates with a very mobile shoulder blade. Muscles developed in the upper limb are supplied by branches from the brachial plexus.

2. Osteology

2.1. Scapular region (Fig. 1)

2.1.1. The clavicle:

- pivots on its sternal attachment, resulting in extensive movement of the scapula on the chest wall
- Moves at the following three joints:
  - **the sternoclavicular joint**
  - **the coracoclavicular ligament**
  - **the acromioclavicular joint**
- keeps the scapula and humerus lateral (**coracoclavicular ligament and medial articular disc**)

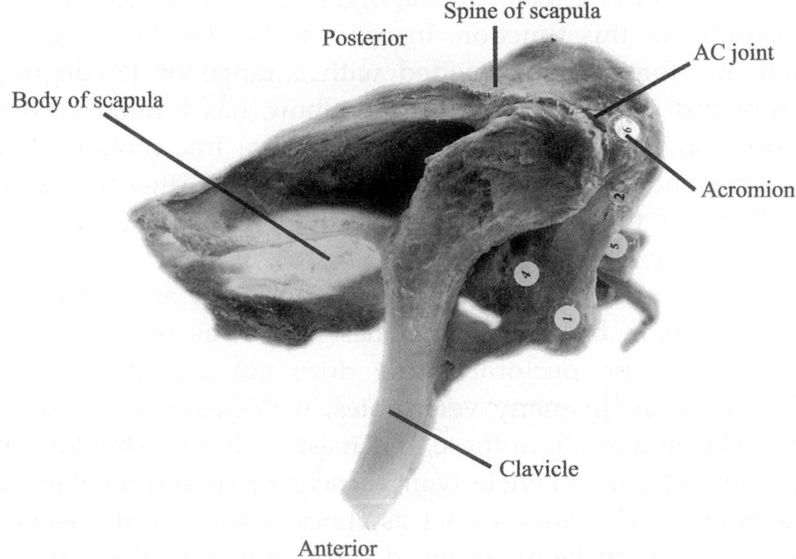

Fig. 1. Superior view of left scapula/clavicle.

2.2. Proximal half of humerus (Fig. 2)

- Head with articular surface
- Anatomical neck
- Lesser tubercle (anterior in anatomical position)
- Intertubercular (bicipital) groove
- Greater tubercle
- Surgical neck
- Deltoid tuberosity
- Posterior spiral groove (for the radial nerve)

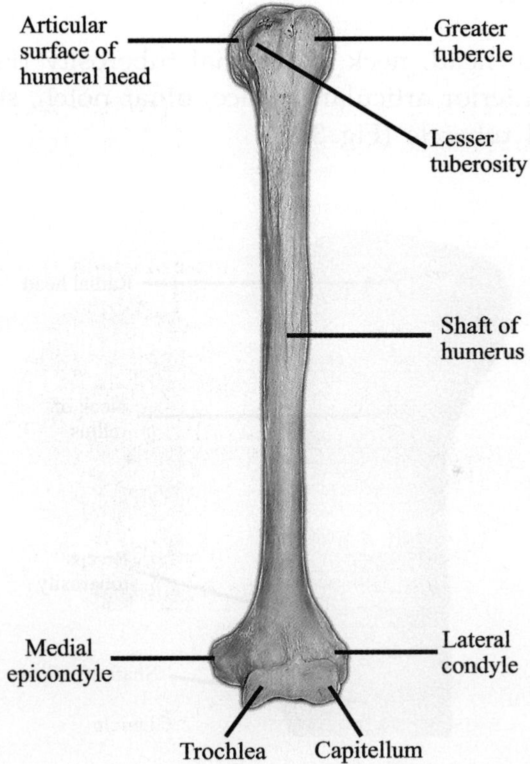

Fig. 2. Anterior view of left humerus.

3. Arm and Cubital Fossa

3.1. Distal half of the humerus (Fig. 2)

- Articular surfaces: **capitellum** and **trochlea**
- Non-articular surfaces: **medial** and **lateral epicondyles** with **medial** and **lateral supracondylar ridges** (attachments for intermuscular septa)
  * The lateral supracondylar ridge ascends to the **spiral groove**.
- Three fossae: **olecranon (posterior), coronoid (anterior)** and **radial fossae**

3.2. Radius

- Proximal end: head, neck and radial tuberosity (Fig. 3(a))
- Distal end: inferior articular surface, ulnar notch, styloid process, dorsal radial tubercle (Fig. 3(b))

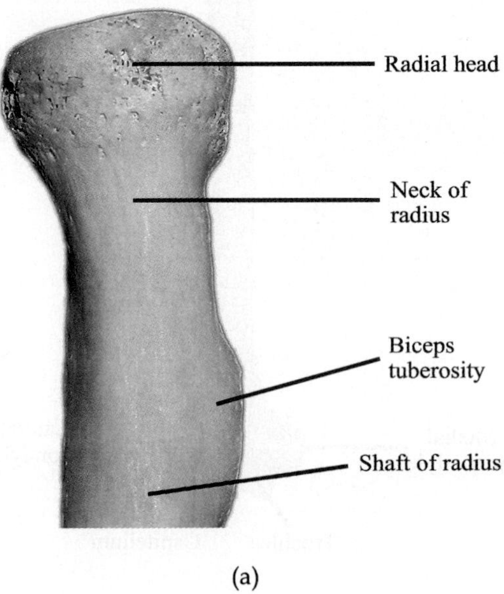

(a)

Fig. 3(a). Proximal end of radius.

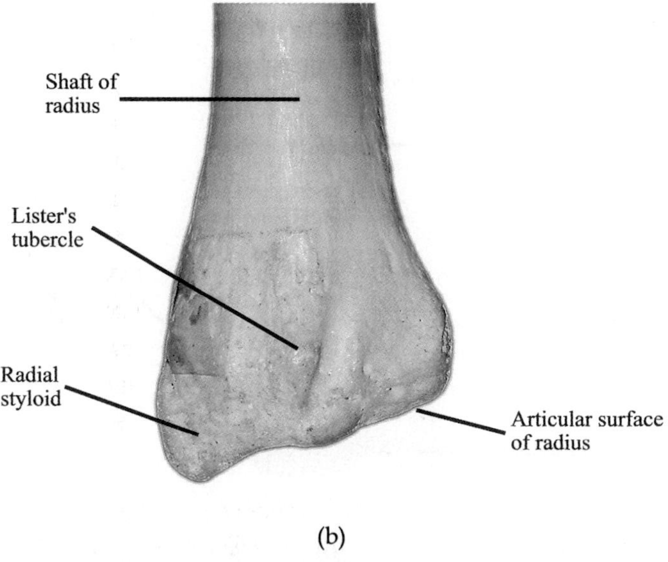

(b)

Fig. 3(b). Distal end of radius (Dorsal view).

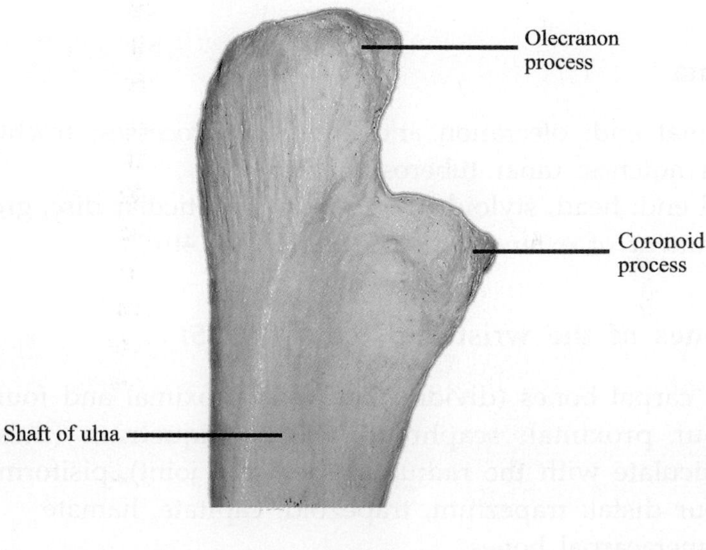

(a)

Fig. 4(a). Proximal end of ulna.

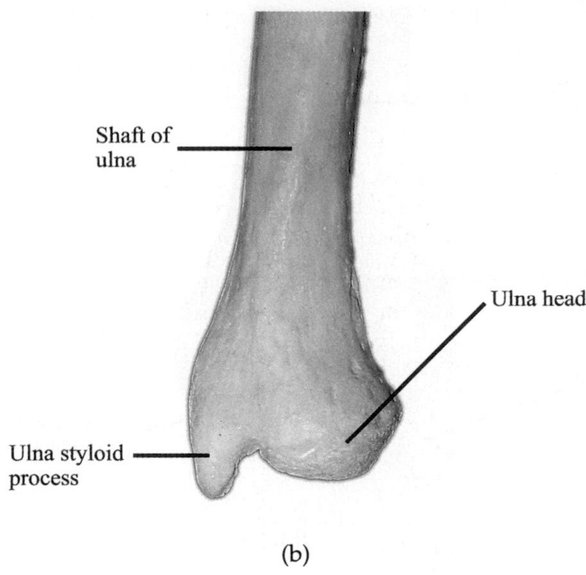

(b)

Fig. 4(b). Distal left ulna.

3.3. Ulna

- Proximal end: olecranon and coronoid processes; trochlear and radial notches; ulnar tuberosity (Fig. 4(a))
- Distal end: head, styloid process, pit for articular disc, groove for attachment of extensor carpi ulnaris (Fig. 4b)

3.4. Bones of the wrist and hand (Fig. 5)

- Eight carpal bones (divided into four proximal and four distal)
  — Four proximal: scaphoid, lunate, triquetrum (these three articulate with the radius at the wrist joint), pisiform
  — Four distal: trapezium, trapezoid, capitate, hamate
- Five metacarpal bones
- 14 phalanges: three on each finger, two for the thumb
  — On each finger, proximal phalanx = 1, middle = 2, and distal = 3

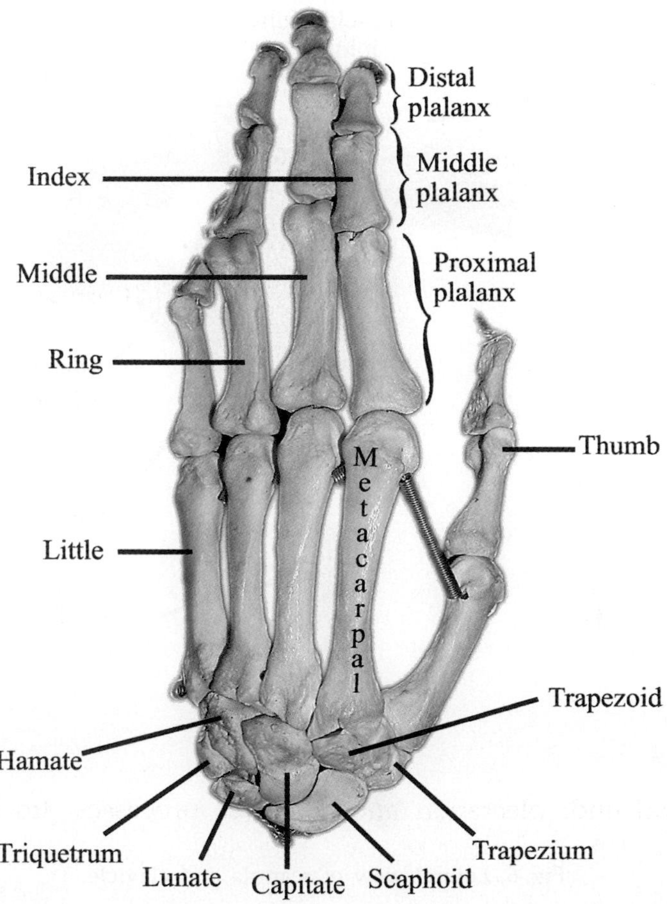

Fig. 5. Dorsal view of left hand-bones.

4. Joints of the Upper Limb

4.1. Shoulder joint (Figs. 1 & 6)

- Multi-axial ball (head of humerus) and socket (glenoid cavity on scapula) joint
- The glenoid labrum (fibrocartilage) runs around the rim of the cavity

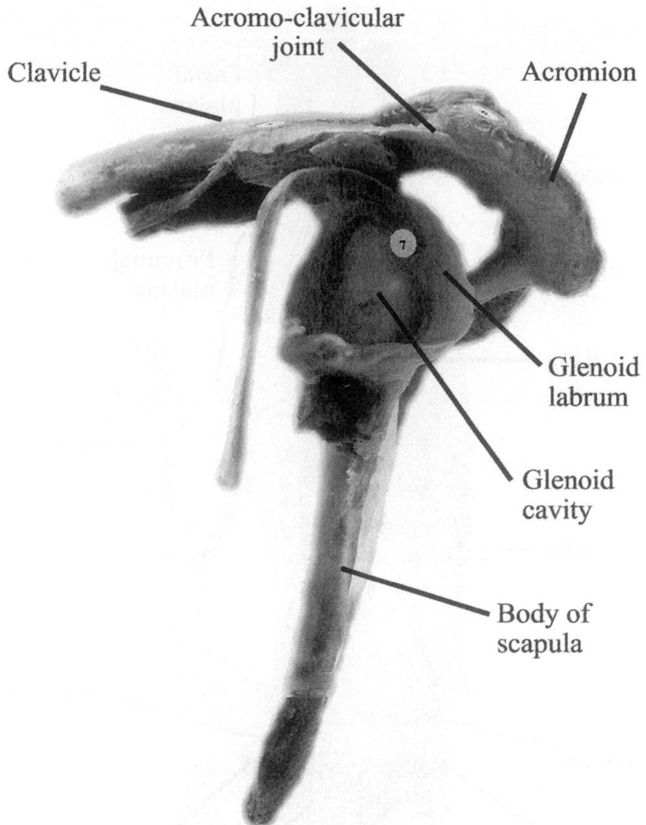

Fig. 6. Lateral view of scapula and clavicle.

- Flex, extend, adduct and abduct (circumduct)
- Medial and lateral rotation

5. The Elbow Joint (Fig. 7)

- Hinge joint
- The capsule is loose anteriorly and posteriorly for flexion and extension
- The collateral ligaments prevent medial and lateral displacement

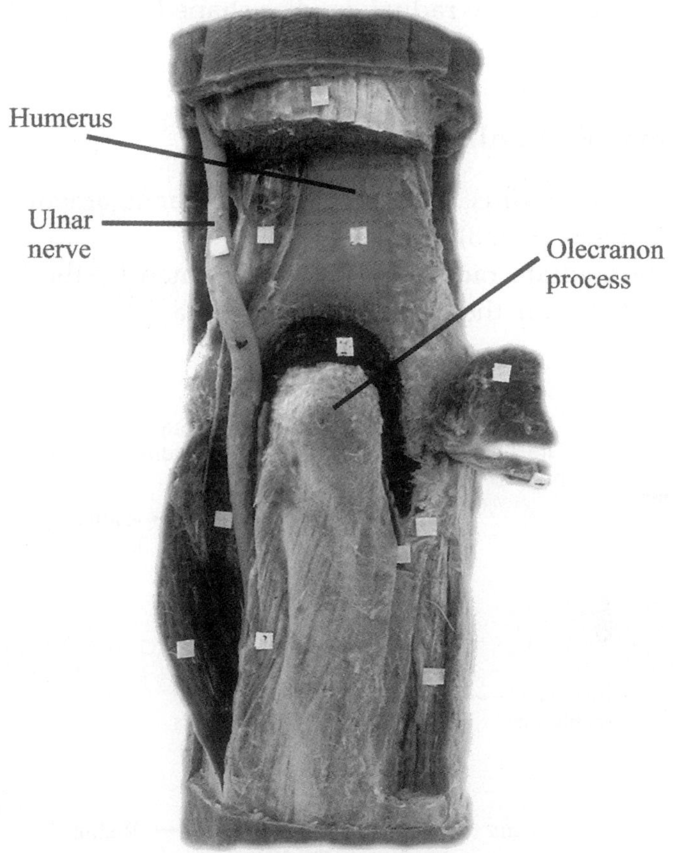

Fig. 7. Posterior view of right elbow.

Distal end of the humerus:

- trochlea and capitellum
- coronoid fossa (anteriorly) and olecranon fossa (posteriorly)

Proximal end of ulna:

- coronoid process (with radial notch laterally and tuberosity anteriorly for attachment of the brachialis tendon)
- olecranon process (subcutaneous olecranon bursa) (Figs. 7 & 8)
- trochlear (semilunar) notch

Proximal head of the radius is disc-shaped and rotates on the capitellum.

6. Proximal Radioulnar Joint

The head of the radius is held by the annular ligament attached to the radial notch (Fig. 8).

The **intermediate radioulnar joint** is formed by the interosseous membrane between the radius and the ulna.

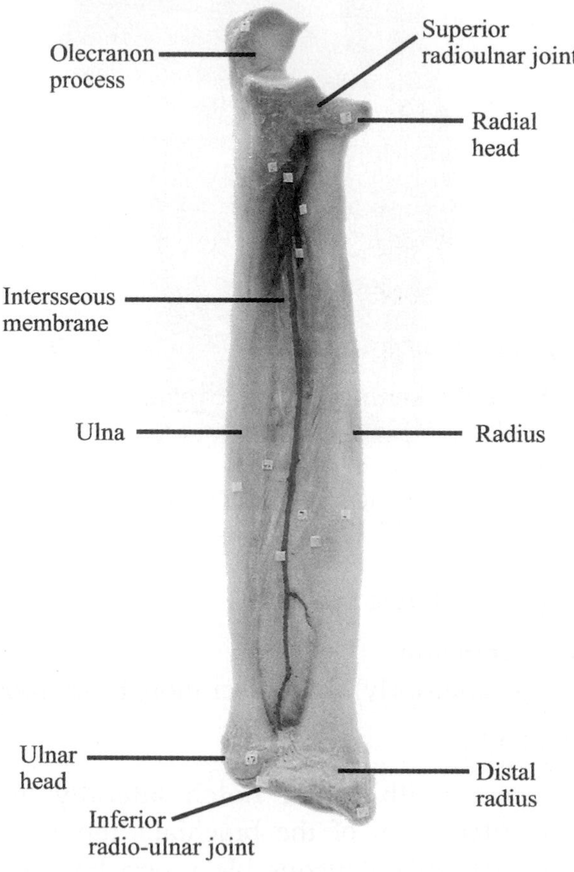

Fig. 8.

7. The Distal Radioulnar Joint (Fig. 8)

- The head of the ulna has a semicircular surface for the ulnar notch of the radius and a distal semilunar surface for the triangular articular disc attached to the fovea, at the base of the styloid process. This articular disc separates the distal radioulnar joint from the radiocarpal joint

8. The Wrist (Radiocarpal) Joint

This is formed by the inferior articular surface of the radius and the articular disc (Fig. 8).

9. Metacarpophalangeal Joints

- can flex and extend
- the collateral ligaments are taut on flexion and slack on extension
- can abduct and adduct only when the joint is extended.

The extensor expansions serve dorsally as ligaments.

The palmar ligaments or plates (volar accessory ligaments)

- are formed by a thickening of the capsule
- are united by the deep transverse metacarpal ligaments
- prevent the metacarpals from spreading

The **carpometacarpal joint of the thumb** allow for flexion, extension, abduction, adduction and some rotation.

Interphalangeal joints are hinge joints.

10. Muscles in the Upper Limb

10.1. Muscles in the shoulder

10.1.1. Deltoid muscle

- from lateral 1/3 of clavicle, lateral border of acromion and spine of scapula

- to deltoid tuberosity
- **axillary nerve (C5, 6)** from the posterior cord of the brachial plexus

10.1.2. The rotator cuff

This is formed by the following muscles (Fig. 9)

- Subscapularis
- Supraspinatus
- Infraspinatus
- Teres minor

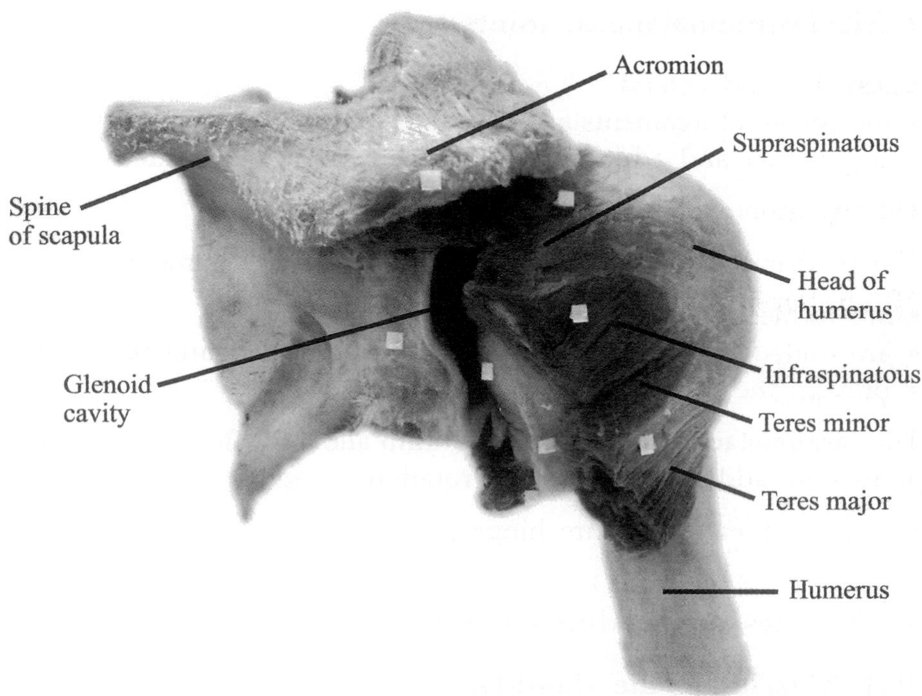

Fig. 9. Posterior view of right shoulder showing rotator cuff muscles.

10.1.3. Muscles of the arm

Anterior compartment

- **coracobrachialis**
- **biceps brachii**
- **brachialis**

All are innervated by the **musculocutaneous nerve (C5, 6)** from the lateral cord of the brachial plexus.

Posterior compartment:
- **triceps brachii** is innervated by the **radial nerve (C5–8, T1)** from the posterior cord of the brachial plexus.

10.1.4. Muscles of the flexor region of the forearm

These are arranged into three layers:

- Superficial layer
- Intermediate layer
- Deep layer

10.1.5. Superficial layer of muscles

- has a common origin from the anterior portion of the medial epicondyle of the humerus
- contains (from medial to ulnar):
  - **pronator teres**
  - **flexor carpi radialis**
  - **palmaris longus**
  - **flexor carpi ulnaris**

10.1.6. Carpal tunnel

- Eight bones of the wrist:
  - proximal (from lateral to medial): scaphoid, lunate, triquetrum, pisiform

— distal (from lateral to medial): trapezium, trapezoid, capitate, hamate
- The flexor retinaculum is attached from the scaphoid and the trapezium on the radial side to the hook of the hamate and the pisiform on the ulnar side

11. Palm of the Hand

11.1. Four layers

- Palmar aponeurosis
- Short muscles of thumb and little finger (for position adjustment and fine movement)
- Long flexor tendons (power of the grip)
- Adductor of the thumb

11.1.1. Surface anatomy of the hand

- The skin of the palm of the hand is ridged and furrowed (fingerprints) for gripping
- Skin creases are due to hand movements
- **Axial line** is the line drawn through the middle finger, capitate and middle metacarpal
- The thumb is set at right angles to four fingers

11.2. Flexor retinaculum

- forms the CARPAL TUNNEL with the carpal bones
- prevents long flexors from bow stringing anteriorly and gives origin to the thenar and hypothenar muscles

11.3. Three thenar muscles

- from flexor retinaculum and tubercles of scaphoid and trapezium
  - **Abductor pollicis brevis** (superficial) to proximal phalanx of thumb

— **Opponens pollicis** to lateral border of thumb metacarpal
— **Flexor pollicis** brevis to base of proximal phalanx of thumb
- innervated by median nerve (C8, T1) and deep branch of ulnar nerve (deep part of flexor pollicis brevis)

11.4. Three hypothenar muscles

- common origin from the flexor retinaculum, pisiform and hook of hamate
  — Abductor digiti V or Minimi to base of proximal phalanx of little digit
  — Flexor brevis digiti V or Minimi to base of proximal phalanx of little digit
  — Opponens digiti V or Minimi to 5th metacarpal bone
- innervated by deep branch of the ulnar nerve

11.5. Lumbricals (four groups)

- arise from flexor digitorum profundus tendons
- lie deep to digital vessels and nerves
- lie radial to fingers
- insert into dorsal extensor expansions beyond interossei
- are innervated by ulnar nerve (medial 2) and by median nerve (lateral 2)
- flex the metacarpophalangeal joints.

12. Extensor Forearm and Dorsum of Hand

12.1. General organisation of muscles in extensor forearm

- Three "outcropping muscles" to thumb divide forearm extensors into lateral and posterior groups, each with its own nerve supply
- An inter-nervous line separates each group of muscles

12.2. Forearm extensors

- From common extensor tendon attached to front of lateral epicondyle, adjacent fascia and supracondylar ridge

12.3. Lateral group

- Brachioradialis
- Extensor carpi radialis longus
- Extensor carpi radialis brevis

Tendons of the extensor carpi muscles cross the snuffbox and pass to bases of the 2nd and 3rd metacarpals, respectively.

12.4. Posterior group

(a) Extensor digitorum (Communis)
 — innervated by posterior interosseous nerve (C7, 8)
(b) Extensor digiti V or minimi
(c) Extensor carpi ulnaris
 — inserts into base of 5th metacarpal
 — innervated by posterior interosseous nerve (C6, 7)
(d) Anconeus
 — from post lateral epicondyle
 — inserts into lateral surface of olecranon and adjacent ulna
 — is innervated by the radial nerve (C7, 8)
 — is a weak extensor of the elbow

12.4.1. Extensor compartment

From lateral to medial
 (i) Abductor pollicis longus and extensor pollicis brevis
 (ii) Extensor carpi radialis longus and brevis
 (iii) Extensor pollicis longus
 (iv) Extensor digitorum communis and extensor indicis

 (v)   Extensor digiti minimi
(vi) Extensor carpi ulnaris

12.5. Interossei muscles

- Innervated by deep ulnar nerve
- Four dorsal (seen on dorsal aspect) arise by double heads from facing sides of bodies of 5 metacarpals. They are abductors (**Dorsal ABduct = DAB**).
- Three palmar interossei arise by single heads from ant. borders of metacarpals 2, 4 and 5, each adducting its own metacarpophalangeal joint (**Palmar ADduct = PAD**).
- Interossei insert into bases of proximal phalanges and into extensor expansions.

13. Upper Limb Arterial Trunk

  (i)   The **subclavian artery** runs to the lateral border of the 1st rib and becomes the **axillary artery**.

 (ii) The axillary artery
     — is enclosed in the axillary sheath (which is continuous with the prevertebral fascia of the neck)
     — is divided into three parts by the pectoralis minor muscle.

(iii) The **brachial artery** begins at the lower border of the teres major and continues to the cubital fossa.

13.1. Axillary artery

This is divided arbitrarily into three parts by the pectoral minor muscle

- one branch from the 1st part: Superior thoracic artery
- two branches from the 2nd part (posterior to pectoralis minor and enclosed by three parts of the brachial plexus
     — thoracoacromial artery (clavicular, acromial, humeral and pectoral branches)
     — lateral thoracic artery (supplying mainly the breast)

- Three branches from the 3rd part
  - subscapular artery
  - posterior humeral circumflex artery
  - anterior humeral circumflex artery

13.2. In the arm

13.2.1. Brachial artery

Throughout the arm, it lies anterior to the triceps brachii and then the brachialis. It divides at the neck of the radius into the **ulnar** and **radial** arteries. Venae comitantes accompany the artery and join the axillary vein.

13.3. Arteries of the hand

Basically, there are four arterial arches in the hand:
  (i) **Superficial palmar arch** (deep to palmar aponeurosis)
  - It is the continuation of the ulnar artery with a variable superficial palmar branch from the radial artery
  - supplies medial 3½ digits (lateral 1½ by deep palmar arch)
  (ii) **Deep palmar arch**
  - Radial artery gives off palmar radial carpal and superficial palmar arteries, then runs lateral to wrist, through anatomical snuffbox, into 1st metacarpal space, through dorsal interosseous muscle and becomes deep palmar arch
  - Completed by deep branch of ulnar artery
  - Two palmar digital branches to lateral 1½ digits
  - Three palmar metacarpal arteries supply interosseous muscles and metacarpals, and form anastomoses with palmar digital branches
  (iii) **Dorsal carpal arch** is applied to dorsal surface of carpal bones
  (iv) **Ventral (palmar) carpal arch** is a network formed by palmar carpal branches of the ulnar and radial arteries, and twigs from the forearm and from the deep palmar arch

14. Innervation of the Upper Limb

In all vertebrates, the skin and muscles of the limbs are supplied by plexuses. The plexuses are formed from the anterior primary rami of spinal nerves. The spinal nerves entering into a limb plexus come from enlarged parts of the cord, the cervical enlargement for the brachial plexus.

The constituents of every limb plexus divide into the anterior and posterior divisions. The anterior divisions of the limb plexus supply the flexor compartment and the posterior divisions supply the extensor compartment of the limb. The flexor compartment has a richer nerve supply than the extensor compartment. The flexor skin is more sensitive than the extensor skin; it has a richer sensory innervation, especially in the distal parts of a limb. Flexor muscles are quicker-acting and under more precise voluntary control. Flexor muscles have a richer innervation than extensor muscles.

In a few cases, muscles near the pre- or post-axial border of a limb receive a double nerve supply. Generally, they are flexor muscles that receive a supply from the nerve of the extensor compartment. The lateral portion of the brachialis (supplied by the radial nerve) is an example of flexor muscles supplied by extensor compartment nerves, and in each case, the remainder of the muscle is in fact supplied by a flexor compartment nerve.

15. Brachial Plexus (Fig. 10)

15.1. Ulnar nerve

- from the medial cord of the brachial plexus [C(7), 8, T1]
- at the elbow, it runs posterior to the medial epicondyle of the humerus and into the forearm. It is accompanied by the superior ulnar collateral artery and the ulnar collateral nerve (a branch of the radial nerve innervating the medial head of the triceps)

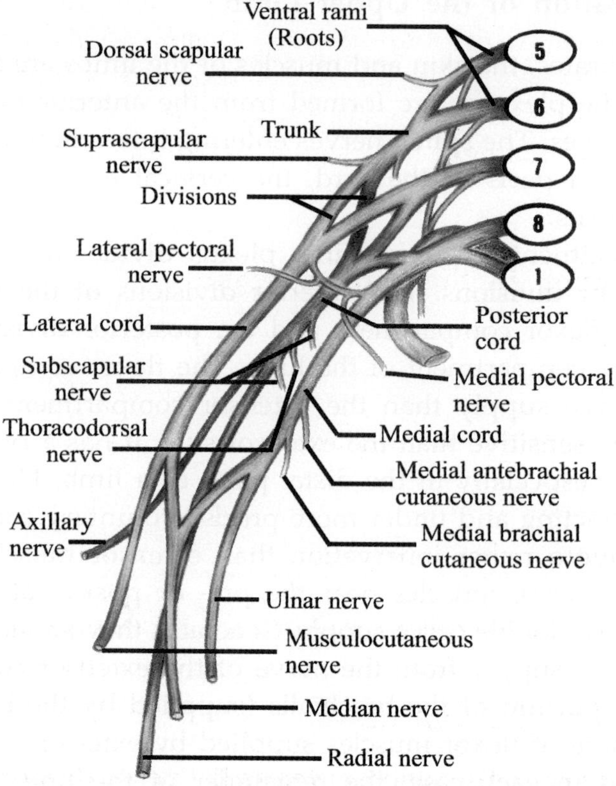

Fig. 10. The brachial plexus.

15.2. Median nerve

- C(5), 6–8, T1 from lateral and medial cords of the brachial plexus unite in the axilla lateral to the brachial artery
- It usually has no branch in the arm

15.3. Radial nerve

- is a continuation of the posterior cord (C 5–8, T1)
- runs posterior to the axillary then brachial artery; runs anterior to the long head of the triceps into the posterior compartment of the

arm; runs in the spiral groove and then into the anterior compartment between the brachioradialis and the brachialis
- lying on the capsule of the elbow joint and then the supinator muscle, it divides into a superficial radial nerve (sensory) and the posterior interosseous nerve (deep radial nerve — mostly motor)

16. Innervation in the Forearm/Hand

16.1. Ulnar nerve

- Innervates:
  — medial 1/2 of flexor digitorum profundus
  — flexor carpi ulnaris
  — elbow joint
- Palmar and dorsal cutaneous branches arise proximal to the wrist
- Ulnar artery accompanies ulnar nerve in most of the forearm.

16.2. Superficial radial nerve

- is the sensory continuation of the radial nerve distal to the origin of the posterior interosseous nerve
- lies deep to the brachioradialis
- runs with the radial artery
- becomes cutaneous about 5 cm proximal to the styloid process of the radius

16.3. Median nerve

- runs deep to the flexor digitorum superficialis and then deep to the flexor retinaculum
- innervates the elbow, wrist joint and all flexor muscles of the forearm, except the flexor carpi ulnaris and the medial 1/2 of flexor digitorum profundus

16.4. Neurovascular pattern in the forearm

- A nerve runs down each border
- The brachial artery divides into two branches: radial and ulnar arteries which approach the nerves but never cross them
- The median nerve, deep to the flexor digitorum superficialis, crosses the ulnar artery and lies between the two arteries

16.5. Ulnar nerve

In the hand:

- passes between pisiform and hook of hamate, in front of the flexor retinaculum and pisohamate ligament
- divides into deep and superficial branch

16.6. Median nerve

- through carpal tunnel, in the midline of skin crease of hand, on the deep surface of flexor retinaculum
- in the palm, it is deep only to the palmar aponeurosis
- divides into "recurrent" and digital branches
- innervates five short muscles, skin of 3½ lateral digits, joints of digits and local vessels

17. Acknowledgements

The author thanks Mr. Luke Tan Boon Kiat for the photography and digital imaging, Mr. Lee Man Hang for the digital imaging, Mr. Leow Eng Lye for the illustration, Prof. Ling Eng Ang, Head of Anatomy, for the kind use of the lab specimens, Ms. Ng May Fong for typing the manuscript and Dr. Alvin Eng for vetting the manuscript.

Advances in Tissue Banking Vol. 5

2 ANATOMY OF THE LOWER LIMB

AZIZ NATHER

NUH Tissue Bank, National University Hospital
Lower Kent Ridge Road, Singapore 119074

1. Bones of Lower Limb

1.1. Femur

The femur or thigh bone is the longest bone in the human body. It consists of a shaft and two extremities. The upper end of the bone comprises a head, a neck, a greater and a lesser trochanter (Fig. 1). The head forms slightly more than half a sphere and is directed upwards, medially and slightly anteriorly. There is a small roughened pit or fovea just below and behind the centre for attachment of the ligamentum teres. The neck of the femur, about 5 cm long connects the head to the shaft at an angle of about 135°. The greater trochanter is a large quandrangular eminence located laterally at the junction of the neck with the shaft. The lesser trochanter is a smaller conical eminence projecting medially and posteriorly from the neck-shaft junction. The intertrochanteric line joining the two trochanters marks the lower attachment of the hip capsule. The shaft of the femur is thinnest in its mid-portion, expanding slightly when traced upwards but widens noticeably towards the lower end of the bone. It has three surfaces, anterior, posterior and lateral surface. The posterior border is formed by a broad, rough ridge, the linea aspera. The lower end of the femur is widely expanded into two prominent masses, the

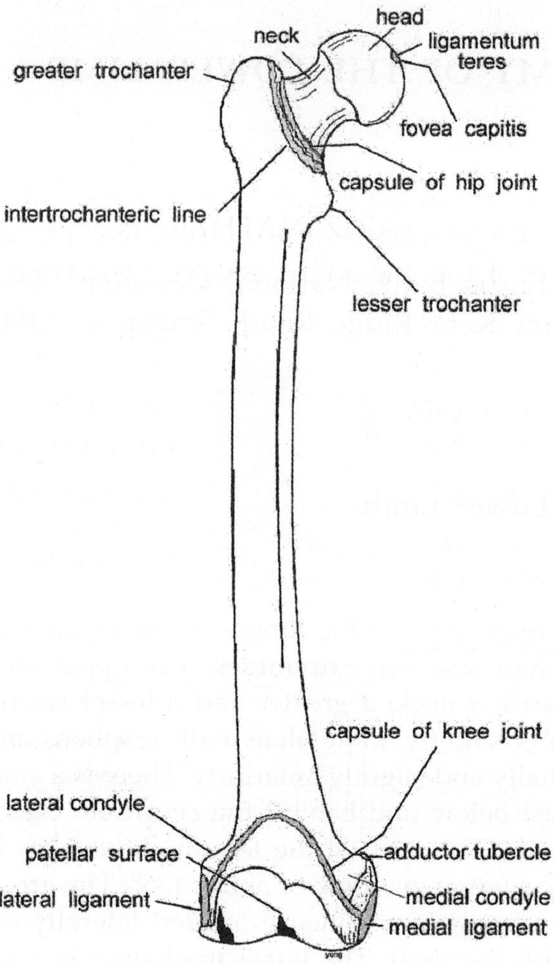

Fig. 1. Femur.

medial and lateral condyles. Anteriorly, the articular surfaces of both
condyles are joined together to form a grooved articular surface, the
patellar surface for articulation with the patella (knee cap). Posteriorly,
the articular surfaces of the two condyles are separated by the
intercondylar fossa (intercondylar notch). The medial condyle bulges
medially with the adductor tubercle in its uppermost part for

insertion of the adductor magnus. The lateral condyle presents a flattened lateral surface in contrast.

1.2. Patella

The patella (knee cap) is the largest of the sesamoid bones situated in front of the knee joint in the quadriceps femoris tendon. It is flat and triangular in shape, the apex pointing inferiorly. The posterior

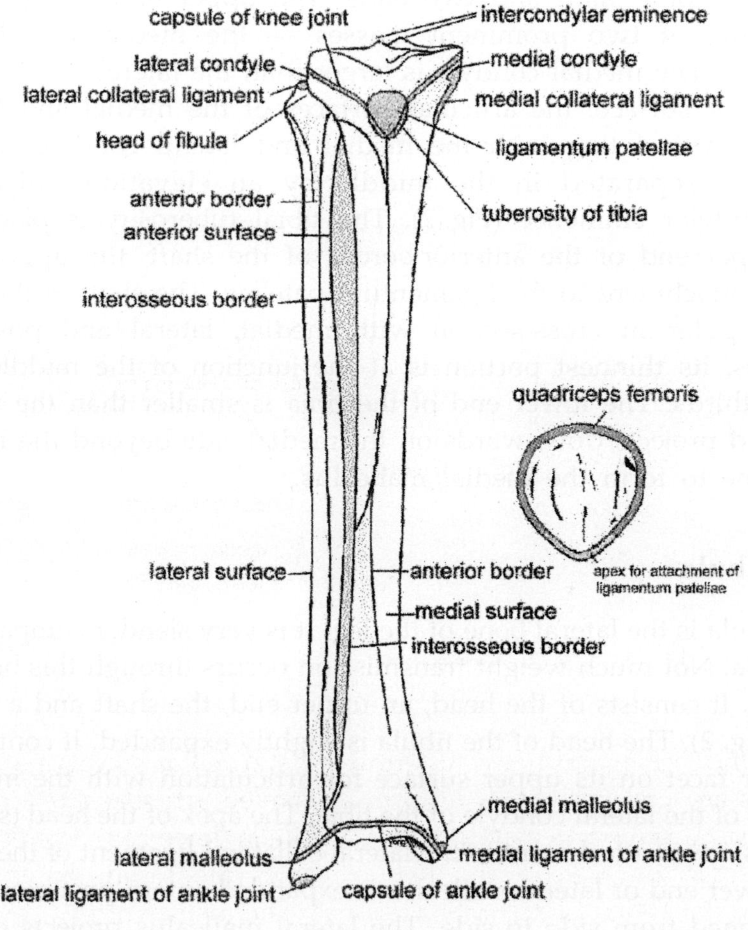

Fig. 2. Tibia.

surface consists of the articular surface above, divided into two facets by a vertical ridge, the lateral facet being larger than the medial facet. The apex is roughened in its lower part to give attachment to the ligamentum patellae (Fig. 2).

1.3. Tibia

The tibia is the larger of the two bones on the medial side of the leg. It is the second longest bone in the body next to the femur. It consists of a shaft and two ends. The upper end is expanded, consisting of two prominent masses — the medial and lateral condyles. The medial condyle is larger than the lateral condyle. On the upper surface, the articular surfaces of the medial and lateral condyle articulating with the medial and lateral condyles of the femur is separated in the middle by an elevation called the intercondylar eminence (Fig. 2). The tibial tuberosity is placed at the upper end of the anterior border of the shaft, the upper part giving attachment to the ligamentum patellae. The shaft of the tibia is triangular in cross-section with medial, lateral and posterior surfaces. Its thinnest portion is at the junction of the middle and lower thirds. The lower end of the tibia is smaller than the upper end and projects downwards on the medial side beyond the rest of the bone to form the medial mallealus.

1.4. Fibula

The fibula is the lateral bone of the leg. It is very slender compared to the tibia. Not much weight transmission occurs through this bone in the leg. It consists of the head, an upper end, the shaft and a lower end (Fig. 2). The head of the fibula is slightly expanded. It contains a circular facet on its upper surface for articulation with the inferior surface of the lateral condyle of the tibia. The apex of the head (styloid process) gives attachment to the lateral collateral ligament of the knee. The lower end or lateral mallealus is expanded antero-posteriorly but is flattened from side to side. The lateral mallealus projects downwards to a lower level than the tibia and on a more posterior plane.

Its inner surface presents a triangular articular surface with its apex pointing downwards to articulate with the lateral surface of the talus.

1.4. Foot

The skeleton of the foot consists of three segments, the tarsal bones, the metatarsal bones and the phalanges or bones of the toes (Fig. 3). The tarsus comprises seven bones, making up the posterior half

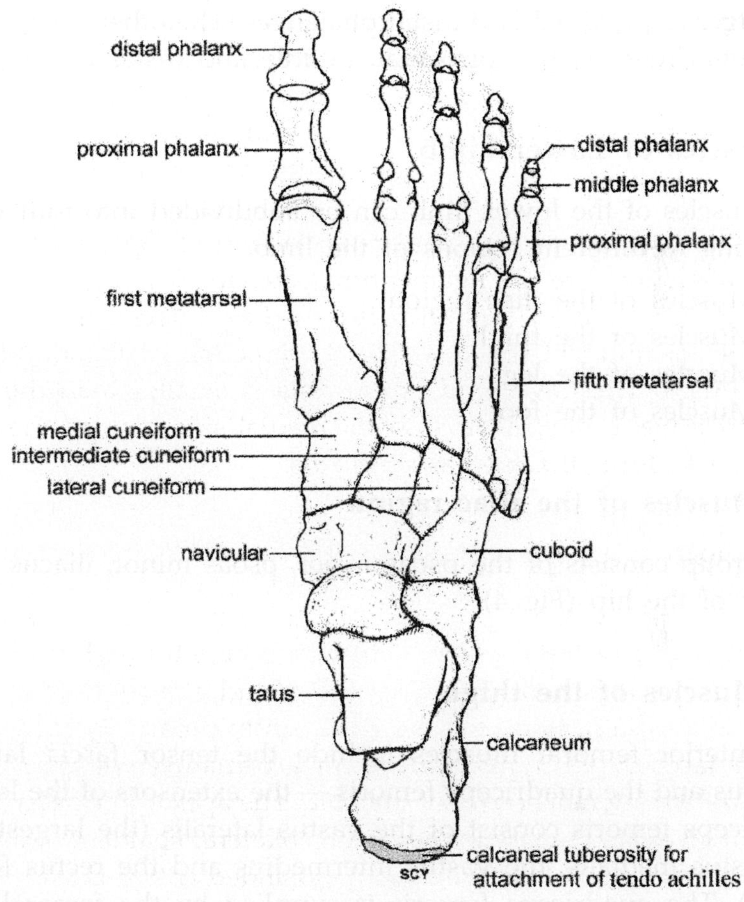

Fig. 3. Foot.

of the foot. The proximal row consists of the talus and the calcaneum. The talus lies above the calcaneum. The distal row contains four bones, the medial cuneiform, the intermediate cuneiform, the lateral cuneiform and the cuboid. These bones lying side by side form the transverse arch of the foot, which is convex dorsally. On the medial side, the navicular bone is interposed between the talus and the medial three bones of the distal row. The calcaneum projects backwards beyond the bones of the leg to form the calcaneal tuberosity which gives insertion to the tendo Achilles. The forefoot consists of five metatarsal bones and phalanges. The big toe has only two phalanges — proximal and distal phalanges. The other four toes has three phalanges each — proximal, middle and distal phalanges.

2. Muscles of Lower Limb

The muscles of the lower limb can be subdivided into four groups according to different regions of the limb:

  (i)   Muscles of the iliac region
  (ii) Muscles of the thigh
 (iii) Muscles of the leg
 (iv) Muscles of the foot

2.1. Muscles of the iliac region

This group consists of the psoas major, psoas minor, iliacus — the flexors of the hip (Fig. 4).

2.2. Muscles of the thigh

The anterior femoral muscles include the tensor fascia lata, the sartorius and the quadriceps femoris — the extensors of the leg. The quadriceps femoris consist of the vastus lateralis (the largest part), the vastus medialis, the vastus intermedius and the rectus femoris (Fig. 4). The quadriceps femoris is supplied by the femoral nerve (L2, L3, L4).

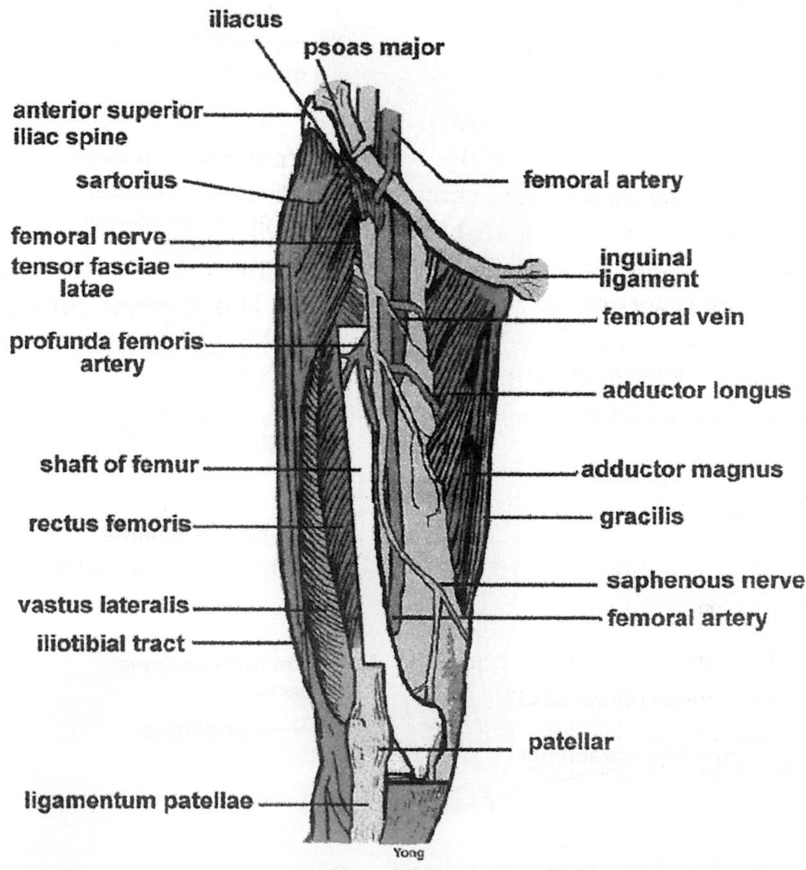

Fig. 4. Muscles of thigh — Anterior aspect.

The muscles of the gluteal region included the gluteus maximus, the gluteus medius and the gluteus minimus. The gluteus maximus, supplied by the inferior gluteal nerve (L5, S1, S2), extends the thigh. The gluteus medius and the gluteus minimus, supplied by the superior gluteal nerve (L5, S1), are abductors of the thigh. They have a stabilising effect on the pelvis during normal gait. Other muscles in this group include the short lateral rotators of the thigh, the piriformis, the obturator internus, and the superior and inferior Gemelli (Fig. 5).

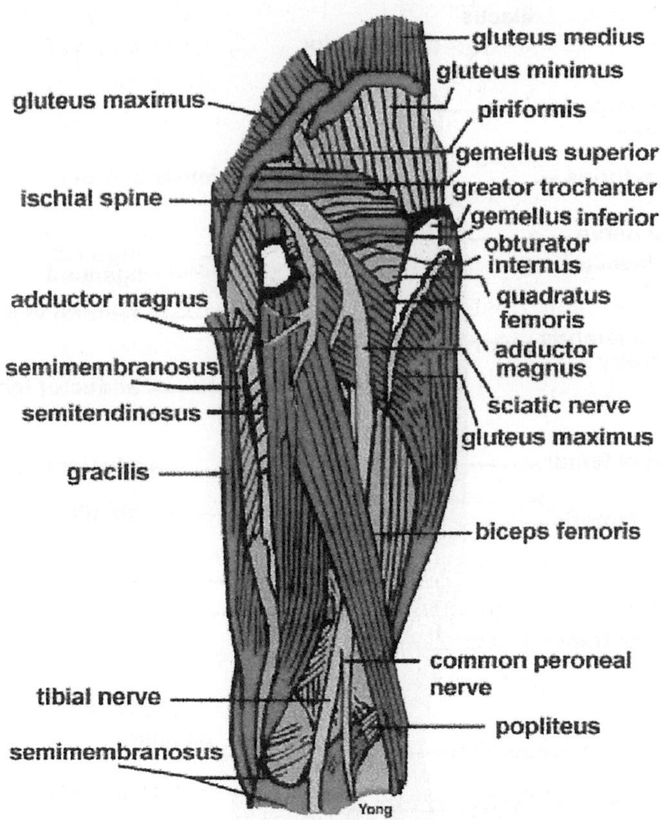

Fig. 5. Muscles of thigh — Posterior aspect.

The posterior femoral muscles consist of the hamstrings, the biceps femoris, the semitendinosus and the semimembranosus (Fig. 5). The hamstrings are supplied by the sciatic nerve (L5 S1, S2). Acting from above, they flex the leg on the thigh. Acting from below, they draw the trunk backwards when it is raised from the stooping position.

2.3. Muscles of the leg

They are divided into three groups: anterior, lateral and posterior. The anterior crural muscles include the tibialis anterior, the extensor hallucis longus, the extensor digitorum longus and the peroneus tertius (Fig. 6). These muscles supplied by the deep peroneal nerve are dorsiflexors of the foot. The tibialis anterior becomes tendinous in the lower third of the leg and passes down the medial side of the foot to be inserted into the undersurface of the medial cuneiform bone and adjoining part of the base of the first metatarsal bone. The lateral crural muscles consist of the peroneus longus and peroneus brevis (Fig. 6). They are supplied by the superficial peroneal nerve and evert the foot. The posterior crural muscles can be subdivided into two groups — superficial and deep. The superficial group forms the muscle mass of the calf of the leg. The superficial group consists of

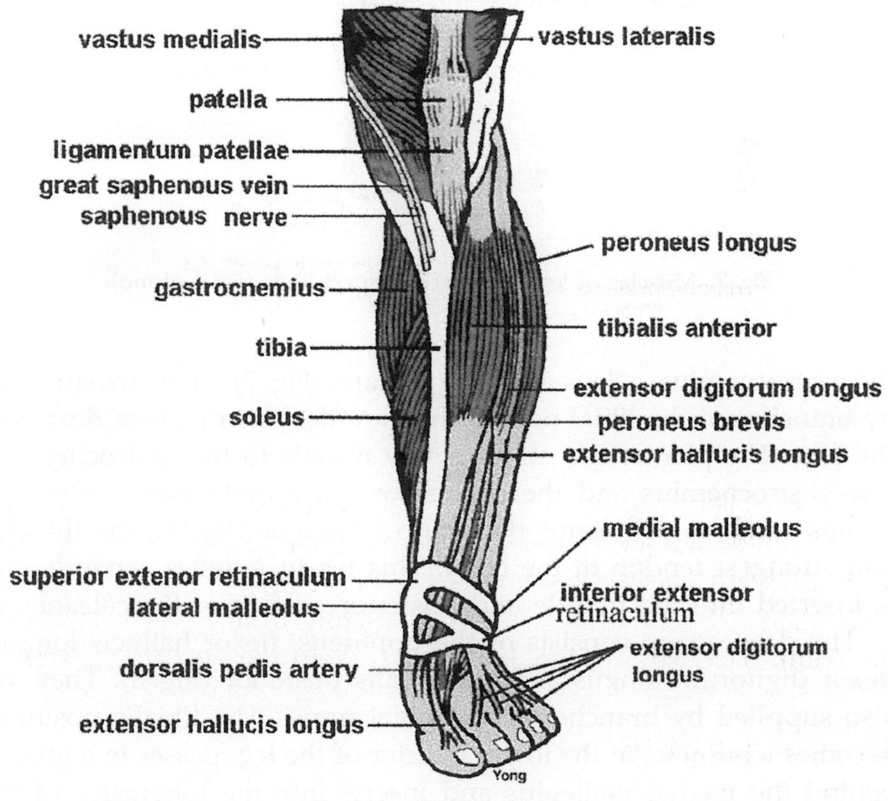

Fig. 6. Muscles of leg — Anterior aspect.

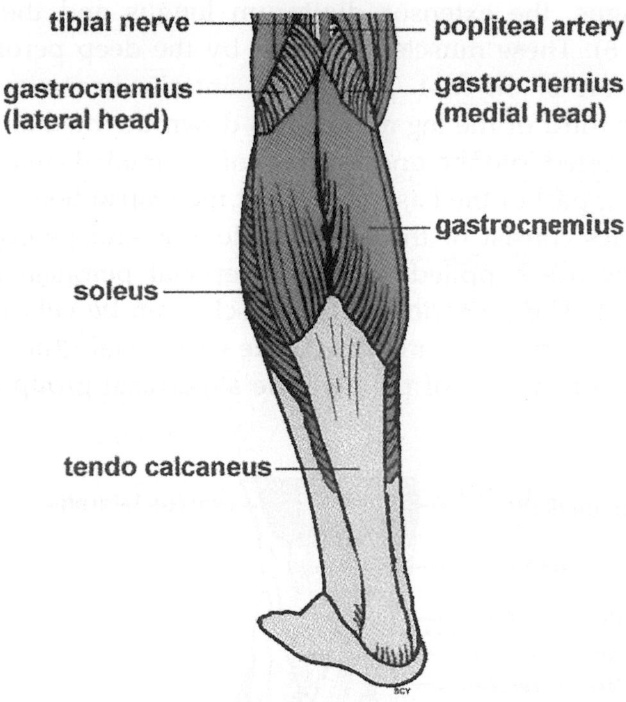

Fig. 7. Muscles of leg — Posterior aspect (superficial group).

the gastrocnemius, soleus and the plantaris (Fig. 7). They are supplied by branches of the tibial nerve. They are the main plantar flexors of the foot. The plantaris is an accessory muscle to the gastrocnemius. The gastrocnemius and the soleus form a muscle mass called the triceps surae, which forms the tendo calcaneus (Fig. 7), the thickest and strongest tendon in the body. This tendo Achilles expands and is inserted into the middle and posterior surface of the calcaneum.

The deep group consists of the popliteus, flexor hallucis longus, flexor digitorum longus and the tibialis posterior (Fig. 8). They are also supplied by branches of the tibial nerve. The tibialis posterior becomes tendinous in the lower quarter of the leg, passes in a groove behind the medial malleolus and inserts into the tuberosity of the navicular bone. It is the principal invertor of the foot.

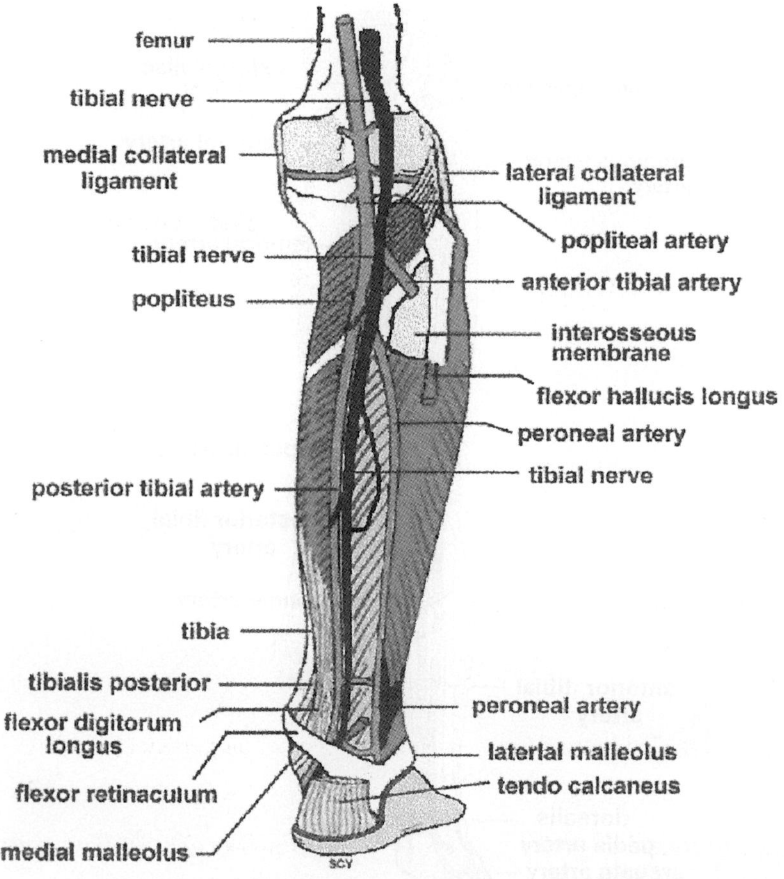

Fig. 8. Muscles of leg — Posterior aspect (deep group).

3. Vessels of Lower Limb

The femoral artery, the continuation of the external iliac artery, enters the thigh beneath the inguinal ligament midway between the anterior superior iliac spine and the symphysis pubis. It is the main arterial supply to the lower limb (Fig. 9). It enters the popliteal fossa through the opening in the adductor magnus muscle as the popliteal artery. The profunda femoris is a large artery arising from the lateral side of the femoral artery. The popliteal artery ends at the lower

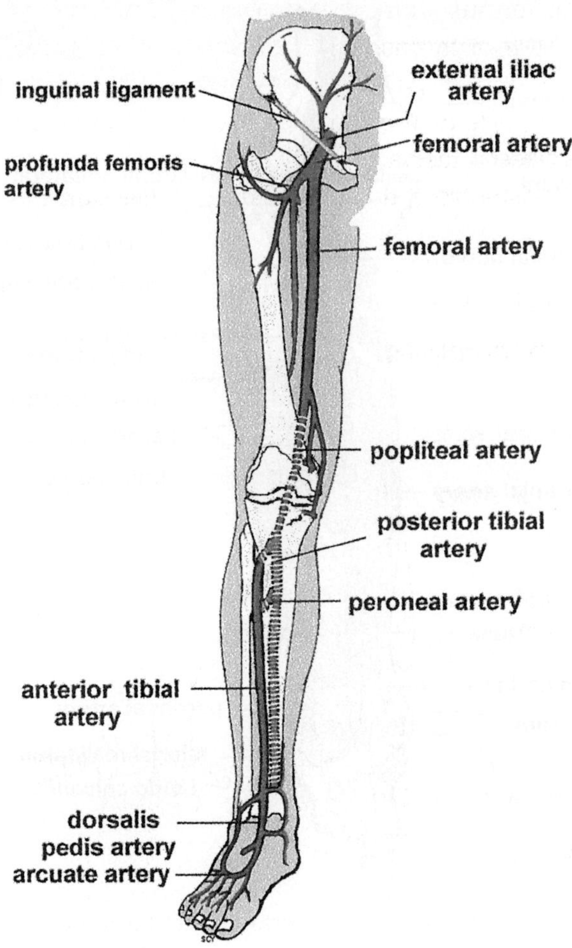

Fig. 9. Arteries of lower limb.

border of the politeus muscle by dividing into the anterior and posterior tibial arteries. The anterior tibial artery continues down the front of the leg to pass behind the superior extensor retinaculum to the front of the ankle joint to become the dorsalis pedis artery. The posterior tibial artery continues down the back of the leg to pass behind the medial malleolus deep to the flexor retinaculum and divides into the medial and lateral plantar arteries.

The great saphenous vein drains the medial end of the dorsal venous arch of the foot to pass upward directly in front of the medial mallealus (Fig. 10). It then passes behind the knee and curves forward around the medial side of the thigh. It passes through the saphenous opening in the deep fascia to join the femoral vein. The small saphenous vein arises from the lateral end of the dorsal venous arch

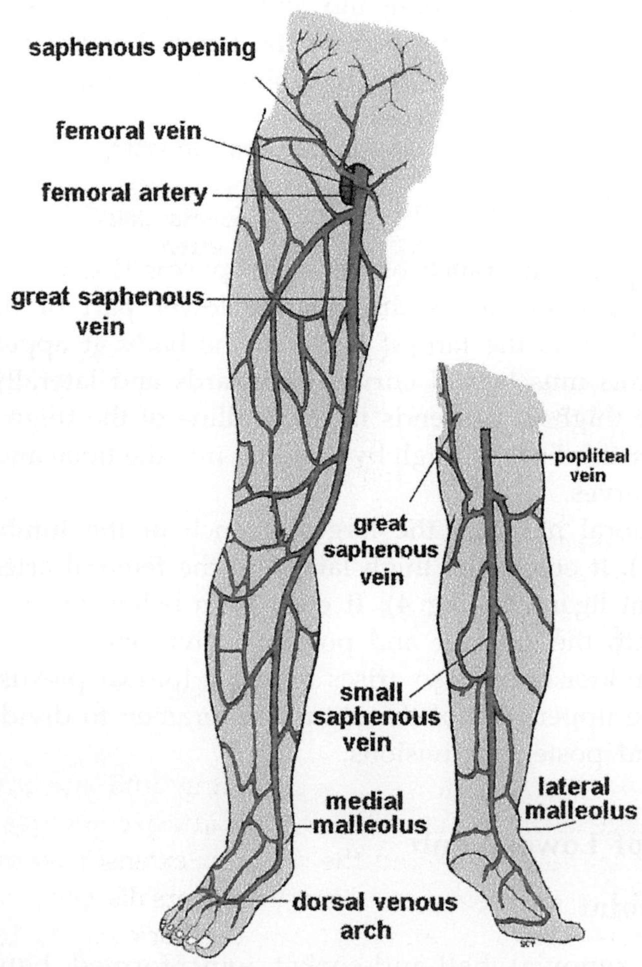

Fig. 10. Veins of lower limb.

of the foot to pass upward behind the lateral malledus up the middle of the back of the leg. It pieces the deep fascia in the middle of the back of the knee to end in the popliteal fossa by joining the popliteal vein. The popliteal vein is formed by the junction of the venae comitantes of the anterior and posterior tibial arteries at the lower border of the popliteus muscle on the medial side of the popliteal artery. It ascends the popliteal fossa crossing behind the popliteal artery to lie on its lateral side. It passes through the opening in the adductor magnus to become the femoral vein. The femoral vein ascends the thigh, crossing behind the femoral artery to be on its medial side. It leaves the thigh behind the inguinal ligament to become the external iliac vein.

4. Nerves of Lower Limb

The sciatic nerve, a branch of the sacral plexus (L4, L5, S1, S2, S3), emerging from the pelvis through the lower part of the greater sciatic foramen, is the largest nerve in the body. It appears below the piriformis muscle and curves backwards and laterally into the back of the thigh. It descends in the midline of the thigh and ends in the lower third of the thigh by dividing into the tibial and common peroneal nerves.

The femoral nerve is the largest branch of the lumbar plexus (L2, L3, L4). It enters the thigh lateral to the femoral artery behind the inguinal ligament (Fig. 4). It ends 4 cm below the ligament by dividing into the anterior and posterior divisions.

The obturator nerve also arises from the lumbar plexus. It enters through the upper part of the obturator foramen to divide into the anterior and posterior divisions.

5. Joints of Lower Limb

5.1. Hip joint

This is a synovial ball-and-socket joint formed between the hemispherical head of the femur and the cup-shaped acetabulum of

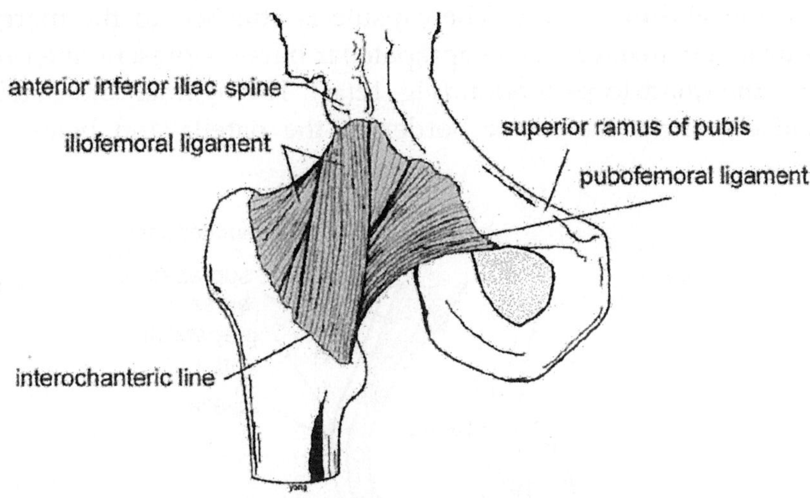

Fig. 11. Hip joint.

the hip bone (Fig. 11). The articular surface of the acetabulum is horseshoe shaped, deficient inferiorly as the acetabular notch. The cavity of the acetabulum is deepened by a fibrocartilaginous rim — the acetabular labrum. The capsule of the joint is attached to the acetabular labrum medially and to the intertrochanteric line anteriorly and halfway along the posterior part of the femoral neck. The condensations of this fibrous capsule form the iliofemoral ligament or Y-shaped ligament and the pubofemoral ligament anteriorly, and the ischiofemoral ligament posteriorly.

5.2. Knee joint

The knee joint is the largest and most complicated joint in the body. It consists of the articulation between the medial and lateral condyles of the femur and the corresponding condyles of the tibia, and a gliding joint, between the patella and the patellar surface of the femur. The articular surfaces of the femur, tibia and patella are covered with hyaline cartilage. The tibio-femoral joint is a synovial joint of the hinge type whilst the patello-femoral joint is a synovial joint of the gliding variety. The capsule is attached to the margins of the articular surfaces. The suprapatellar bursa is present anteriorly beneath the quadriceps tendon (Fig. 12(a)). The ligamentum patellae is attached above the lower border of the patella and below the

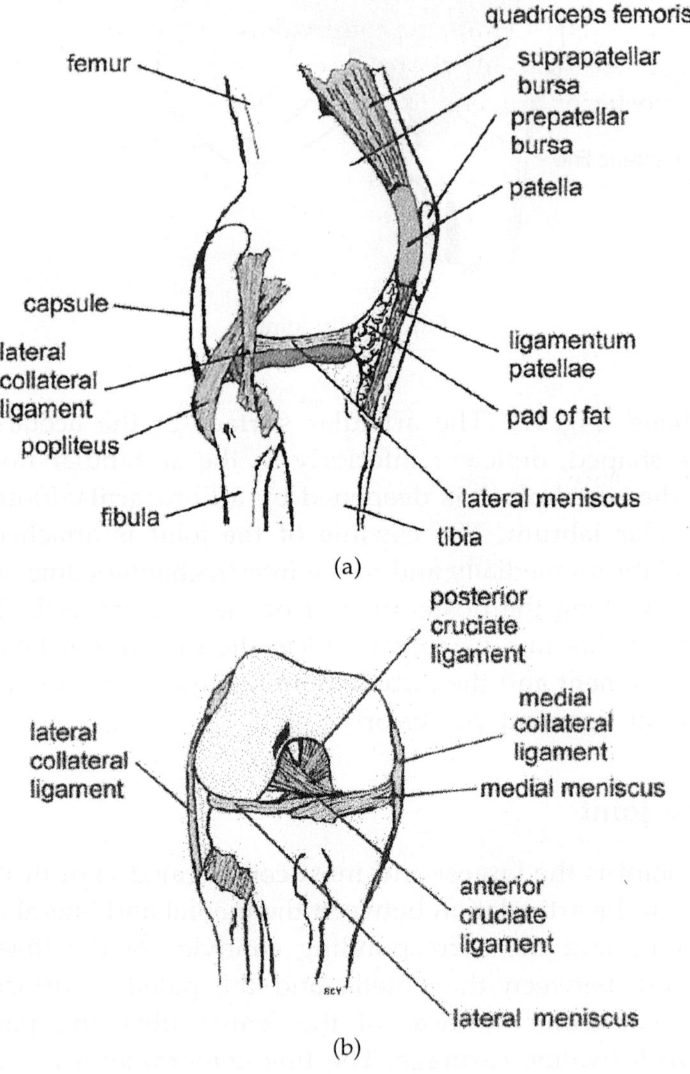

Fig. 12. Knee joint.

tuberosity of the tibia. The lateral collateral ligament is attached above the lateral condyle of the femur and below the head of the fibula. The medial collateral ligament is attached above the medial condyle of the femur and below the medial surface of the tibial shaft. Both ligaments are extracapsular.

The cruciate ligaments are two very strong intracapsular ligaments crossing each other within the joint cavity (Fig. 12(b)). The anterior cruciate ligament prevents posterior displacement of the femur on the tibia. The posterior cruciate ligament presents anterior displacement of the femur on the tibia. The meniscus or semi-lunar cartilages within the joint act as cushions between the femur and the tibia. The medial meniscus is nearly semi-circular in shape whilst the lateral meniscus is nearly circular in shape.

6. Acknowledgements

The author would like to record his gratitude to Mr. S.C. Yong for drawing all the illustrations and also Dr. Wang Lihui and Mrs. D.P. Vathani for the secretarial assistance provided.

Advances in Tissue Banking Vol. 5
© 2001 by World Scientific Publishing Co. Pte. Ltd.

3 ANATOMY OF THE SPINE

JOSEPH THAMBIAH

Department of Orthopaedic Surgery
National University Hospital
Lower Kent Ridge Road, Singapore 119074

Abstract

The spine or vertebral column forms the axial or central skeleton of the body. It serves the functions of protection the spinal cord and nerve roots, supporting the weight of the head and trunk transmitting this to the lower limbs via the pelvis as well as providing a base from which the upper and lower limbs can function via the shoulder and pelvic girdles. The great strength of the spine comes from the size and architecture of the vertebrae as well as the intrinsic strength of the ligaments binding them together.

The spine is a multisegmented structure which comprise essentially repeating segmental units. These units comprise in turn irregularly-shaped bones called vertebra separated by fibrocartilaginous stuctures called discs. The multisegmented nature of the spine provides flexibilty. Incremental motion at each segment combine to provide significant mobility.

There are essentially 33 vertebrae arranged in five groups. These are:

cervical (7)
thoracic (12)

lumbar (5)
sacral (5, fused to form the sacrum)
coccygeal (4; the lower three are commonly fused)

1. General Characteristics of a Vertebra

Although vertebrae in the different anatomical regions show certain differences, they all possess a common pattern (Fig. 1).

A *typical vertebra* consists of a rounded or kidney-shaped body anteriorly and a vertebral arch posteriorly. These enclose a space called the spinal canal, within which lie the thecal sac and its contents — the spinal cord and nerve roots (cauda equina). The vertebral arch consists of a pair of cylindrical pedicles, which form the sides of the arch, and a pair of flattened laminae, which complete the arch.

The vertebral arch gives rise to seven processes, one spinous, two transverse, and four articular.

The spinous process is formed at the junction of the two laminae. The transverse processes are directed laterally from the junction of

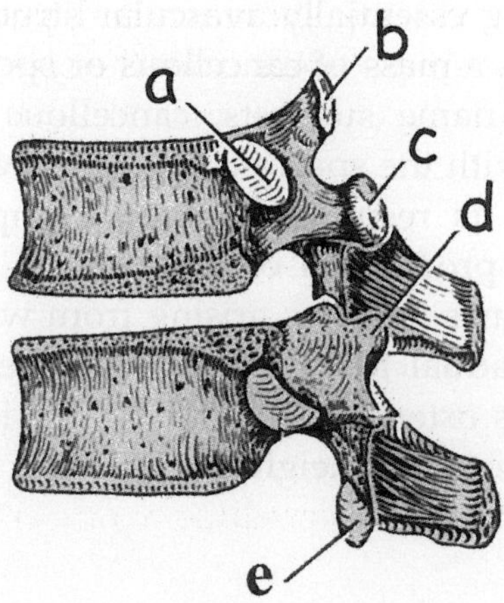

Fig. 1. a — Costal facet; b — Superior articular facet; c — Tubercle for rib; d — Mamillary process; e — Inferior articular facet.

the laminae and the pedicles. The spinous and transverse processes receive the attachments of various muscles and ligaments. It is through the action of these muscles that spinal motion is achieved.

The articular processes are vertically arranged and consist of two superior and two inferior processes. Their articular surfaces are covered with hyaline cartilage. The superior articular processes of one vertebral arch articulate with the inferior articular processes of the arch above, forming a synovial joint.

The space between the superior aspect of one pedicle and the inferior aspect of the pedicle above form the intervertebral foramen. The foramina transmit the spinal nerves.

2. Internal Architecture

The body of the vertebra is designed to provide great strength while maintaining a low mass. The body comprises a shell of cortical bone thickest at the superior and inferior aspects forming the end-plates. These end-plates are covered by hyaline cartilage and are in intimate contact with the intervertebral discs, transmitting forces directly to adjacent vertebrae through the discs. The nutrition of the discs depends on the diffusion of nutrients through perforations in the end-plates, the discs being essentially avascular structures. This shell of cortical bone encloses a mass of cancellous or spongy bone arranged in lamellae. As the name suggests, cancellous bone resembles a sponge in structure with the spaces being filled with haematogenous bone marrow which is responsible for the important function of haemopoeisis — the production of blood cells. The trabeculae are arranged along the lines of stress arising from weight-bearing. With ageing, there is a gradual loss of the trabeculae and bone mass — a condition known as osteoporosis. This results in weakening of the bone with a loss of vertebral height as well as a propensity towards compression fractures.

3. Development of the Spine

In the foetus *in utero*, the spinal column has only one kyphotic curve resembling a large letter "C". This is the primary curvature of the spine. As the child develops head support and begins to hold up its head, a lordotic curvature develops in the cervical spine. With the development of the standing posture and ambulation, the lumbar lordosis begins to develop. The cervical and lumbar curvatures are referred to as secondary curvatures. The remnant primary curves are the thoracic and sacral curves. These are essentially immobile curves. The spine at this stage, therefore, no longer resembles a large "C" but rather forms a series of gentle lordotic and kyphotic curves.

4. Cervical Vertebrae

These are the vertebrae in the neck. The cervical spine can broadly be divided into the atlanto-axial articulation and the subaxial spine. The atlanto-axial articulation comprises the atlas (or C1) and the axis (or C2). These are atypically-shaped cervical vertebrae which are designed to provide support for the skull as well as allow nodding and rotational movements of the neck.

The atlas or C1 vertebra has no body and no spinous process — it comprises only a ring of bone consisting of the anterior and posterior arches and a lateral mass on either side. The atlas articulates with the occipital condyles of the skull, forming the atlanto-occipital joints, as well as with the axis, forming the atlanto-axial joints.

The axis or C2 vertebra has a peglike odontoid process which articulates with the a notch on the anterior arch of the atlas.

The vertebrae below the atlanto-axial articulation form the subaxial cervical spine. These are more typically shaped and have the characteristics of all vertebrae. In addition, they also possess a foramen transversarium to allow for the passage of the vertebral artery as well as an additional set of synovial joints anteriorly — the uncovertebral joints or the Joints of Lushka.

5. Thoracic Vertebrae

The thoracic spine is a relatively immobile portion of the spine. The thoracic vertebrae increase in size from above downwards. There are costal facets present for articulation with the heads of the ribs, and on the transverse processes for articulation with the tubercles of the ribs. The facet joints have a more coronal orientation than the lumbar facet joints. This pattern changes at the thoraco-lumbar junction, which forms a transitional zone.

6. Lumbar Vertebrae

The five lumbar vertebrae form a smooth anteriorly-directed curvature, the lumbar lordosis. The major spinal movements of flexion and extension occur in this portion of the spine with spinal rotation taking place mainly at the thoraco-lumbar junction. The body of each lumbar vertebra is large and kidney-shaped. The pedicles are strong and directed backward. The laminae are thick and the vertebral foramina are triangular in shape. The transverse processes are long and slender. The spinous process is short, flat and quadrangular in shape (Fig. 1) and projects directly backward. The contents of the lumbar canal comprise the spinal cord up to the lower border of the L1 vertebra and subsequently, the contents comprise the nerve roots which make up the cauda equina. This has implications in lumbar spinal injuries as there may be a combination of cord and nerve root injuries, depending on the level of involvement.

7. Sacrum

The sacrum consists of five vertebrae fused together to form a wedge-shaped bone, which is concave anteriorly. The upper border, or base, of the bone articulates with the fifth lumbar vertebra. The narrow inferior border articulates with the coccyx. Laterally, the sacrum articulates with the two innominate, or hip, bones to form the sacro-iliac joints. The anterior and upper margin of the first sacral vertebra bulges forward as the posterior margin of the pelvic inlet, and is known as the sacral promontory. The contents of the sacral canal are the sacral and coccygeal nerve roots.

8. Coccyx

The coccyx consists of four vertebrae fused together to form a small triangular bone, which articulates at its base, with the lower end of the sacrum at the fibrocartilaginous sacro-coccygeal joint.

9. Intervertebral Discs

The intervertebral discs are semi-elastic structures which are thickest in the cervical and lumbar regions, where the movements of the vertebral column are the greatest. They function effectively as shock absorbers when the load on the vertebral column is suddenly increased as in running or jumping. Their elasticity diminishes with age as the water content progressively diminishes.

Each disc consists of an outer part, the annulus fibrosus, and a central part, the nucleus pulposus (Fig. 2). The annulus fibrosus is

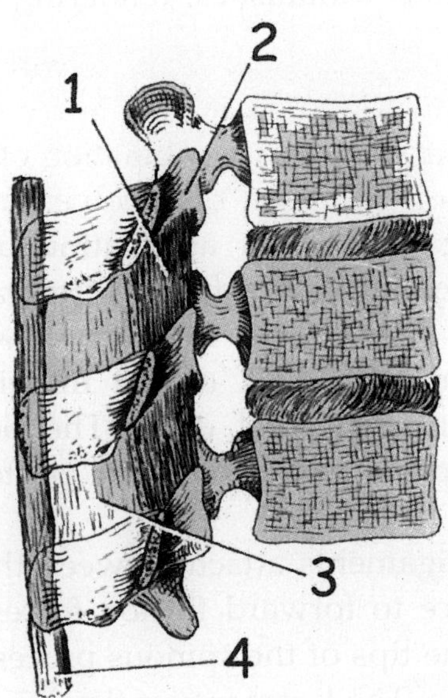

Fig. 2. 1 — Ligamentum flavum; 2 — Lamina; 3 — Interspinous ligament; 4 — Supraspinous ligament.

composed of fibrocartilage, in which the collagen fibres are arranged in concentric lamellae.

The nucleus pulposus in a child is an ovoid mass of gelatinous material containing a large amount of water, a small number of collagen fibres and a few cartilage cells. It is normally under pressure and situated slightly nearer to the posterior than to the anterior margin of the disc.

The upper and lower surfaces of the bodies of adjacent vertebrae that abut onto the disc are covered with thin plates of hyaline cartilage. The semi-fluid nature of the nucleus pulposus allows it to change shape and permits one vertebra to rock forward or backward on another, as in flexion and extension of the vertebral column. When the nucleus pulposus is tense, it therefore functions as a ball bearing. Due to the repetitive strains on the annulus fibrosus, tears may sometimes develop resulting in herniation of the inner nuclear material — a condition known as herniated nucleus pulposus or prolapsed intervertebral disc. With advancing age, the water content of the nucleus pulposus diminishes, rendering the disc more prone to injury.

10. Ligaments

The longitudinal ligaments run as continuous bands down the anterior and posterior surfaces of the vertebral column from the skull to the sacrum. The anterior ligament is wide and is strongly attached to the front and sides of the margins of the vertebral bodies and to the intervertebral discs. The posterior ligament is weak and narrow, and is attached to the posterior borders of the discs.

The interspinous ligaments attach between the spinous processes and provide resistance to forward flexion forces. The supraspinous ligaments attach to the tips of the spinous processes. They are strong bands of fibrous tissue. The ligamentum flavum (or yellow ligament) is located in the interlaminar spaces. These ligaments are rich in elastic tissue and provide great flexibility.

11. Articulations Between Vertebrae

The articulations between the vertebrae may be divided into an anterior articulation between the bodies and a posterior articulation between the neural arches.

11.1. Articulations between the bodies

The vertebral bodies are bound together by the intervertebral discs. This forms a very strong secondary cartilaginous joint or symphysis. The lamellar anatomy of the outer covering of the disc, the annulus fibrosus, provides the strength required to resist bending and torsional forces.

11.2. Articulations between the neural arches

The articulation between the neural arches takes place at the junction of the superior and inferior articular processes. These are covered with hyaline cartilage and form a pair of synovial joints on either side of the midline — the facet joints.

12. Musculature of the Vertebral Column

There is a large mass of muscles which run along the posterior aspect of the whole length of the spine from the skull to the sacrum. These are collectively known as the erector spinae. The action of these muscles is aided by gravity in a manner which can best be described as "paying out rope".

The erector spinae is divided into three layers:

(i) *A superficial layer* comprising the ilio-costalis, the costalis, longissimus, the spinalis and the splenius,

(ii) *An intermediate layer* comprising the multifidus, the semispinalis and the levatores costarum,

(iii) *A deep layer* comprising the interspinales, the intertransversales and the rotatores.

These erector spinae muscles produce extension and are able to effect flexion with the aid of gravity by "paying out rope". Flexion is primarily, however, produced by the action of the prevertebral muscles — the longus capiti, the longus colli and the psoas.

Rotation is produced indirectly by the action of the abdominal wall musculature.

4 ANATOMY OF THE PELVIS

AZIZ NATHER

National University Hospital Tissue Bank
National University Hospital
Lower Kent Ridge Road, Singapore 119074

1. Surface Anatomy

The iliac crest is palpable through its entire length. The anterior superior iliac spine is located at the anterior end of the crest. It lies at the upper and lateral end of the groin fold. The posterior superior iliac spine lies below a small skin-dimple–sacral-dimple at the level of S2 spine. The pubic tubercle is felt at the upper border of the pubis. The symphysis pubis is in the midline between the bodies of the pubic bones. The pubic crest is the ridge felt on the superior surface of the pubic bone medial to the pubic tubercle. The inferior end of the coccyx is palpable in the natal cleft.

2. Bones of the Pelvis

The bony pelvis consists of four bones: the two innominate bones forming the lateral and anterior wall, and the sacrum and coccyx, which are the continuation of the vertebral column forming the posterior wall (Fig. 1). The pelvic brim, consisting of the sacral promontory behind, the iliopectineal lines laterally and the pubis symphysis anteriorly, divides the pelvis into the false or greater pelvis above the brim and the true or lesser pelvis below.

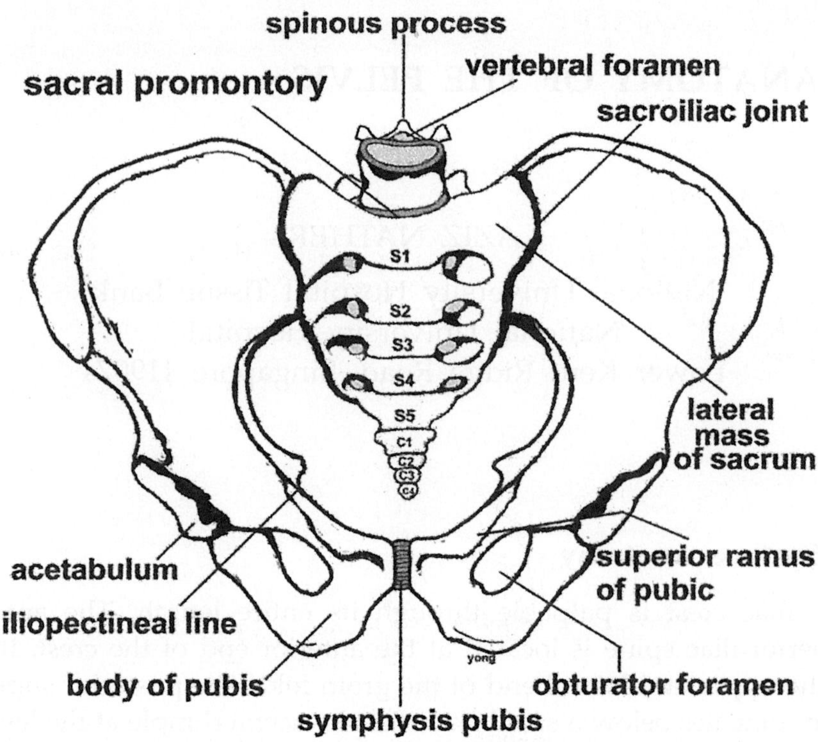

Fig. 1. Bones of pelvis.

The innominate or hip bone consists of the ilium, the ischium and the pubis (Fig. 2). The outer surface is marked by a deep depression, the acetabulum, which forms the socket for the head of the femur in the hip joint. The upper flat part of the bone is formed by the ilium. The iliac crest is a prominent ridge running between the anterior superior iliac spine and the posterior superior iliac spine. The ischium is the inferior and posterior part of the hip bone marked inferiorly by the prominent ischial tuberosity. The anterior part of the bone is the pubis. Medially, the pubic crest articulates with the opposite side to form the symphysis pubis. The pubis is marked by the prominent obturator foramen between the superior and inferior pubic ramus.

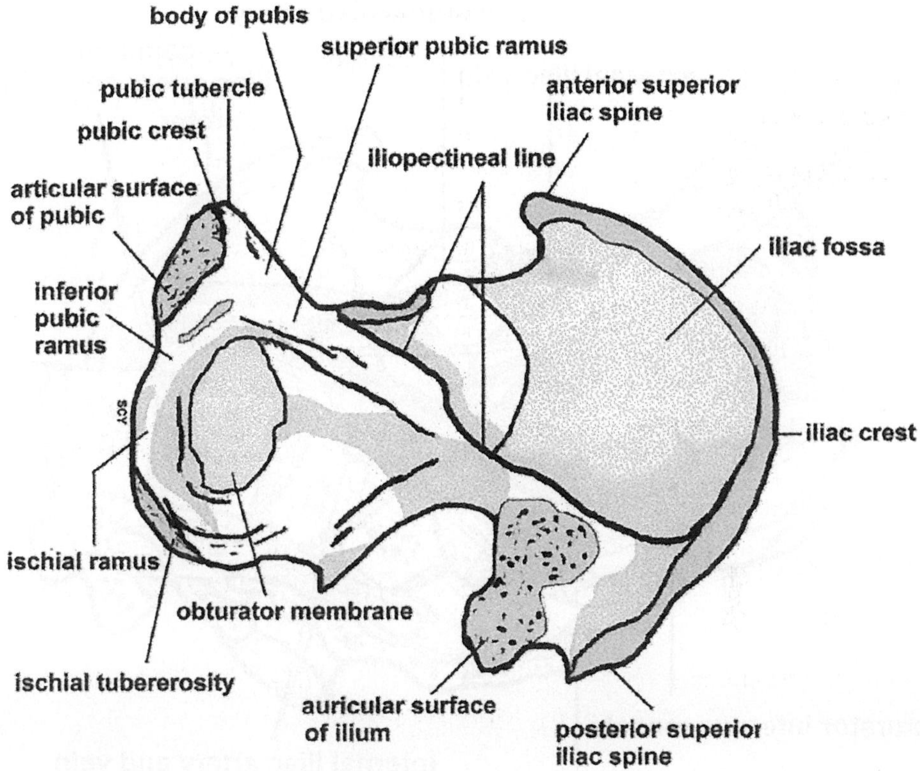

Fig. 2. Innominate bone.

The sacrum is made up of five rudimentary vertebrae fused together to form a wedge articulating with two innominate bones by the sacro-iliac joints (Fig. 1). The coccyx is formed from four rudimentary fused vertebrae to form a small triangular bone at the lower end of the sacrum.

3. Muscles of the Pelvis

These are divided into two groups: (i) the piriformis and the obturator internus (Fig. 3), which form part of the muscles of the lower limb; and (ii) the levator ani and the coccygeus, which form the pelvic diaphragm.

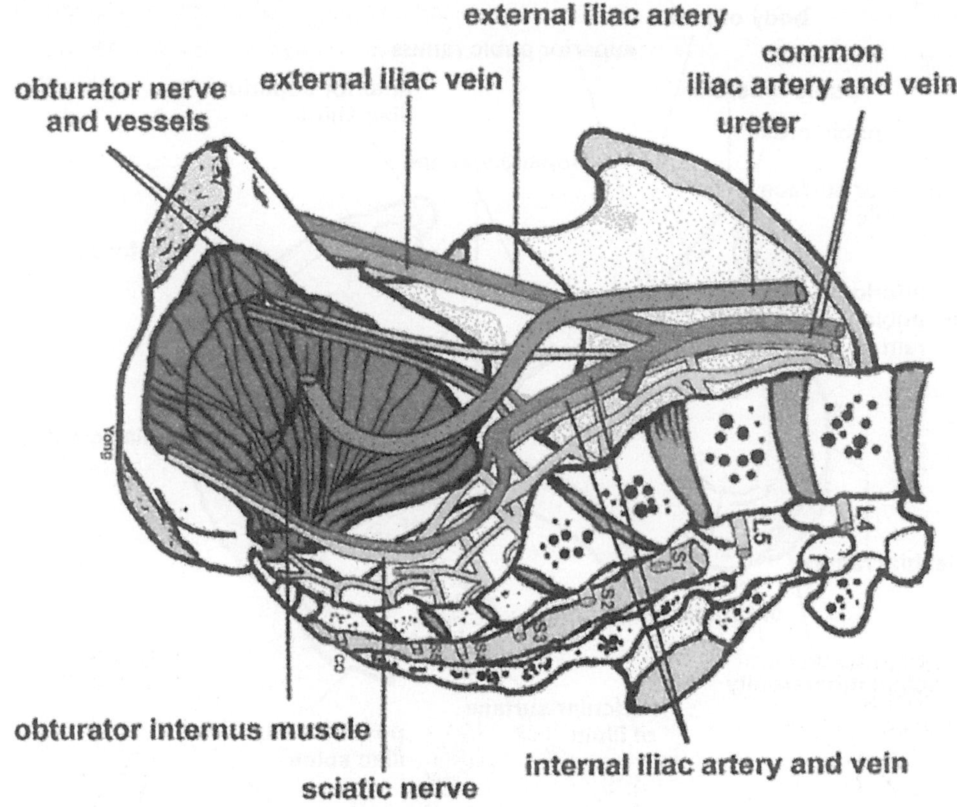

Fig. 3. Vessels of pelvis.

In the iliac region, the iliacus muscle arises from the inside of the iliac bone and the fibres are inserted into the lateral side of the tendon of the psoas major to be inserted into the lesser trochanter.

4. Vessels of the Pelvis

The common iliac artery ends at the pelvic inlet in front of the sacro-iliac joint by dividing into the external and internal iliac arteries (Fig. 3). The external iliac artery runs along the border of the psoas major muscle. It leaves the greater pelvis under the inguinal ligament to become the femoral artery. The internal iliac artery passes down into the pelvis to the greater sciatic foramen to divide into anterior and posterior divisions.

The external iliac vein is the continuation of the femoral vein. It begins behind the inguinal ligament and runs on the medial side of the artery. It is joined by the internal iliac vein to become the common iliac vein.

5. Nerves of the Pelvis

The sacral plexus lies on the posterior pelvic wall in front of the piriformis muscle. It is formed by the anterior rami of L4 L5, S1, S2, S3 and S4 nerves. The ramus of L4 joins the ramus of L5 to form

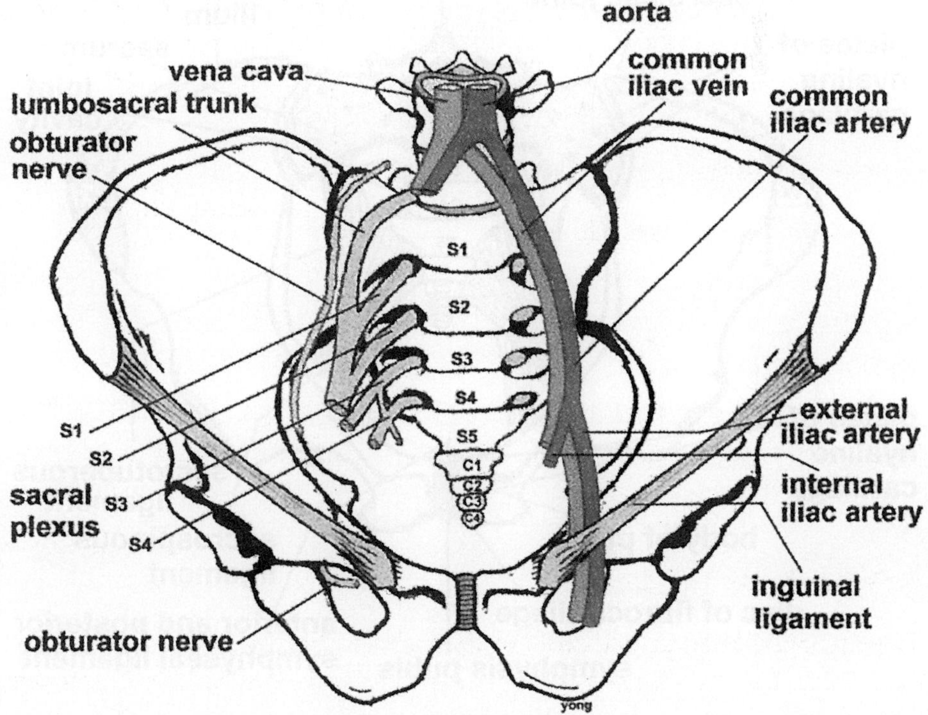

Fig. 4. Nerves of pelvis.

the lumbo-sacral trunk which passes over the alar of the sacrum (Fig. 4).

6. Joints of the Pelvis

The sacro-iliac joints are very strong synovial joints formed between the articulating surfaces of the sacrum and the iliac bone. They are held by very strong posterior and interosseos sacro-iliac ligaments (Fig. 5). The pubis symphysis is a cartilaginous joint between the articulating surfaces of both bodies of pubis, which are covered by hyaline cartilage and joined together by a fibrocartilaginous disc.

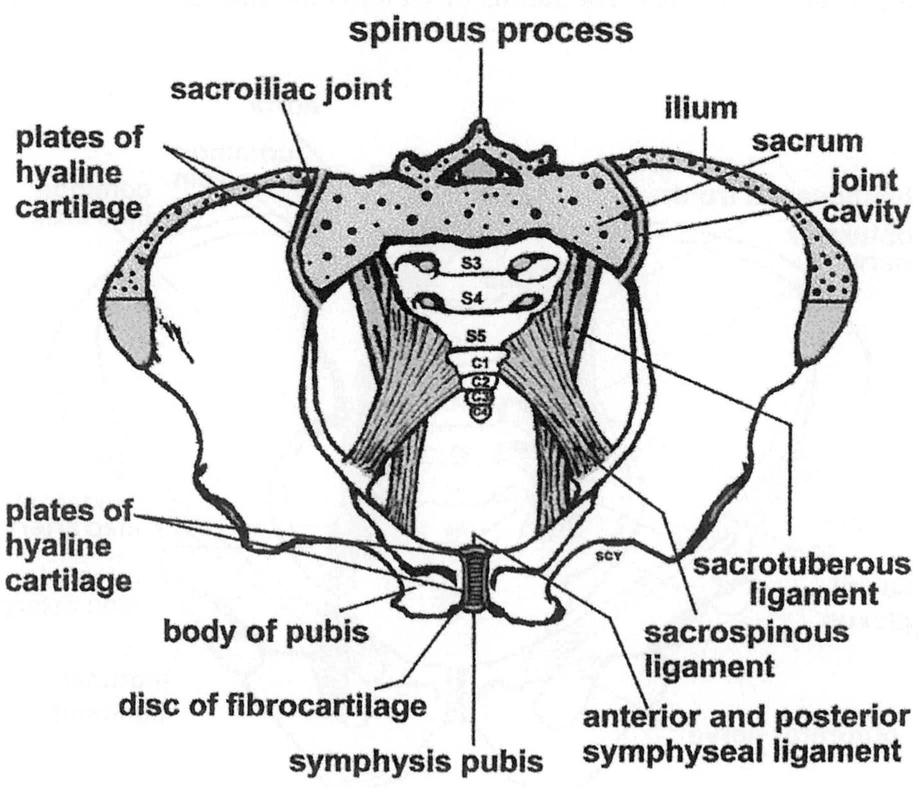

Fig. 5. Joints of pelvis.

7. Acknowledgements

The author would like to record his gratitude to Mr. S.C. Yong for drawing all the illustrations, and also Dr. Wang Lihui and Mrs. D.P. Vathani for the secretarial assistance provided.

5 ANATOMY OF THE ORAL MAXILLOFACIAL REGION

HO KEE HAI

Department of Oral and Maxillofacial Surgery
National University Hospital
Lower Kent Ridge Road, Singapore 119074

1. Introduction

The skull can be divided into thirds. The upper third lies between the calvarium to the horizontal joining the two fronto-zygomatic sutures. The mid-third is from the fronto-zygomatic sutures to the

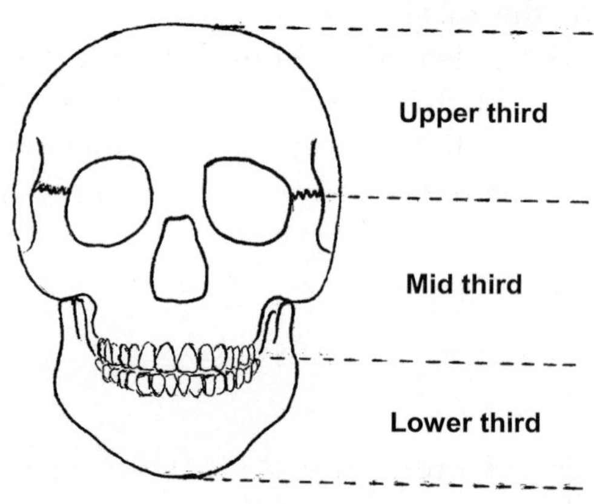

Fig. 1. Skull.

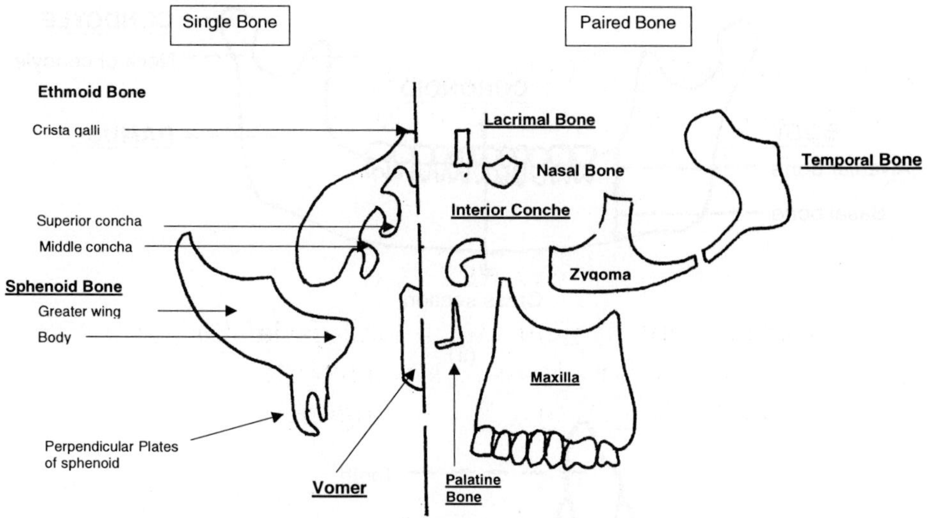

Fig. 2. Exploded view of middle third of facial skeleton.

occlusal surfaces of the maxillary dentition. The lower third is from the mandibular occlusal surface to the lower border of the mandible.

The lower third consists of only one bone, the mandible. The mandible is a strong U-shaped tubular body with two flat vertical bones at each end, the rami.

The middle third consists of 17 bones of which seven are paired and three are single. The paired bones are the maxilla, the zygoma, the lacrimal, the nasal, the inferior concha, the palatine and the temporal (pterygoid plates). The sphenoid, ethmoid and vomer are the single bones.

The frontal bone forms the upper third.

2. The Mandible

The mandible consists of a tubular body that flares vertically upwards as two flat rami. The superior end of the ramus are the condyle and the coronoid, connected by the sigmoid notch. The condyle articulates with the base of the skull at the glenoid fossa of the temporal bone.

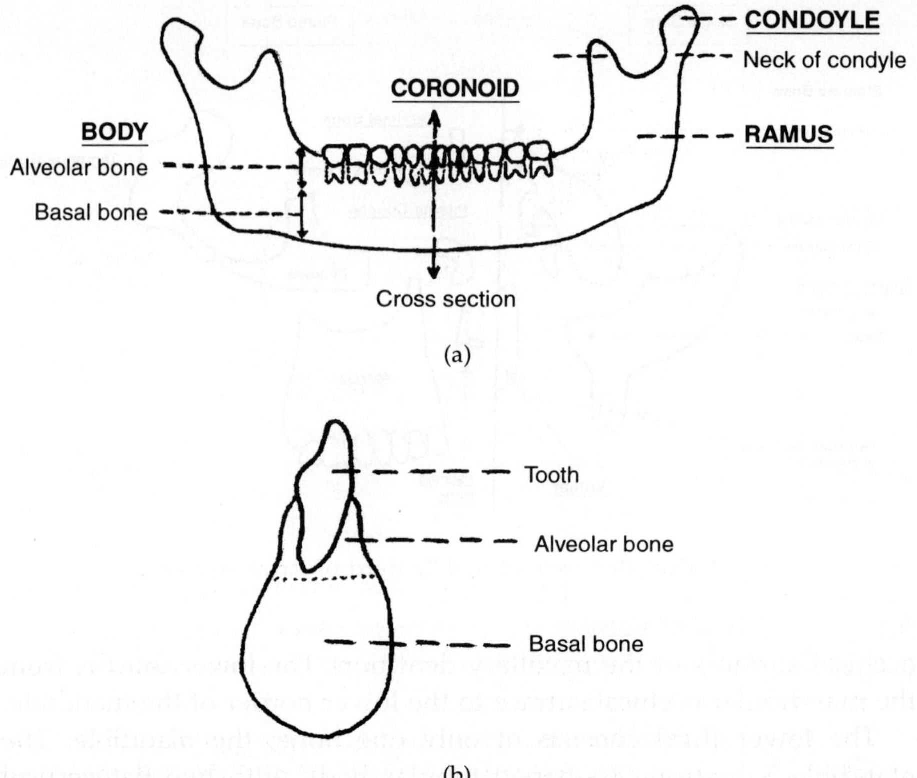

Fig. 3. (a) Parts of mandible — Panoramic view. (b) Cross section of body of mandible.

The body of the mandible can be divided into the strong basal bone (body proper) and the alveolar bone that carries the teeth. This alveolar bone will undergo resorption when the teeth are lost.

2.1. The temporo-mandible joint (TMJ)

The mandible is the only mobile bone in the facial skeleton. It articulates to the base of the skull at the temporo-mandible joint (TMJ).

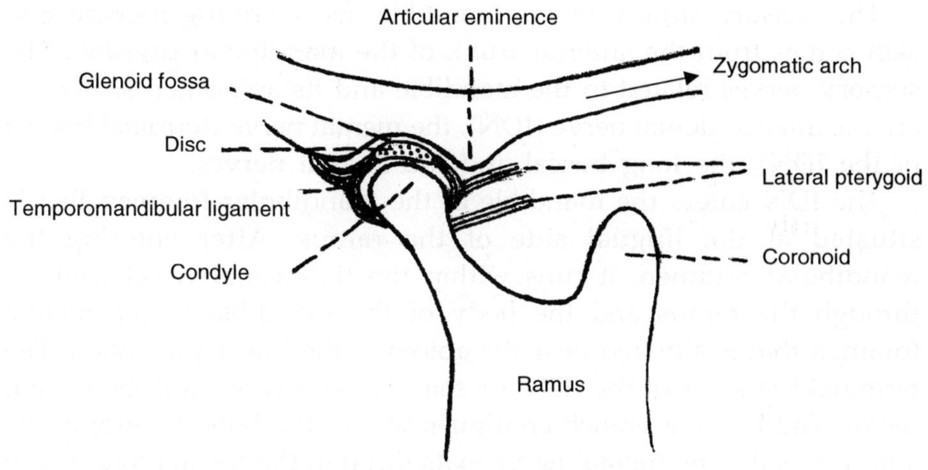

Fig. 4. Temporo-mandibular joint.

The TMJ is made up of the condyle of the mandible, the glenoid fossa with a disc in between. The TMJ is a synovial joint enclosed by a capsule. The joint cavity is divided by the cartilaginous disc into an upper and a lower compartment.

The upper and lower heads of the lateral pterygoid muscles are attached to the disc and the condyle, respectively. The two heads of the lateral pterygoid act antagonistically. Contraction of these muscles moves the condyle and the disc. The TMJ is stabilised by its capsule and the ligaments, namely spheno-mandibular and the stylo-mandibular ligaments, as shown in Fig. 4.

The condyle and the glenoid fossa are covered by fibrocartilage. This fibrocartilage of the condyle contributes to the growth of the mandible. Damage to this TMJ cartilage in a growing child can lead to retrognathia, as seen in Still's disease and TMJ ankylosis.

2.2. Sensory nerves related to the mandible

The main sensory nerves to the mandible are from the mandibular division of the trigelminal nerve. As the mandibular division exits through the foramen ovale, it divides into an anterior and a posterior trunk.

The sensory supply to the mandible, its overlying mucosa and skin comes from the anterior trunk of the mandibular division. The sensory nerves related to the mandible and its associated structures are the inferior dental nerve (IDN), the mental nerve (terminal branch of the IDN), the long buccal and the lingual nerves.

The IDN enters the mandible at the mandibular foramen that is situated at the lingual side of the ramus. After entering the mandibular foramen, it runs within the IDN canal which courses through the ramus and the body of the mandible to the mental foramen that is situated near the apices of the lower premolars. The terminal branches of the IDN are the incisive nerves and the mental nerve. The incisive branch continues within the bone to supply the anterior teeth. The mental nerve exits through the mental foramen to supply the lower lip and the adjacent mucosa.

The lingual mucosa and the anterior two-third of the tongue receive their sensory supply from the lingual nerve. The buccal mucosa behind the premolar is supplied by the long buccal nerve while that anterior to the premolar is supplied by the mental nerve.

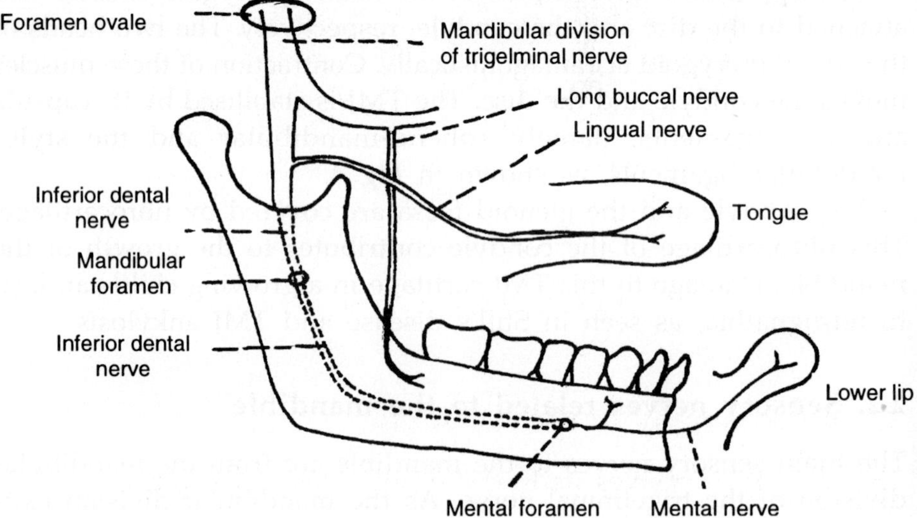

Fig. 5. Nerve supply of the mandible, lip and tongue.

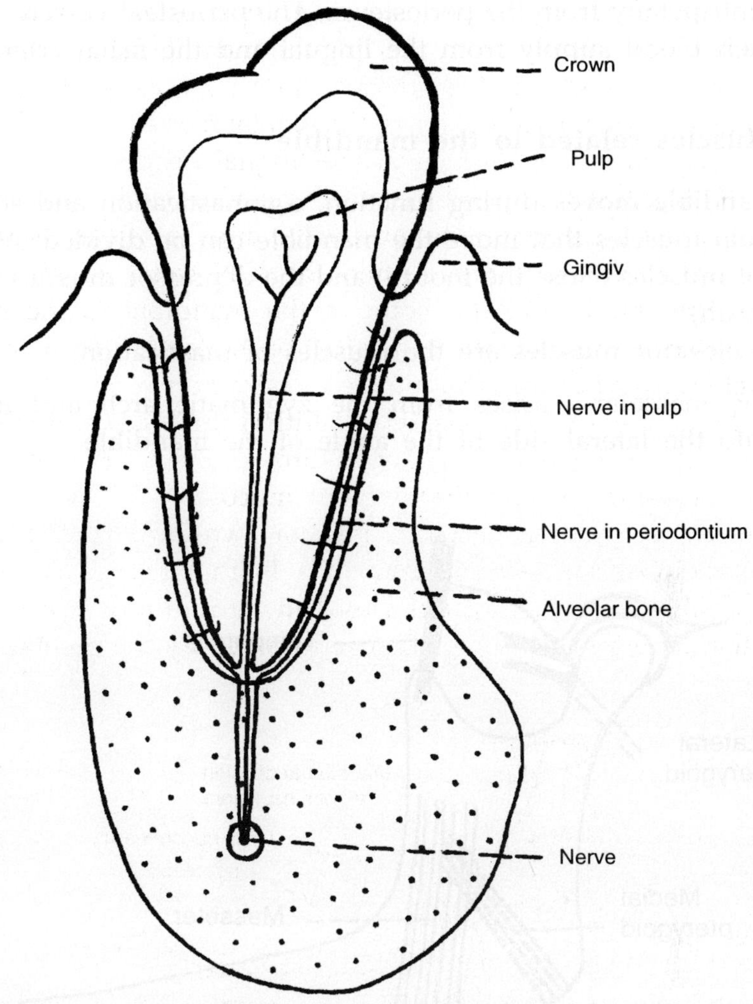

Fig. 6. Nerve supply of the teeth.

2.3. Blood supply of the mandible

The mandible receives its blood supply from two sources:

(i)   centrifugally from the inferior dental artery which accompanies the inferior nerve bundle

(ii)   centripetally from the periosteum. The periosteal vessels derive
       their blood supply from the lingual and the facial arteries

2.4. Muscles related to the mandible

The mandible moves during function, e.g. mastication and speech.
The main muscles that move the mandible can be divided into the
elevator muscles (close the mouth) and the depressor muscles (open
the mouth).

   The elevator muscles are the muscles of mastication:

(i)   the masseter — arises from the zygomatic arch and inserts
      into the lateral side of the angle of the mandible

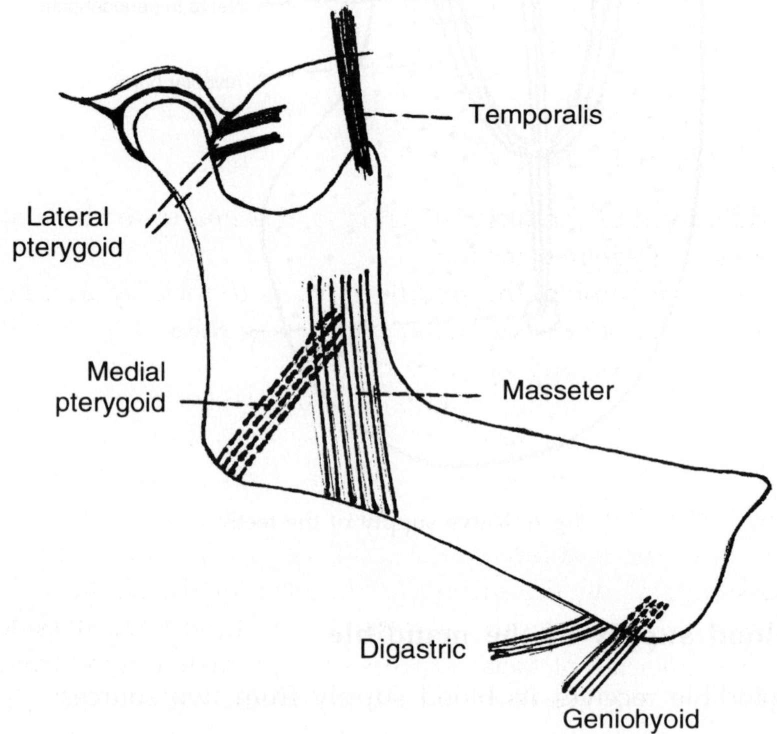

Fig. 7. Muscles associated with the mandible.

(ii) the medial pterygoid — arises from the medial aspect of the medial pterygoid plate and attaches to the medial side of the angle of the mandible

(iii) the temporalis — originates from the temporal crest and fossa of the temporal bone, and inserts into the coronoid process of the mandible

These muscles are supplied by the motor branches from the posterior trunk of the mandibular division.

The depressor muscles are:

(i) the lateral pterygoid — attaches to the lateral side of the medial pterygoid plate and inserts into the neck of the condyle

(ii) the digastric muscle — arises from the hyoid bone and attaches to the lower border of the mandible

(iii) the geniohyoid — arises from the hyoid bone and inserts onto the genial tubercle

3. The Middle Third

The middle third of the facial skeleton is attached to the base of the skull along a 45-degree incline.

Unlike the mandible, the middle third is formed by thin bones. These bones are further weakened by bony cavities — the maxillary sinuses, the nasal cavity and the orbits.

However, these thin bones are strengthen by vertical struts at the zygomatic buttress and pyriform fossa regions. These vertical struts allow the mid-third to take the vertical forces of mastication. The mid-third is unable to withstand horizontal shearing force. Trauma to the front of the mid-face would displace the mid-third downward and backward along the incline of the base of the skull.

No strong muscle is attached to the mid-third facial skeleton. Only small muscles of facial expression take their origins from the mid-third and are inserted into the skin. Most of the muscles of facial expression are innervated by branches of the facial nerve. Some muscles of facial expression are not innervated by the facial

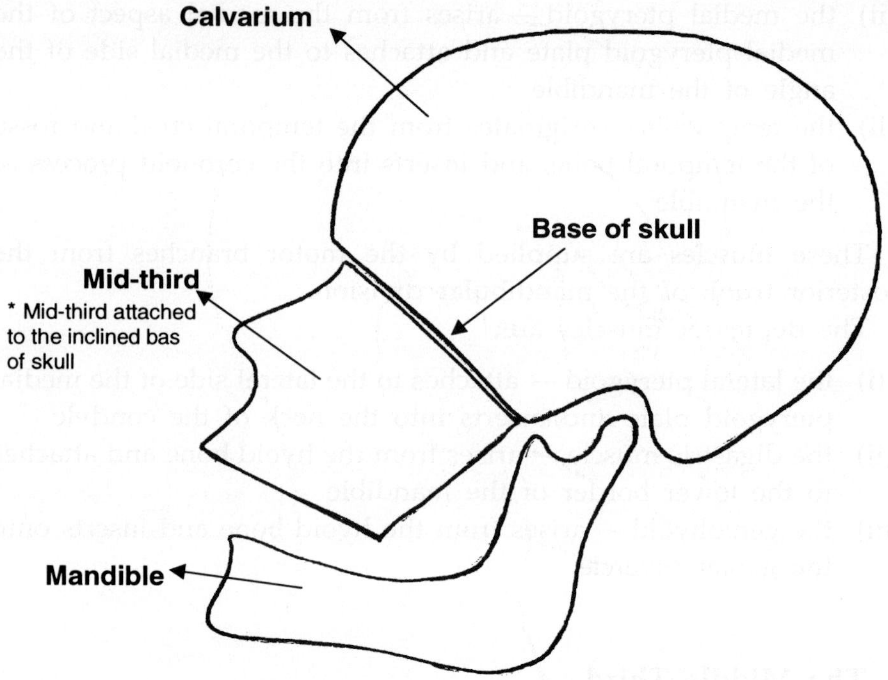

Fig. 8. Base of skull, calvarium and mid-third.

nerve, e.g. the levator palpebral superioris and the muscles of the eye are supplied by the ocular nerve.

3.1. Sensory supply of the middle third

The maxillary division of the trigelminal nerve is the main sensory nerve of the mid-third.

The hard palate is supplied by the incisive nerve anteriorly and the greater palatine nerve posteriorly. The soft palate is innervated by the lesser palatine nerve.

The maxilla carries the upper dentition. Posterior to the last molar is the tuberosity, a mass of cortico-cancellous bone which sometimes serves as a donor site for autogenous bone for orofacial reconstruction.

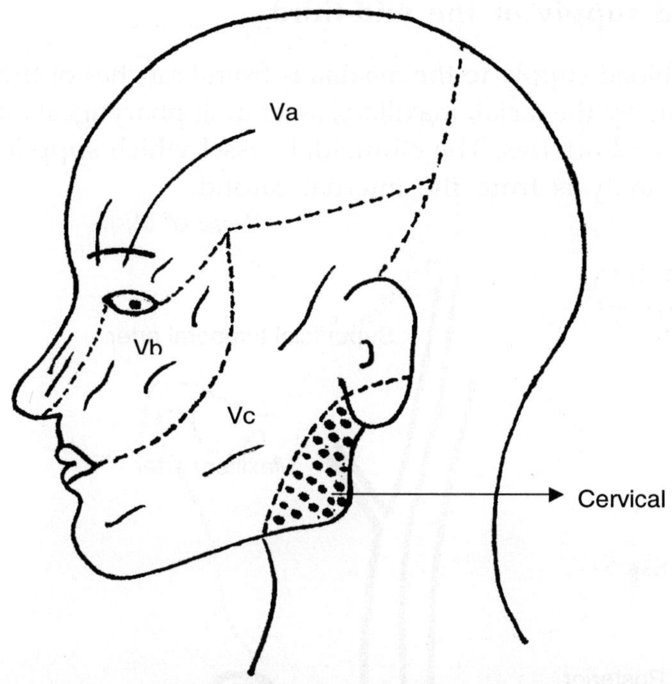

Fig. 9. Cutaneous sensory nerve of the face (5, 3, 3).

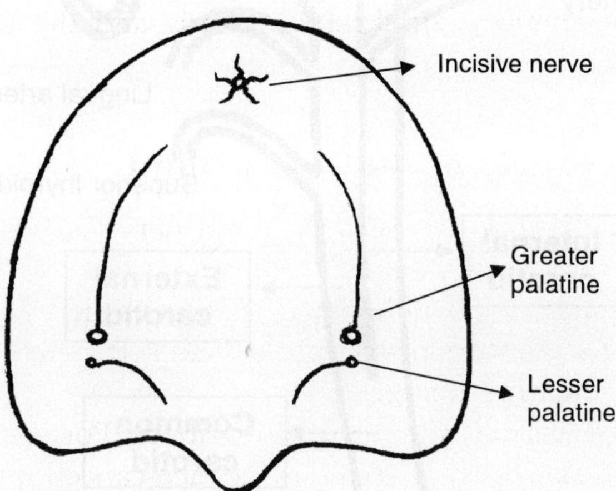

Fig. 10. Sensory nerve supply of palate.

3.2. Blood supply of the mid-third

The main blood supply to the maxilla is from branches of the external carotid, namely the facial, maxillary, ascending pharyngeal and superficial temporal arteries. The ethmoidal vessel which supplies part of the nasal cavity is from the internal carotid.

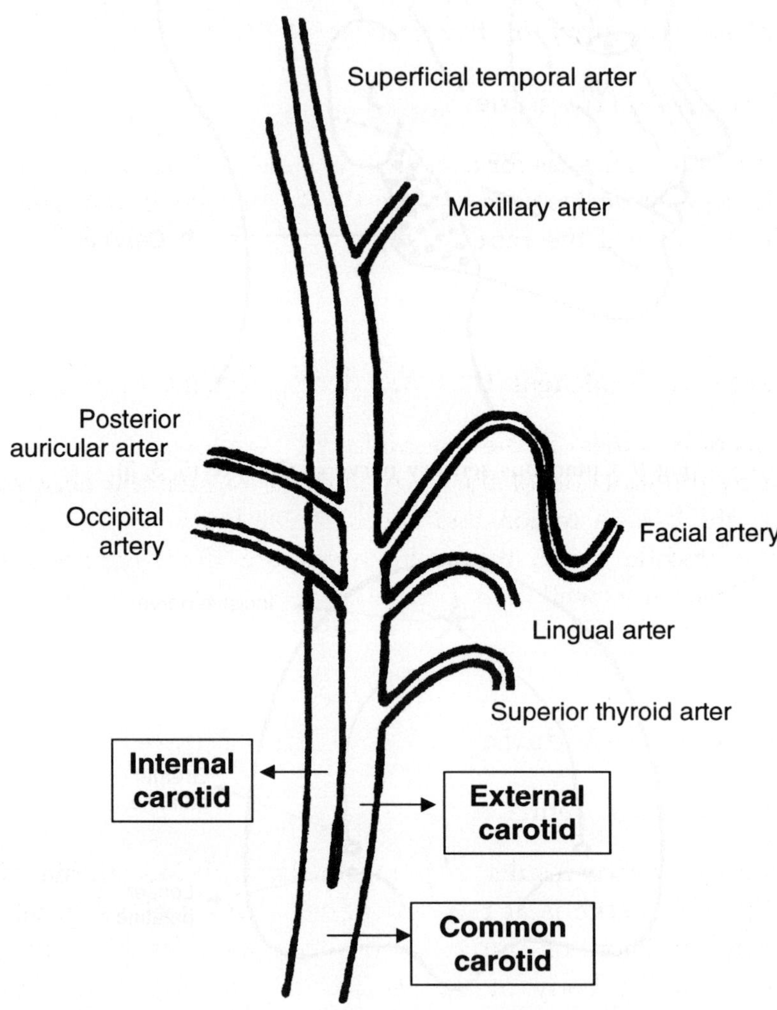

Fig. 11. Main blood supply of OMS region.

4. Upper Third

The upper third of the facial skeleton is formed by the frontal bone. The frontal bone contributes to the superior part of the orbital rim. The zygomatic bone and the maxilla forms the lateral and infero-medial parts of the rim, respectively.

5. Applied Anatomy of the Orofacial Area

5.1. Donor sites for bone graft

The common donor sites for autogenous bone in orofacial reconstruction are from the calvarium (upper third), the maxillary tuberosity (middle third), and the retromolar and symphysis of the mandible (lower third).

5.2. Areas of weakness that are prone to fractures

The areas of weakness in the mandible are the angles of the mandible formed by the junction of the body and the ramus; the neck of the condyle; the canine region and the alveolar bone.

In the middle third, the weak areas are the zygomatic arch, lateral and middle wall of the maxillary sinus, the nasal bones and the alveolus.

5.3. Nerves at risk during surgical procedures

5.3.1. The inferior dental nerve

Injury to this nerve results in paraesthesia and anaesthesia of the lower lip. This nerve is at risk during procedures like sagittal split osteotomy; excision of impacted wisdom teeth and insertion of implants into the body of the mandible posterior to the mental foramen.

5.3.2. Lingual nerve

Injury to this nerve will give rise to numbness of the anterior two-thirds of the tongue. This nerve is particularly at risk during removal of impacted wisdom teeth and submandibular gland surgery.

5.3.3. Mandibular branch of the facial nerve

This nerve exits at the anterior border of the parotid and travels along the deep cervical fascia towards the lower border of the mandible and loops up to supply the lower lip. This nerve is at risk during submandibular incision and parotid surgery.

5.3.4. Branches of the facial nerve

Damage to the facial nerve will cause facial palsy. The facial nerve is at risk during temporo-mandibular joint surgery or parotid surgery.

5.3.5. The olfactory nerve

Fibres of the olfactory nerve traverse the cribriform plate of the ethmoid. Injury to this nerve will cause anosmia. Injury can occur during fracture of the facial skeleton involving the ethmoid.

SECTION II:

MATRIX BIOLOGY AND PHYSIOLOGY OF TISSUES

Advances in Tissue Banking Vol. 5
© 2001 by World Scientific Publishing Co. Pte. Ltd.

6 THE ORGANISATION OF THE EXTRACELLULAR MATRIX

GARETH J. THOMAS and MALCOLM DAVIES

Institute of Nephrology
University of Wales College of Medicine
Heath Park, Cardiff CF14 4XN
Wales, UK

1. Introduction

The last decade has witnessed a rapid increase in our knowledge of
the extracellular matrix (ECM) (Hay, 1999). This is largely due to
advances in molecular biology that have greatly contributed to our
understanding of the composition and the function of this matrix.
In mesenchymal cells, the ECM can be conveniently divided into
the pericellular matrix, close to or adjacent to the cell surface, and
an intercellular matrix, which is more distant and surrounds the
cell. The intercellular matrix can also form specialised structures,
such as cartilage, tendon, and (with secondary deposition of calcium
phosphate) bone and teeth. In addition, the matrix that underlies all
epithelia and endothelia has a different chemical composition and
organisation from the mesenchymal matrix, and is referred to as the
basement membrane (Timpl and Brown, 1996). In the pre-molecular
era of matrix research, the ECM was merely thought to provide
inert scaffolding upon which cellular and tissue development could
take place. It is now recognised that the ECM is a prerequisite for

the existence of multicellular organisms since it maintains tissue form and cellular polarisation, and also plays a pivotal role in a number of different cellular processes, including cell migration, cell growth and differentiation and wound healing. Also, different components of the ECM have been shown to act as antigens in immunopathological processes, and as defective components in certain pathological conditions. The literature concerned with ECM is extensive and since this review is brief and somewhat arbitrarily selective, only recent key papers and reviews are included.

2. Structure of ECM in Normal Tissue

The extracellular matrix of connective tissue represents a complex material made up of insoluble fibres, microfibres and a wide range of soluble proteins and glycoproteins (Hey, 1993). The macro-molecules that make up the ECM are synthesised and secreted by local cells. Both biochemical and molecular biological investigations have identified four major classes of macromolecules, namely collagens, proteoglycans and glycosaminoglycans, structural glycoproteins, and elastin (Ayad *et al.*, 1996).

3. Collagens

The collagens represent a large heterogeneous family of proteins that form supramolecular protein structures to support the integrity of a tissue (Bateman *et al.*, 1996). They also play a pivotal role in embryonic development and tissue regeneration. At present, at least 19 different types of collagens, which composed of at least 33 individually genetically different polypeptide α-chains, are known. A central feature of all collagen molecules is the triple-stranded helix. This helix comprises three α-chains, each with a left-handed polyproline-II-type helical configuration, wound round each other to form a right-handed superhelix. The α-chains have the general composition of $(Gly-X-X)_n$, where X and Y are frequently the amino acid proline and hydroxyproline. This repeating triplet is an absolute requirement for the stability of the triple-helix. Glycine is small enough to occupy the crowded interior of the collagen triple-helix, while hydroxyproline is important for stabilising the structure of the collagen by the formation of hydrogen bonds. Lysine and hydroxylysine residues are also important for the stability of inter-molecular collagen, and as sites for sugar attachment.

The collagens can be divided into four subfamilies: (a) fibril-forming collagens, (b) fibril-associated collagens, (c) non-fibrillar and finally, (d) a group of collagens detected from cDNA and genomic sequencing (see Table 1 and Fig. 1).

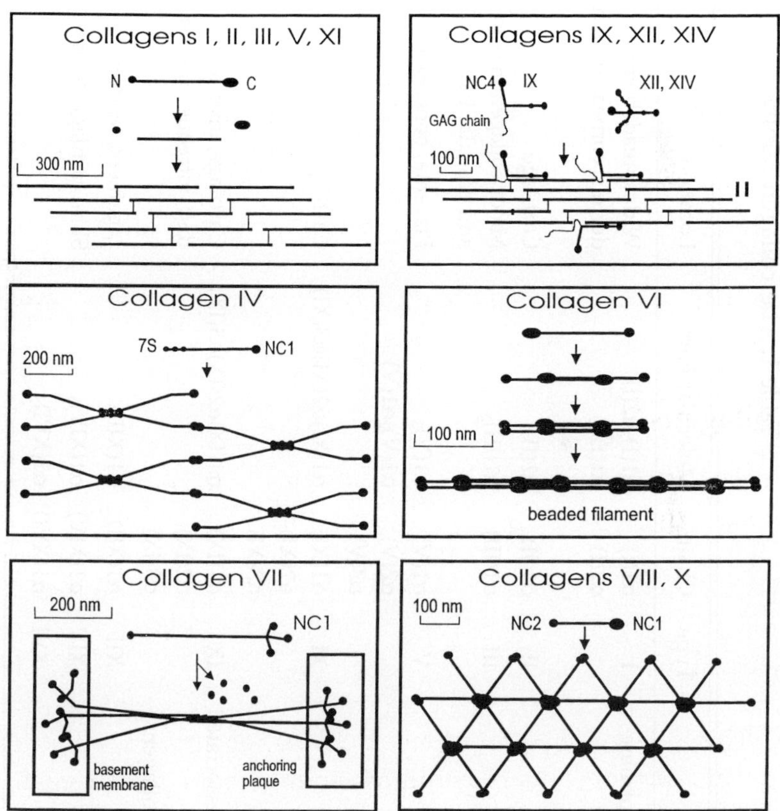

Fig. 1. Collagen molecular assemblies. Reprinted with permission from Bateman, J., Lamande, S. and Ramshaw, J. Collagen superfamily. In: *Extracellular Matrix*, W.C. Comper, ed. Copyright © 1996 Harwood Academic Publications, Amsterdam.

Table 1. The collagen family.

Class	Type	Chain	Molecular Form	Location	Comment
1. Fibril-forming collagens	I	$\alpha1(I)$ $\alpha2(I)$	$\alpha1(I)_2\alpha2(I)$ $\alpha1(I)_3$	Widespread; bone, dermis, cornea, tendon	Most abundant collagen type Frequently referred to as the interstitial collagen
	II	$\alpha1(II)$	$\alpha1(II)_3$	Cartilage	Cross-linked to type IX collagen
	III	$\alpha1(III)$	$\alpha1(III)_3$	Major collagen in skin and vascular tissue	Frequently found with type I collagen in interstitium
	V	$\alpha1(V)$ $\alpha2(V)$ $\alpha3(V)$	$\alpha1(V)_3$ $\alpha1(V)_2\alpha1(V)$	Placenta, bone, skin	Quantitatively minor fibrillar collagen. Forms heterotypic fibrils with types I and III
	XI	$\alpha1(XI)$ $\alpha2(XI)$ $\alpha3(XI)$	$\alpha1(XI)\alpha2(XI)\alpha3(XI)$	Cartilage	Quantitatively minor fibrillar collagen. Forms heterotypic with types II and IX
2. Fibril-associated collagens (FACIT collagens)	IX	$\alpha1(IX)$ $\alpha2(IX)$ $\alpha3(IX)$	$\alpha1(IX)\alpha2(IX)\alpha3(IX)$	Cartilage, invertebral disc, vitreous humour	Associates with type II collagen The $\alpha2(IX)$ can be substituted with CS/DS chains
	XII	$\alpha1(XII)$	$\alpha1(XII)_3$	Ligament, tendon	Loosely linked to ECM
	XIV	$\alpha1(XIV)$	$\alpha1(XIV)_3$	Skin, cartilage, tendon	Found with type I collagen
	XVI	$\alpha1(XVI)$	$\alpha1(XVI)_3$		

Table 1. (*Continued*)

Class	Type	Chain	Molecular Form	Location	Comment
3. Non-fibrillar collagens	IV	$\alpha 1(IV)$ $\alpha 2(IV)$ $\alpha 3(IV)$ $\alpha 4(IV)$ $\alpha 5(IV)$ $\alpha 6(IV)$	$\alpha 1(IV)_2\alpha 4(IV)$ $\alpha 3(IV)_2\alpha 4(IV)$ $\alpha 5(IV)_2\alpha 6(IV)$	Basement membranes	Self-assembles to form a scaffold for the assembly of other basement membrane components
	VIII	$\alpha 1(VIII)$ $\alpha 2(VIII)$	$\alpha 1(VIII)_2\alpha 2(VIII)$	Descemet's membrane	Assembles into hexagonal lattice
	X	$\alpha 1(X)$	$\alpha 1(X)_3$	Foetal tissue	
	VI	$\alpha 1(VI)$ $\alpha 2(VI)$ $\alpha 3(VI)$	$\alpha 1(VI)\alpha 2(VI)\alpha 3(VI)$	All connective tissue	Contains a short collagenous domain Essentially a glycoprotein
	VII	$\alpha 1(VII)$	$\alpha 1(VII)_3$	Specialized epithelia	Large collagen which anchors BM to stromal tissue
	XVII	$\alpha 1(XVII)$	Not known	Dermal-epidermal junction	Bullous pemphigoid antigen
4. Other types	XIII	Not known			Characterized by cDNA
	XV	Not known		Expressed in fibroblasts	Type XVI may be a FACIT collagen
	XVI	Not known		Expressed in fibroblasts	
	XVIII	Not known		Expressed in fibroblasts	
	XIX	Not known			

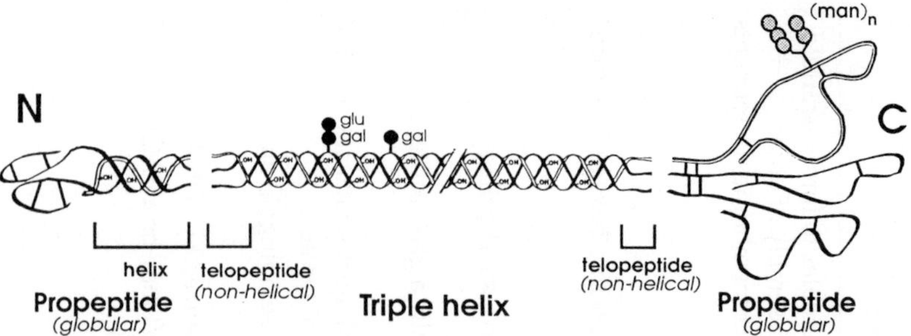

Fig. 2. The structure of type 1 procollagen molecule. Reprinted with permission from Bateman, J., Lamande, S. and Ramshaw, J. Collagen superfamily. In: *Extracellular Matrix*, W.C. Comper, ed. Copyright © 1996 Harwood Academic Publications, Amsterdam.

3.1. Fibril-forming collagens

The fibril-forming collagens represent the main collagen form in different tissues. They are synthesised in precursor (procollagen) forms from which N- and C-terminal propeptides are selectively cleaved off by specific endopeptidases. The resulting mature molecule has a 300 nm helical rod with short non-collagenous sequences at the N- and C-terminal and is resistant to proteolysis by the majority of proteinases, including trypsin (Fig. 2). The processed monomers are spontaneously assembled head to tail longitudinally and aggregate longitudinally to form the fibrils. The individual molecules are staggered by 234 amino acids (67 nm) so that adjacent molecules are displaced longitudinally by approximately one-quarter of their length. This staggered arrangement maximises the number of interchain electrostatic and hydrophobic interactions between molecules and allows specific lysine and hydroxylysine residues in the helix to form stable cross-links. It also gives rise to the striated appearance of interstitial collagens observed with negatively-stained fibrils.

3.2. Fibril-associated collagen

The members of this subgroup are frequently referred to as the FACIT collagens (Fibril-Associated Collagens with Interrupted Triple-helices). They have small triple-helical domains (30 nm) interrupted by short non-helical domains (Fig. 1). Furthermore, much of the molecule (> 90%) is non-collagenous. FACIT collagens do not form fibrils but they are found along the surface of fibril-forming collagen. Collagen IX is associated with collagen type II while types XII and XIV molecules with types I and III collagen fibrils. Collagens IX, XII and XIV can also exist with chondroitin sulphate glycosaminoglycan side chains.

3.3. Non-fibrillar collagen

The third group of collagens includes type IV collagen, which is the principle protein of mammalian basement membranes (Kuhn, 1995). The monomer of this collagen comprises three structurally distinct domains in which a long central triple-helix domain is flanked at its C-terminus by the globular NC1 domain and at its N-terminus by a short (30 nm) triple-helical 7S domain. The central domain contains up to 25 interruptions of the Gly–X–Y amino acid triplet repeats that determines the formation of the triple-helix. These discontinuities also results in a higher flexibility of collagen IV as compared to fibrillar collagens. In contrast to the fibril-forming collagens, procollagen type IV assembles to flexible three-dimensional network by tetramerisation of its N-terminus and by dimerisation of its C-terminus (Fig. 1). The resulting meshwork forms the scaffold of the basement membrane and provides an anchorage for other basement membrane components (laminin, entactin and perlecan) and for adjacent cells.

3.4. Other collagen types

Very little is known about the structure of the fourth group. The existence of these collagen chains is based on cDNA and genomic sequencing and their structure, molecular composition remain to be resolved. Recent studies suggest collagens XVI and XIV may be related to the FACIT group of collagens.

4. Proteoglycans

Proteoglycans are a diverse superfamily of proteins found on cell surfaces, basement membranes and incorporated into extracellular matrices. By definition, they are complex glycoproteins containing at least one covallently attached glycosaminoglycan chain (GAG) (Jackson *et al.*, 1991; Hardingham and Fosang, 1992; Iozzo and Murdoch, 1996). This definition encompasses a wide range of macromolecules that vary in their molecular size, core protein and GAG chain as well as function. Protein and cDNA sequencing has established that the proteoglycan superfamily now contains more than 30 macromolecules that fulfil this definition (Table 2) (Iozzo and Murdoch, 1996). They have been implicated in a wide variety of processes, such as tissue organisation, biological filters, cell adhesion and migration, cell proliferation and the maturation of specialised tissue, regulation of collagen fibrillogenesis and growth factor sequestration and regulation.

The glycosaminoglycan moieties of proteoglycans are sulphated linear polysaccharide chains composed of repeating disaccharide units consisting of one amino sugar (D-glucosamine or D-galactosamine) and one hexuronic acid (D-glucuronic or iduronic acid). Both units are variably N- and O-sulphated. An exception to this rule is keratan sulphate in which galactose replaces the hexuronic acid. There are four main types of GAGs: (i) chondroitin sulphate or its epimerised homologue dermatan sulphate, (ii) heparan and heparin, (iii) keratan sulphate and (iv) hyaluronan (Table 3). Chondroitin, dermatan and heparin/heparan GAGs are linked to protein via the tetrasaccharide linkage sequence composed of xylose, two galactose residues and glucuronate. The actual linkage is between xylose and the amino acid serine in the protein cores. Keratan sulphate is either N-linked to asparagine via mannose and N-acetylglucosamine residues (e.g. corneal keratan sulphate), or O-linked to serine/ threonine via N-actylgalactosamine (skeletal keratan sulphate). Hyaluronan (hyaluronic acid) is a non-sulphated GAG that consists of repeating glucuronic acid and N-acety-glucosamine disaccharides,

Table 2. Proteoglycans.

Proteoglycan	Gene Product	Protein Core (~ kDa)	GAG	Tissue Distribution	Comments
1. SLRPs	Decorin	36	CS/DS (1)	Widespread, bone, teeth mesothelia	Binds to collagen Interact with TGF-β Controls collagen fibril formation
	Biglycan	38	CS/DS (1–2)	Interstitium, cell surface	
	Fibromodulin	42	KS (2–3)	Cartilage	
	Lumican	38	KS (2–3)	Cornea, aorta, muscle intestine	
	PRELP	44	KS (2)		
	Keratocan	38	KS(3–5)	Cornea, sclera, skin, ligament, artery	
	Osteoadherin	42	(2–3)	Bone	Involved in cell attachment
	Epiphycan	35	DS/CS (2–3)	Epiphyseal cartilage	
	Osteoglycin	35	KS (2–3)		
	Chondroadherin			Bone	
2. Aggrecan family: (Hyalectins or Hyaladherins)	Aggrecan	220	CS (approx. 100) KS (20)	Found in cartilage	Interacts with HA to form large aggregates containing 100 PGs per HA molecule.
	Versican	260–370	CS (20)	Found in vascular tissue	Binds to CD44 at cell surface.
	Neurocan			Brain	
	Brevican			Brain	

Table 2. (*Continued*)

Proteoglycan	Gene Product	Protein Core (~ kDa)	GAG	Tissue Distribution	Comments
3. Basement membrane proteoglycans	Agrin	250	HS	Major proteoglycan of neuromuscular junction and renal basement membranes	
	Perlecan	400–500	HS/CS	Provides charge-selectivity of BM Interacts with laminin and collagen IV	
	Bamacan	138	CS	Mesangial matrix, skin	Abnormally expressed in glomerulus of diabetic rats
4. Cell surface proteoglycans	Syndecans		HS	Major proteoglycans of cell surface Four sub-types; syndecan-1 (epithelial cell), syndecan-2 (fibroblasts), syndecan-3, neuronal cells and syndecan-4, widely expressed	Interact with cytokines and growth factors (e.g. FGF) Syndecan-4 found in focal adhesions
	Glypicans		HS	Attached to cell membrane via GPI-linkage Five sub-types	

Table 3. Structure of glycosaminoglycan chains.

GAG Type	Basic Structure	Major Disaccharide	Sulphate Content (per disaccharide)
Hyaluronan	[GlcA β1–3 GlcNAc β1–4]n	GlcA – GlcNAc	0
Chondroitin sulphate	[GlcA β1–3 GalNAc β1–4]n	GlcA – GalNAc (4S)	0–2
		GlcA – GalNAc (6S)	
		GlcA – GalNAc (4S,6S)	
Dermatan sulphate	[IdoA α1–3 GalNAc β1–4]n	IdoA – GalNAc (4S)	0–2
		IdoA(2S) – GalNAc (4S)	
		IdoA(2S) – GalNAc (6S)	
Heparan sulphate	[GlcA β1-4 GlcNAc α1-4]n	GlcA – GlcNAc	0–3
		GlcA – GlcNAc (6S)	
		IdoA – $GlcNSO_3$	
		IdoA – $GlcNSO_3$ (6S)	
		IdoA(2S) – $GlcNSO_3$	
Heparin	[Ido α1-4 GlcNAc α1-4]n	IdoA(2S) – $GlcNSO_3$ (6S)	0–4
		IdoA(2S) – $GlcNSO_3$ (3S)	
Keratan sulphate	[GlcNAc β1-3Gal β1-4]n	GlcNAc(6S) – Gal	0–2
		GlcNAc(6S) – Gal (6S)	

is synthesised without a protein core and therefore does not strictly conform to the definition of a proteoglycan.

4.1. Proteoglycan nomenclature

Originally, the main criterion for the classification of proteoglycans was the nature of their GAG chains. This approach was adopted because of the lack of an underlying feature of the protein core, such as the triple-helix of collagens. However, cDNA sequencing, as well as information on their distribution in tissues, established that proteoglycans could be placed in a number of sub-families that share structural properties of their protein core (Table 2). It must be borne in mind that there is no formal nomenclature for proteoglycans.

4.2. Small leucine-rich proteoglycans (SLRPs)

This family of proteoglycans currently comprises nine relatively well-documented members that are grouped together on the basis of a central domain containing leucine-rich repeats flanked at either side by small cysteine clusters (Hocking *et al.*, 1998). They are, in addition, commonly found in most connective tissue. The proteoglycans in this sub-family have all been given names based on their putative function (see Table 2). The prototype member, decorin, is so named because it "decorates collagen fibres". Decorin and biglycan are the best known and studied sub-group of the SLRP family. Decorin contains a single GAG chain attachment at a serine located four amino acids from the N-terminus. Normally, biglycan contains two chains (hence its name) which are linked with serine 5 and serine 10 of the mature protein. In decorin, biglycan, and also epiphycan, the GAG chains can either be dermatan or chondroitin sulphate. In contrast, fibromodulin and lumican contain N-linked keratan sulphate chains in the central domain. In addition, these molecules contain, towards the N-terminus, a tyrosine-sulphate-rich region which is absent from decorin and biglycan. Thus, despite the absence of chondroitin/dermatan sulphate, fibromodulin and lumican are strongly anionic molecules and their N-termini are involved in interactions with cationic domains of the extracellular matrix.

4.3. Modular proteoglycans

4.3.1. Hyalectins or hyaladherins; proteoglycans that bind to hyaluronan

The proteoglycans that make up this sub-family were originally referred to as large aggregating chondroitin sulphate proteoglycans (Heinegard *et al.*, 1998). The members include the cartilage-derived aggrecan, versican (and its chicken homologue PG-M) and two smaller proteoglycans expressed in nervous tissue, named brevican and neurocan. Common features of these four molecules are a highly homologous hyaluronan-binding domain at the N-terminus and a set of epidermal growth factors, a lectin-like domain and a complement regulatory protein element in the C-terminus. A glycosaminoglycan attachment domain that bears between 3 (brevican) and 100 (aggrecan) chondroitin sulphate chains interrupts these shared structural modules. In aggrecan, a short proline-rich region N-terminal to the chondroitin sulphate region is substituted with up to 30 keratan sulphate chains.

4.3.2. Basement membrane proteoglycans

Basement membranes are specialised extracellular matrices that contain varying amounts of collagen types IV and V, laminin, nidogen and at least one type of proteoglycan. The best characterised is the large proteoglycan normally referred to as perlecan, whose core protein is approximately 400–460 kDa in size, and is usually substituted with three heparan sulphate chains, but in some cases, may alternately or additionally bear chondroitin chains (Iozzo *et al.*, 1994). The core protein of perlecan is one of the most complex structures identified in the extracellular matrix. It is made up of five domains with only one (Domain I at the N-terminus) comprising a unique sequence, the SEA module, named after the three proteins—sperm protein, enterokinase and agrin (Iozzo, 1998). Domain II has homology with low-density lipoprotein receptor. Domain III has the highest homology to the α1-laminin chain and is composed of three globular domains with alternating cysteine-rich regions (epidermal-growth-factor-like repeats). Domain IV consists of immunoglobulin-like repeats which resemble the cell adhesion molecule N-CAM, and is likely to be involved in cell adhesion or self-assembly. The final Domain (V) resembles the C-terminal globular region of the α-laminin chain, but it also homologous to the C-terminus of agrin. Agrin is a second heparan sulphate PG constituent located in basement membranes. It is the major proteoglycan of neuromuscular junctions, and renal tubular and glomerular basement membranes. Like perlecan, it is a multi-domain protein that shares similarities with perlecan and laminin and can be divided into four distinct domains; Domain I contains a novel laminin-binding domain (or NtA, N-terminal in agrin); Domain II is characterised by 9-follistatin-like protease inhibitors interrupted by two laminin-like EGF repeats; Domain III, as in perlecan, contains a central SEA motif flanked by two serine/threonine-rich domains; Domain IV contains three sequences sharing homology with globules of the α-laminin chains interrupted by EGF-like repeats. The agrin molecule also contains two regions in Domain II favourable for heparan sulphate attachment. Agrin is essential for synaptic formation at the neuromuscular junction. Its modular components indicate that agrin plays an important role in cell matrix adhesion. Another important putative function for agrin is that, because it contains nine proteinase-inhibiting domains, it protects the basement membrane proteins against extracellular proteinase degradation.

The detection of chondroitin sulphate in basement membranes led to the isolation and characterisation of a third proteoglycan named bamacan. This proteoglycan was first isolated from embryonic rat tissue and adult rat kidney. The core protein of bamacan is the product of a single gene that is different from any other basement membrane proteoglycan. The secondary structure analysis of the protein reveals a sequential organisation of three globular regions interconnected by two alpha-helix coils. Bamacan mRNA levels are low in normal cells and markedly reduced during quiescence but are highly increased when cells resume growth upon serum stimulation. In contrast, in all transformed cells tested, bamacan is constitutively overexpressed, and its levels do not change with cell cycle progression. This suggests that bamacan is involved in the control of cell growth and transformation.

4.4. Cell membrane HSPGs

Heparan sulphate proteoglycans are present at the plasma membrane of virtually all mammalian cells (Carey, 1997; Zimmermann and David, 1999). To date, nine have been identified that are divided into two major families, the syndecans and glypicans (Table 2). All the four members of the syndecan family (numbered 1 to 4 in chronological order of their discovery) have highly homologous transmembrane and cytoplasmic domains, except for a short variable region at the centre of the latter domain. The highly-conserved cytoplasmic protein sequence contains tyrosine residues that provide phosphorylation sites for protein kinases, which are key enzymes in many transduction pathways and sites for cross-linkage with cytosketal elements. In contrast, the ectodomain of these molecules exhibit little homology apart from the amino sequences in the region of HS glycanation. The majority of the GAG chains added to syndecan core proteins are HS, but some of the core proteins bear chondroitin sulphate chains as well (Table 2). The glypican family consists of glycosylphosphatidylinositol (GPI)-anchored proteoglycans bearing 2–3 heparan sulphate chains. To date, six such proteoglycans have been identified, all of which consist of highly-conserved protein cores that share GPI-anchorage mechanism, a unique cysteine motif and glycanation sites that contain carboxyl termini, close to the anchor structure that links the protein to the cell surface.

The syndecans and glypicans are involved in cell-extracellular and cell-to-cell interactions through their heparan chains, since heparan sulphate GAGs are able to interact with a wide range of molecules, including enzymes and proteinase inhibitors, extracellular molecules, and cytokines and growth factors. Of particular importance amongst these interactions is that HS is an essential co-receptor for the expression of the biological activity of bFGF, in addition to αFGF, FGF-4, IL-8 and hepatocyte growth factor.

5. Hyaluronan (Hyaluronic Acid, Hyaluronate)

Hyaluronan is a linear non-sulphated glycosaminoglycan consisting of alternating N-acetylglucosamine and glucuronic acid disaccharides, with GlcNAc(β 1–4) GlcUA (β 1–3) GlcNac linkages (Laurent and Fraser, 1992). Unlike other glycosaminoglycans, hyaluronan is not found covalently bound to a protein core. It is synthesised at the plasma membrane, through which the growing chain is extended into the extracellular space. Hyaluronans have very high molecular weights and single molecules can reach up to 10 million (i.e. approximately 25,000 repeat disaccharides) in size. To date in vertebrates, three hyaluronan synthase genes (*HAS 1*, *HAS 2* and *HAS 3*) that control the synthesis of hyaluronan have been identified, but the precise interrelationship of these genes has yet to be determined. Interestingly, initial studies suggest clear differences between the three enzymes indicating the synthesis of three different sized hyaluronan polymers. For example, the *HAS 3* gene generates significantly shorter chains than *HAS 2*. This finding could be of biological significance because the size of the hyaluronan polymer may be an important factor in the regulation of cellular function.

The cellular function of HA is based on its ability to entrap large amounts of fluids and so create hydrous channels that facilitate cell migration. In addition, hyaluronan specifically binds to cell surface receptors such as CD44, indicating that hyaluronan effects cell migration by specific ligand–receptor interactions (Toole, 1990).

6. Fibronectin, Laminin and Other Extracellular Glycoproteins

6.1. Fibronectin

Fibronectin is a class of multifunctional modular glycoproteins present on the cell surface and in the pericellular and intercellular matrix (Hymes, 1990). The fibronectin molecule is a dimer composed of two similar homologous subunits covalently linked together in an antiparallel manner by a pair of disulphide bonds near their C-termini. Each monomer consists of three types of structurally independent units called Type I, Type II and Type III (Fig. 3). Differential splicing of the units EIIIA, EIIIB, and the variable region can produce theoretically 20 isoforms. Each fibronectin polypeptide bears a series of functional domains that are specialised for binding to the extracellular matrix or cell membranes. Fibronectin exists in a soluble dimeric form in the plasma and as an insoluble (fibrillar) multimeric form in the ECM. The mechanism responsible for the

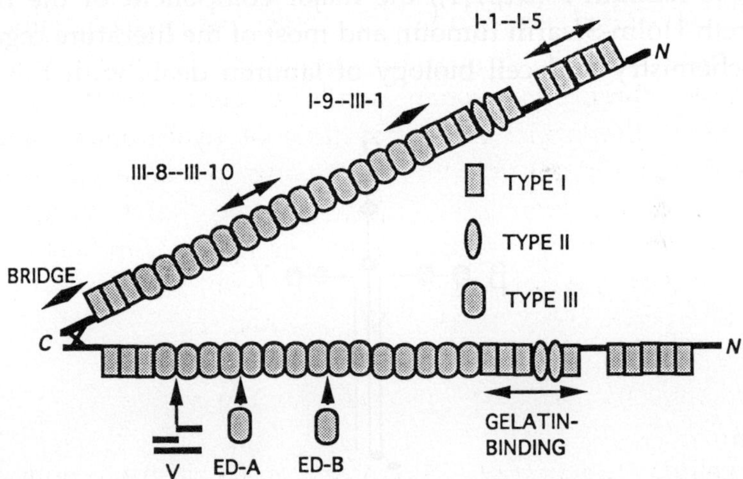

Fig. 3. Domain structure of fibronectin dimer. Reprinted with permission from Peters, D.M.P. and Mosher, D.F. Formation of fibronectin extracellular matrix. In: *Extracellular Matrix Assembly and Structure*, P.D. Yurchenco, D.E. Birk and R.P. Mecham, eds. Copyright © 1994 Academic Press, Amsterdam and San Diego.

assembly of fibronectin fibrils is not completely understood but appears to involve multiple fibronectin-binding integrins and components of the cytoskeleton. The insoluble form in the ECM is cross-linked by transglutaminase.

6.2. Laminin

Laminin refers to a family of three genetically distinct but structurally related polypeptides, α1, β1 and γ1, with M_r of 200–400, 215 and 200 kDa, respectively (Beck *et al.*, 1990; Timpl and Brown, 1994). These chains are linked together by disulphide bonds to form a cruciform or Y-shaped heterotrimer made up of three short arms and a long arm (Fig. 4). The amino termini of each chain extend to form three short arms, which consist of several sub-domains. There are currently 12 reported laminins assembled from five α, three β and three γ chains that have been shown to be distinct gene products. As with the collagens, laminin heterotrimers are named with Arabic numerals essentially in the order of their discovery. The most studied laminin isoform is laminin-1 (α1β1γ1), the major component of the murine Engelbreth-Holm-Swarm tumour, and most of the literature regarding the biochemistry and cell biology of laminin deals with this form.

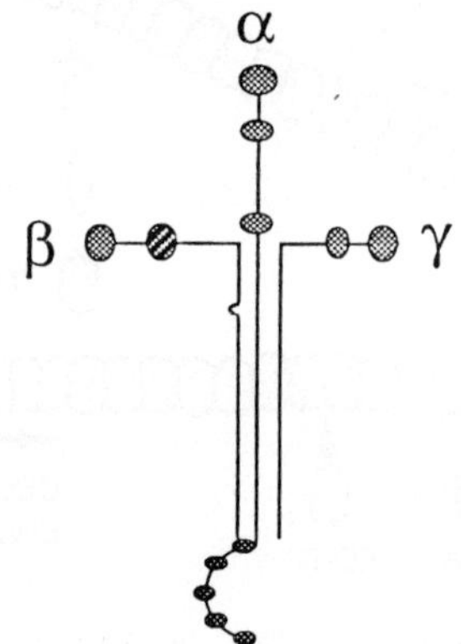

Fig. 4. Structure of laminin trimer. Reprinted with permission from Lindholm, A. and Paulson, M. Basement membranes. In: *Extracellular Matrix*, W.C. Comper, ed. Copyright © 1996 Harwood Academic Publications, Amsterdam.

Laminins are distributed ubiquitously in all basement membranes, with the possible exception of laminin-1 ($\alpha 2\beta 1\gamma 3$), which contains the recently reported novel $\gamma 3$ chain. Two major functions have been ascribed to laminin. Firstly, it functions as a structural molecule that forms a polymer essential for basement membrane architecture, providing mechanical support to adjacent cells. Secondly, it acts as a ligand for cell membrane receptors (integrins) and matrix receptors, such as type IV collagen, entactin and perlecan. Laminin stimulates neurite outgrowth, promotes cell attachment, chemotaxis, cell differentiation and neural survival. These distinct biological events have been assigned to specific amino acid sequences within the laminin polypeptides. For example, the peptides YIGSR and RYVVLPR are recognition sequences for many cells and heparin, respectively.

6.3. Entactin nidogen

Entactin/nidogen is an elongated sulphated glycoprotein of approximately 150 kDa that serves as a link between laminin and

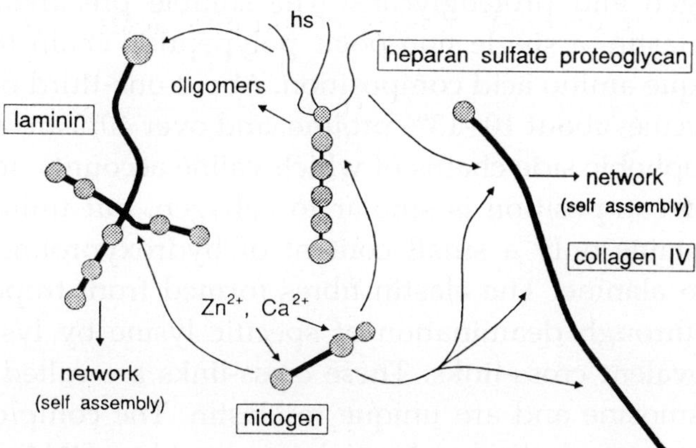

Fig. 5. Interaction of nidogen, laminin, perlecan and type IV collagen in the supramolecular organisation of the basement membranes. Reprinted with permision from Mayer, U. and Timpl, R. Nidogen: A versatile binding protein of basement membrane. In: *Extracellular Matrix Assembly and Structure*, P.D. Yurchenco, D.E. Birk and R.P. Mecham, eds. Copyright © 1994 Academic Press, Amsterdam and San Diego.

collagen in all basement membranes (Chung and Durkin, 1990). It has a dumb-bell shape with globular ends connected by two linear segments (Fig. 5). The amino acid sequence reveals that nidogen contains six EGF-like repeats, one cysteine repeat found in thyroglobulin, and a region with homology to the LDL receptor. The C-terminus (G3) globule contains the binding site for laminin, whereas the G1 (N-terminus) independently binds collagen IV and perlecan core protein. Thus, nidogen serves as a link between laminin, collagen IV and perlecan in basement membranes (Fig. 5).

7. Elastin Fibres

Elastin fibres consist of two protein compounds, the more abundant elastin, which appears as an amorphous mass on electron microscopy, and elastin microfibrils (Mecham and Davis, 1994).

7.1. Elastin

Elastin is an extremely insoluble protein found in the ECM, associated with collagen and proteoglycans. The soluble precursor of elastin is α-tropoelastin, a single non-polar polypeptide chain (65–70 kDa) with a unique amino acid composition. About one-third of the amino acids is glycine, about 10–13% proline, and over 40% are amino acids with hydrophobic side chains of which valine accounts for 17%. The amino acid composition is similar to collagen, but unlike collagen, elastin contains only a small content of hydroxyproline. Elastin is also rich in alanine. The elastin fibres formed from tropoelastin are stabilised through deamination of specific lysine by lysyl oxidases to form covalent cross-links. These cross-links are called desmosine and isodesmosine and are unique to elastin. The complete primary structure of tropoelastin has been determined by cDNA cloning and the predicted structure indicates that elastin consists entirely of two structurally distinct domains: (a) hydrophobic regions, rich in glycine, proline and valine, and (b) cross-linking regions which contain alanine together with two or three lysine residues.

7.2. Elastin-associated microfibrils

An increasing number of elastin-associated microfibrils have been described. The molecules are glycoproteins ranging in molecular weight from 31 kDa (i.e. Microfibril Associated GlycoProtein, MAGP) to 350 kDa (i.e. fibrillins 1 and 2). Other proteins associated with elastin include Microfibrillin Proteins, MP25, MP78 and MP70, emulin, fibrillin-like protein and TGF-β1 binding protein. The best characterised of the these proteins are fibrillins 1 and 2, both of which have been cloned. The predicted domain structure indicated that these molecules are rod-like structures containing 56 cysteine-rich repeat sequences, 47 of which are similar to motifs found in epidermal growth factor (EGF). Immunoelectron microscopy studies reveal that the fibrils occur as ordered aggregates in tissues which include skin, aorta, cartilage, lung connective tissue, placenta and Descement's membrane of the cornea. It has been suggested that the two fibrillin molecules have distinct, but related, functions in the formation and maintenance of the extracellular elastin associated microfibrils. The aggregates function to influence biochemical properties in a variety of tissues and organs.

7. Summary

The ECM is now recognised as a complex but highly organised structure containing multiple members of families of macromolecules. An understanding of this matrix is important if such processes as cell shape, cell migration and the control of cell growth and differentiation are to be comprehended. Over the last decade considerable progress has been made in the identification and characterisation of the components that make up the ECM, and many of the interactions between them. Several human diseases involve perturbation of the ECM, particularly to the basement membrane. Increasingly, molecular and biochemical analysis will help us to understand the basis of diseases such as diabetic vascular disease, Goodpasture's disease and Alport's syndrome. The utilisation of mutant cell lines and the generation of animal models with perturbed matrix metabolism will enable investigators to unambiguously define the individual roles of the different matrix components in many human pathologies.

8. References

AYAD, S., BOOT-HANDFORD, R., HUMPHRIES, M.J., KADLER, K.E. and SHUTTLEWORTH, A. (1996). *The Extracellular Matrix. Facts Book.* 2nd edn., Academic Press, London.

BATEMAN, J., LAMANDE, S. and RAMSHAW, J. (1996). Collagen superfamily. In: *Extracellular Matrix.*, W.C. Comper, ed., Harwood Academic Publications, Amsterdam, pp. 22–67.

BECK, K., HUNTER, I. and ENGEL, J. (1990). Structure and function of laminin: Anatomy of a multidomain glycoprotein. *FASEB J.* **4**, 148–160.

CAREY, D.J. (1997). Syndecans: Multifunctional cell-surface co-receptors. *Biochem J.* **327**, 1–16.

CHUNG, A.E. and DURKIN, M.E. (1990). Entacin: Structure and function. *Am. J. Respir. Cell. Mol. Biol.* **3**, 275–282.

HARDINGHAM, T.E. and FOSANG, A.J. (1992). Proteoglycans: Many forms and many functions. *FASEB J.* **6**, 861–870.

HAY, E.D. (1999). Biogenesis and organisation of extracellular matrix. *FASEB J.* **13**(Suppl 2), S281–283.

Hay, E.D. (1993). *Cell Biology of the Extracellular Matrix.* Plenum Press, New York.

HEINEGARD, D. BJORNSSON, S., MOREGELIN, M., and SOMMARIN, Y. (1998). Hyaluronan-binding matrix proteins. In: *The Chemistry, Biology and Medical Applications of Hyaluronan and its Derivatives*, T.C. Laurent, ed., Portland Press, London. pp. 113–122.

HOCKING, A.M., SHINOMURA, T. and MCQUILLAN, D.J. (1998). Leucine-rich repeat glycoproteins of the extracellular matrix. *Matrix Biol.* **17**, 1–19.

HYMES, R.O. (1990). *Fibronectins*, Springer-Verlag, New York.

IOZZA, R.V. (1998). Matrix proteoglycans: From molecular design to cellular function. *Ann. Rev. Biochem.* **67**, 609–652.

IOZZO, R.V., COHEN, I.R., GRASSEL, S. and MURDOCH, A.D. (1994). The biology of perlecan: The multifaceted heparan sulphate proteoglycan of basement membranes and pericellular matrices. *Biochem J.* **302**, 625–639.

IOZZO, R.V. and MURDOCH, A.D. (1996). Proteoglycans of the extracellular environment: Clues from the gene and protein side offer novel perspectives in molecular diversity and function. *FASEB J.* **10**, 598–614.

JACKSON, R.L., BUSCH, S.J. and CARDIN, A.D. (1991). Glycosamino-glycans: Molecular properties, protein interactions, and role in physiological processes. *Physiol. Rev.* **71**, 481–539.

KUHN, K. (1995). Basement membrane (type IV) collagen. *Matrix Biol.* **14**, 439–445.

LAURENT, T.C. and FRASER, J.R. (1992). Hyaluronan. *FASEB J.* **6**, 2397–2404.

MECHAM, R.P. and DAVIS, E.C. (1994). Elastin fiber structure. In: *Extracellular Matrix Assembly and Structure*, P.D. Yurchenco, D.E. Birk and R.P. Mecham, eds., Academic Press, San Diego.

TIMPL, R. (1996). Macromolecular organization of basement membranes. *Curr. Opin. Cell Biol.* **8**, 618–624.

TIMPL, R. and BROWN, J.C. (1994). The laminins. *Matrix Biol.* **14**, 75–81.

TOOLE, B.P. (1990). Hyaluronan and its binding proteins, the hyaladherins. *Curr. Opin. Cell Biol.* **2**, 839–844.

ZIMMERMANN, P. and DAVID, G. (1999). The syndecans, tuners of transmembrane signaling. *FASEB J.* **23**(Suppl), S91–S100.

7 HISTOLOGY OF BONE

CHARANJIT KAUR

Department of Anatomy, Faculty of Medicine
National University of Singapore
4 Medical Drive, MD10, Singapore 117597

Abstract

Bone is a specialised type of connective tissue consisting of
cells and an intercellular matrix (ground substance and fibres).
It is a highly vascular, living and constantly changing tissue
supplied richly with blood vessels and nerves, and its
architecture (internal and external) can change in response to
stresses and strains to which it is subjected during life. It is
in a continuous state of dynamic growth. Despite its hardness
and unyielding character, bone possesses elasticity.

1. Functions

— It protects the soft tissues and organs in the cranial, thoracic and
pelvic cavity.
— It provides attachment to muscles and transmits the force of
contraction of muscles from one part of the body to another.
— It constitutes a reservoir for calcium and actively participates in
calcium homeostasis of the body.
— It contains the haematopoetic tissue.

2. Classification of Bones

Bones are classified as long, short, flat, irregular and sesmoid. Long bones are the bones found in limbs, e.g. humerus, femur and tibia. Carpal and tarsal bones are examples of short bones. Vertebrae are irregular bones. Bone found in some tendons are the sesmoid bones, e.g. patella.

3. Terms Used in the Description of Bone Histology

3.1. Parts of a long bone (Fig. 1)

It is useful to know parts of a long bone, since long bones serve as classical models for studying the macroscopic and microscopic features of bone. A typical adult long bone consists of a cylindrical shaft or diaphysis and two rounded ends or epiphyses. Metaphysis connects the diaphysis with the epiphysis in developing long bones.

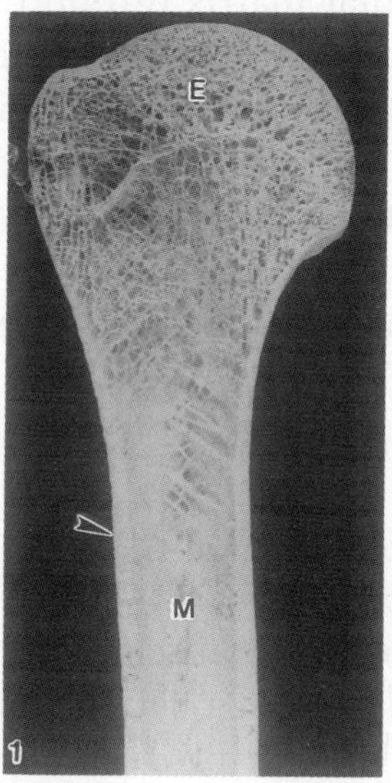

Fig. 1. Longitudinal section through the adult humerus showing compact bone (arrowhead) in the diaphysis Bond trabecular or spongy bone in the epiphysis E. M, bone marrow cavity in the diaphysis. (Magnification 2×)

3.2. Macroscopic organisation

When the cut surface of a mature bone is viewed, the following can be seen.

(i) Compact (cortical) bone — dense, outer layer of bone (Fig. 1).
(ii) Spongy (cancellous or trabecular) bone — a network of small bony spinules or bars in the interior of mature bones (Fig. 1). It is surrounded by compact bone. Primary bone is also spongy.

3.3. Microscopic organisation

Based on microscopic features, bone tissue is of two types:

(i) Woven bone (primary or non-lamellar or immature bone) — collagen fibres are arranged irregularly.
(ii) Lamellar bone (secondary or mature, i.e. compact and spongy) — collagen fibres are arranged in parallel or concentric layers.

3.4. Development of bone

There are two modes of bone development:

(i) Endochondral — takes place in a preformed hyaline cartilage model.
(ii) Intramembranous — takes place by direct transformation of mesenchyme (embryonic connective tissue).

3.5. Ossification centres

(i) Primary ossification centre (e.g. diaphysis of long bones) — where bone formation begins first of all in the embryo.
(ii) Secondary ossification centres (e.g. epiphyses of long bones) — appear later.

3.6. Surfaces of bone

(i)   Periosteal or outer — covered by periosteum.
(ii) Endosteal or inner — lined by endosteum.

The articular surfaces of bones are not covered by the periosteum.

4. Bone Cells

4.1. Osteoprogenitor cells

These are stem cells of mesenchymal origin which can proliferate and differentiate into osteoblasts prior to bone formation.

4.2. Osteoblasts (Fig. 2)

These are bone-forming cells. They are responsible for the synthesis of the organic components of bone matrix (collagen fibres, proteoglycans and glycoproteins, etc). The cells are cuboidal with a rounded nucleus and basophilic cytoplasm. They are located at the surface of bone tissue lying side by side (resembling simple cuboidal epithelium). When they are actively engaged in matrix synthesis, they are cuboidal to columnar in shape and have high alkaline phosphatase activity which is thought to be involved in the calcification of the matrix. When their synthesising activity declines, they flatten and their alkaline phosphatase activity also declines. When an osteoblast is surrounded by newly synthesised matrix, it is called an osteocyte.

At the electron microscopic level, osteoblasts show a large amount of rough endoplasmic reticulum and a well-developed Golgi complex.

Osteoblasts of young bone have protrusions which bud off as vesicular structures known as matrix vesicles. These vesicles are important in mineral deposition in the matrix.

The newly synthesised, not yet calcified matrix is called osteoid or prebone.

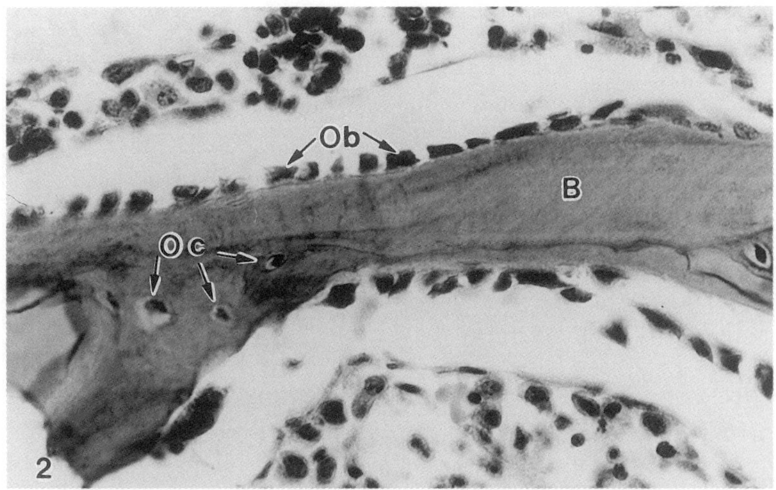

Fig. 2. Section of a developing long bone showing spicules of bone. Active osteoblasts (Ob) are seen arranged in rows on the surface of the bony spicule (B). Osteocytes (Oc) can be seen in the lacunae in the bony spicule. (Magnification 340×)

4.3. Osteocytes (Figs. 2 and 3)

Osteocytes are found in lacunae (cavities or spaces) in the bone matrix. They have long thin cytoplasmic processes called filopodia. Thin, cylindrical spaces in the matrix, called canaliculi, are occupied by the filopodial processes of the osteocytes. Osteocytes are separated from one another by the impermeable bone matrix, only the tips of their filopodia are joined by gap junctions. By this arrangement, nutrients and oxygen can be passed between blood vessels and distant osteocytes. Osteocytes maintain the bone matrix near to them. Osteocytes can also break down the bone matrix near them by a process called *osteocytic osteolysis* to release calcium.

4.4. Osteoclasts (Fig. 3)

These are large, multinucleated cells (formed by fusion of many monocytes) that lie on bony surfaces in shallow depression called

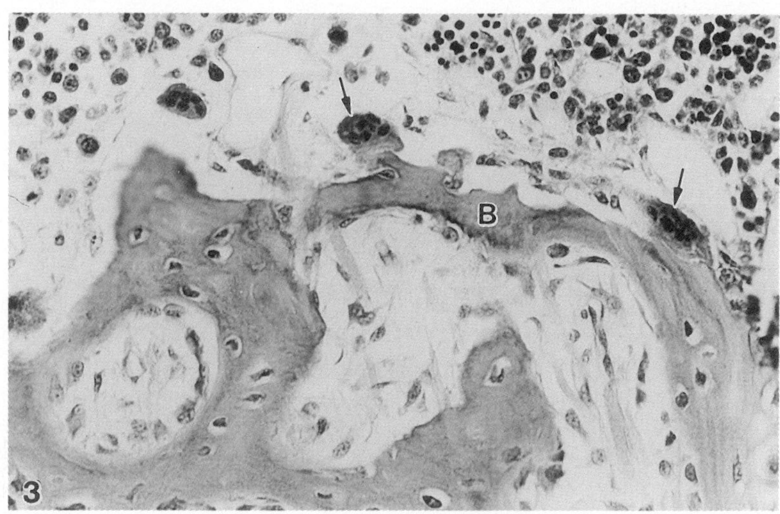

Fig. 3. Osteoclasts (arrows) lying on the surface of bony spicules (B) can be seen in a developing vertebra. Osteocytes occupy lacunae embedded in the bone spicule. (Magnification 340×)

Howship's lacunae. The osteoclast surface facing the depression exhibits a ruffled border of plasma-membrane infoldings. These cells are involved in bone resorption, i.e. breaking down of bone matrix and releasing minerals. They secrete an enzyme called collagenase which helps in breaking down the bone matrix. Osteoclasts respond to the hormones parathormone and calcitonin, secreted by the parathyroid and thyroid gland, respectively. Low serum calcium level stimulates the secretion of parathormone which increases the osteoclastic activity (bone resorption to release calcium) and calcium absorption in the intestines, and decreases excretion of calcium from the kidneys. High serum calcium level stimulates the secretion of calcitonin which inhibits osteoclastic activity, decreases calcium absorption in the intestines and increases excretion of calcium from the kidneys.

5. Bone Matrix

Bone matrix consists of inorganic and organic matter. Inorganic matter consists of abundant calcium phosphate in crystalline form (hydroxyapatite crystals). In addition to calcium phosphate, several other ions are present, e.g. magnesium, potassium, sodium, carbonate and citrate ions.

Organic matter consists of collagen fibres (Type I) embedded in a ground substance which contains proteoglycans and glyco-proteins, etc.

The association of hydroxyapatite with collagen fibres is responsible for the hardness of the bone. After the bone is decalcified, it becomes flexible. Removal of the organic part of the matrix (collagen) leaves the bone with its original shape, but it becomes fragile and breaks easily.

6. Periosteum and Endosteum

The external and internal surfaces (bone marrow cavity and spicules of spongy bone) of bone are covered by layers of bone-forming cells and connective tissue called periosteum and endosteum, respectively.

Active periosteum, as in developing bones (Fig. 4), consists of two layers: an outer layer of collagen fibres and fibroblasts, and an inner layer which is more cellular and is composed of flattened cells (osteoprogenitor cells) with the potential to divide by mitosis and differentiate into osteoblasts. The periosteum is connected to the bone matrix by collagen fibres called Sharpey's fibres.

The endosteum lines all the internal surfaces of bone and is composed of osteoprogenitor cells and a very small amount of connective tissue.

Periosteum and endosteum provide a continuous supply of new osteoblasts for repair or growth of bone.

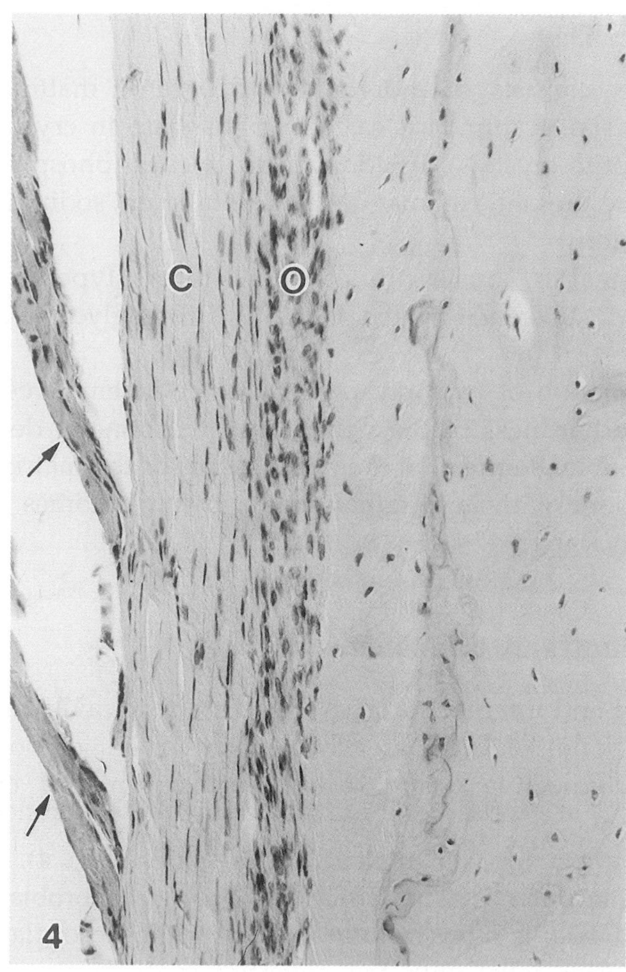

Fig. 4. Section of a developing long bone showing two layers of the periosteum — inner layer of osteoblasts (O) and an outer layer of collagen fibres (C). Some skeletal muscle fibres (arrows) can be seen attached to the outer layer of the periosteum. (Magnification 170×)

7. Types of Bone Tissue

Bone exists in two main forms: immature (primary or woven bone) and mature (secondary or lamellar bone). Both varieties contain the same structural components but in the immature bone, collagen bundles are randomly placed, while in mature bone, these bundles are organised into bone lamellae (membranes or sheets).

7.1. Primary bone tissue

Primary bone tissue is the first to appear in the formation of each bone as well as in the repair process. It is temporary and is replaced in adults by secondary bone tissue. Besides the irregular arrangement of collagen fibres, primary bone consists of a smaller content of minerals and a higher number of osteocytes. In the adult, primary bone tissue may be found in the sockets of teeth.

7.2. Secondary bone tissue

Secondary bone tissue is usually found in adults and consists of two types: compact and spongy (cancellous or trabecular bone). In the spongy bone, collagen fibres are arranged in parallel lamellae. In the compact bone (Figs. 5 and 6), the lamellae of collagen fibres are arranged concentrically around a canal (Haversian canal) which contains blood vessels, nerves and loose connective tissue. The concentric lamellae and the canal are collectively called a Haversian system or an osteon. Lacunae containing osteocytes are found between the lamellae. Surrounding each Haversian system is a deposit of amorphous material called cementing substance, which consists of mineralised matrix with a few collagen fibres.

In compact bone (e.g. diaphysis of long bones) the lamellae exhibit a typical organisation consisting of Haversian systems, outer circumferential lamellae, inner circumferential lamellae and interstitial lamellae (Fig. 7). The principal function of Haversian systems is to bring nutrients to compact bone. Since Haversian systems are longitudinal cylinders, they provide mechanical support to the bone.

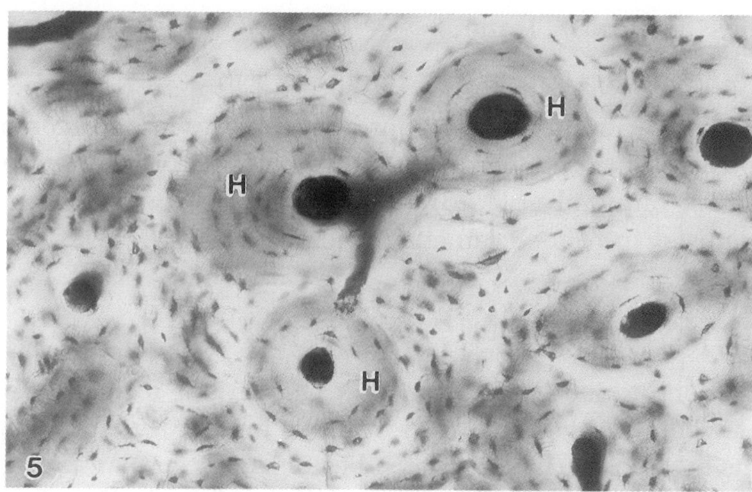

Fig. 5. Unstained ground section of compact bone showing Haversian (H) systems. Concentric rings of flattened lacunae can be seen surrounding the Haversian canals. Details of the osteocytes cannot be seen with this preparation. (Magnification 140×)

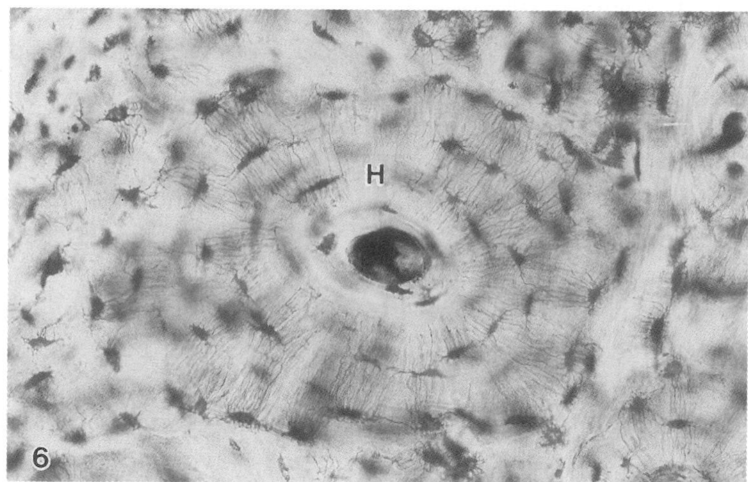

Fig. 6. A Haversian system (H) in ground section of compact bone at high magnification showing concentric arrangement of lacunae. Canaliculi can be seen extending from the lacunae. Osteocytes cannot be seen in this preparation. (Magnification 340×)

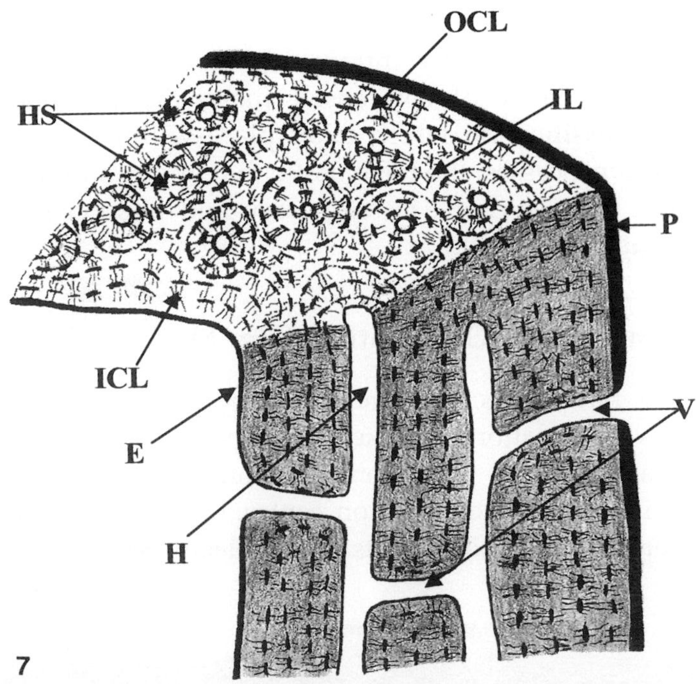

Fig. 7. Diagram of compact bone showing periosteum (P), endosteum (E) Haversian systems (HS), outer circumferential lamella (OCL), inner circumferential lamella (ICL), Haversian canals (H) and Volkman's canals (V).

Haversian systems are absent in thin spicules of spongy bone since nutrients can diffuse into the bony tissue from surrounding capillaries. Each Haversian system is a long cylinder which runs parallel to the long axis of the diaphysis. It consists of a central canal lined by endosteum. The canal contains blood vessels, nerves and loose connective tissue, and is surrounded by 4–20 concentric lamellae. The Haversian canals communicate with the marrow cavity, with the periosteum and with each other through transverse or oblique canals called Volkman's canals.

8. Histogenesis

Bone tissue arises either by intramembranous ossification, which occurs within a layer of condensed mesenchymal tissue or by endochondral ossification which takes place within a cartilaginous model. In both processes, the bone tissue that appears first is primary or immature. Primary bone is temporary and is soon replaced by lamellar or mature bone.

9. Intramembranous Ossification (Fig. 8)

Most of the flat bones, e.g. the skull bones, develop by intramembranous ossification. It takes place within condensations of mesenchymal tissue. In these condensations, the starting point for ossification is called an ossification centre. Groups of mesenchymal cells differentiate into osteoblasts. Osteoblasts begin the synthesis

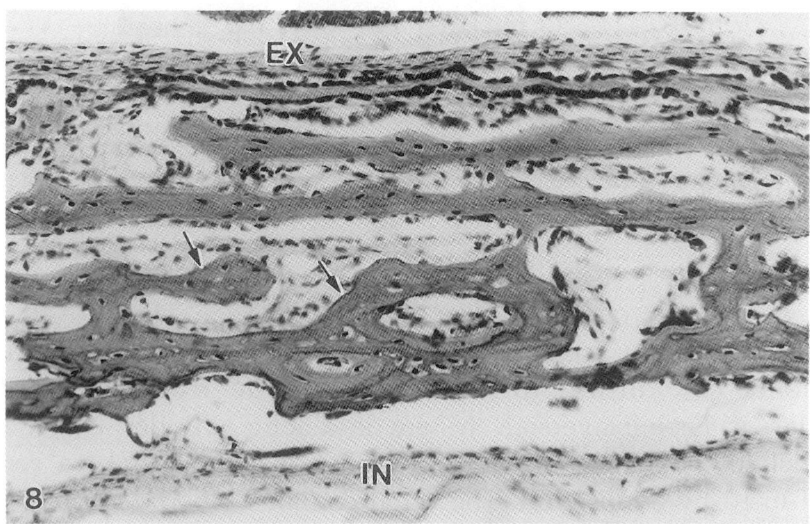

Fig. 8. Skull of a kitten showing the process of intramembranous ossification. The external (EX) and internal (IN) surfaces of the skull are invested with the periosteum. Many developing trabeculae (arrows) of bone can be seen between the external and internal periosteum. (Magnification 220×)

of osteoid, which is followed by calcification. Calcification of the osteoid results in the encapsulation of some osteoblasts which then become osteocytes. These areas of developing bone are called spicules or trabeculae. There are several such spicules developing simultaneously at the ossification centers. Fusion of these spicules results in the formation of bone which is spongy in appearance. This is immature or woven bone. The connective (mesenchymal) tissue that remains in between the spicules is penetrated by growing blood vessels and additional undifferentiated mesenchymal cells which give rise to bone marrow cells. The woven bone undergoes progressive remodelling by osteoclastic resorption and osteoblastic deposition to form mature compact and spongy bone. The portion of connective tissue layer that does not undergo ossification gives rise to the endosteum and the periosteum of intramembranous bone.

10. Endochondral Ossification (Fig. 9)

Endochondral ossification takes place within a piece of hyaline cartilage whose shape resembles a small model of the bone to be formed. All long and short bones are developed by this type of ossification.

Endochondral ossification is most easily understood if we consider the process in one of the long bones of the limbs, for example, the femur. The first sign of bone formation is seen near the middle of the future shaft by the formation of primary ossification centre. Here, the chondrocyctes hypertrophy and the lacunae become bigger. The cartilage matrix is reduced to thin septa. These septa then undergo calcification and the chondrocytes degenerate and die possibly due to prevention of diffusion through the matrix because of its calcification.

Simultaneous with these changes in the cartilage cells, the cells in the perichondrium surrounding the middle of the deep part of the periosteum undergo transformation to osteoprogenitor cells and then to osteoblasts. They rapidly form a thin layer of bone around the middle of the shaft called the periosteal bone collar. At the same

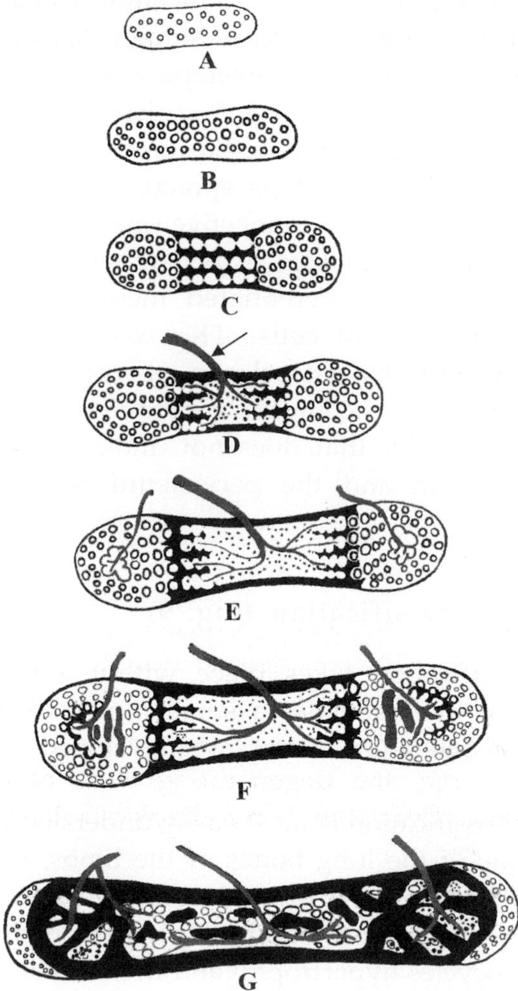

Fig. 9. Diagram showing the process of endochondral ossification. (A) cartilage model, (B) hypertrophy of the cartilage cells at the primary ossification center, (C) formation of the periosteal bone collar, calcification of the bone matrix and degeneration of hypertrophied cartilage cells, (D) invasion of the spaces left by dead cartilage cells by blood vessels (periosteal bud, arrow) and mesenchymal cells, (E) formation of bone spicules and secondary ossification centres, (F) formation of the epiphyseal growth plate, (G) replacement of the epiphyseal growth plate at physical maturity by bone.

time, primitive mesenchymal cells and blood vessels (periosteal bud) invade the spaces left by degeneration of chondrocytes. The primitive mesenchymal cells differentiate into osteoblasts and blood-forming cells of the bone marrow. The osteoblasts make use of the calcified cartilage trabeculae (septa) as a framework and start the deposition of bone matrix on the calcified cartilage trabeculae.

11. Growth in Length of Long Bones

After the formation of the primary ossification centre in the diaphysis, the primitive medullary cavity (marrow cavity), formed by confluence of the cartilage lacunae, begins to expand in the direction of the future epiphyses (ends of a long bone). The expansion of the marrow cavity takes place in such a way that the first formed bone trabeculae are rapidly resorbed by osteoclasts. Concurrent with the extension of the narrow cavity to the epiphyseal ends of the cartilage, the chondrocytes are arranged in longitudinal columns. The interface between the diaphysis and each epiphysis constitutes a growth or epiphyseal plate. Within the growth plate, the cartilage cells proliferate continuously, resulting in progressive elongation of the bone. At the diaphysial aspect of each growth plate, the chondrocytes mature and then die, the degenerating zone of cartilage being replaced by bone. Thus, the bony diaphysis lengthens and the epiphyses are pushed further and further apart.

In the meantime, secondary ossification centres appear in the epiphysis and bone formation similar to that in the diaphyseal cartilage occurs. A thin layer of hyaline cartilage always remains at the surface as articular cartilage.

12. Epiphysial Growth Plate (Plate of Cartilage Separating the Epiphysis from the Diaphysis) (Fig. 10)

In this plate, there is continuous formation of cartilage which is replaced by bone. This is responsible for growth in the length of growing bones. The transition between the cartilage and bone occurs in the following stages:

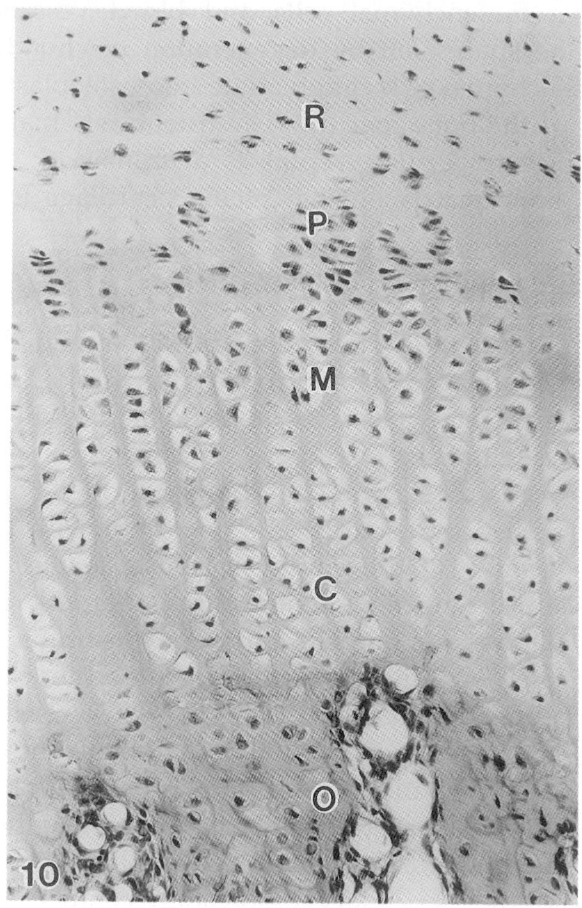

Fig. 10. Section through the epiphyseal plate in a developing tibia showing various zones: R, zone of reserve cartilage; P, zone of cell proliferation; M, zone of maturation and hypertrophy; C, zone of cell degeneration; and O, zone of ossification. (Magnification 140×)

  (i)   Zone of reserve cartilage
 (ii)   Zone of proliferation of cartilage cells
(iii)   Zone of maturation and hypertrophy of cartilage cells
(iv)   Zone of cartilage degeneration or cell death (zone of calcification)

(v) Osteogenic zone or zone of bone formation (also called metaphysis)

At physical maturity, cartilage proliferation ceases, and the cartilage is replaced by bone with the result that the diaphysis is bound to the epiphysis by a bony union (fusion of epiphysis and diaphysis). Injury to the growth plate may cause severe disturbances of growth and hence is of great clinical importance.

13. Growth in Diameter of Long Bones

The shaft of the long bones grows in diameter by the activity of osteoblasts in the deeper layers of periosteum which lay down bone at the periphery of the shaft by sub-periosteal (intramembranous) ossification. At the same time, activity of the osteoclasts causes resorption of bone from the internal surface of the shaft, but at a slightly slower rate than the deposition of the bone on the external surface.

14. Factors Affecting Bone Growth

14.1. Nutrional factors

(a) Vitamins

Vitamins D, C and A are important for bone growth. Deficiency of vitamin D leads to poor absorption of calcium in the intestines and hence reduced blood calcium levels, leading to incomplete calcification of bone matrix. Vitamin C is required for normal collagen synthesis. In vitamin A deficiency, synthesis of the bone matrix by osteoblasts is slow so that the balance between bone deposition and resorption is disturbed.

(b) Hormones

Bone growth is influenced by hormones. The role of parathormone and calcitonin has already been mentioned (see Sec. 4.4). Growth hormone from the anterior pituitary is important for normal bone growth. Increased production of growth hormone in childhood leads to gigantism whereas lack of growth hormone causes dwarfism. In adults, excessive production of growth hormone leads to the development of acromegaly. Sex hormones (androgens and oestrogens) are related to the appearance of ossification centres and closure of epiphyses.

15. Bone Fracture and Healing

Bones undergo regeneration following a fracture. Under favourable conditions, there can be complete restoration of bone to as that before the injury. Whenever there is a fracture, there is haemorrhage at the site of fracture (between the broken ends of bone) because of tearing of blood vessels in the periosteum, Haversian and Volkman's canals, leading to the formation of a blood clot. This is invaded by macrophages and fibroblasts from the periosteum. The macrophages remove the blood clot whereas the fibroblasts form the connective tissue. Some fibroblasts in the connective tissue transform into chondroblasts which lay down cartilage, thus forming a soft callus. The cartilage in the soft callus undergoes endochondral ossification and forms woven bone (hard callus). Cells from the deep part of the periosteum also lay down woven bone at the periphery. Woven bone is then remodelled to form lamellar bone.

16. Acknowledgements

The author expresses deep gratitude to Prof. E.A. Ling for his valuable comments during the preparation of this chapter. The technical assistance of Ms. L.S. Ng and Mr. P. Gobalakrishnan and the secretarial help of Mrs. M. Singh is gratefully acknowledged.

8 HISTOLOGY OF CARTILAGE

CHARANJIT KAUR

Department of Anatomy, Faculty of Medicine
National University of Singapore
4 Medical Drive, MD10, Singapore 117597

Abstract

Cartilage is a semi-rigid, specialised kind of connective tissue
consisting of cells and extracellular components. The cells are
called chondrocytes and the extracellular components are called
the matrix. The matrix consists of fibres (collagen and elastic)
and abundant ground substance which is firm and gel-like. It
forms most of the foetal skeleton which is gradually replaced
by bone in the growing individual.
There are three types of cartilages:

  (i)   hyaline
 (ii)   elastic
(iii) fibrocartilage

1. Functions of Cartilage

  (i) Hyaline cartilage covers the articular surfaces of bones,
providing a smooth surface for them and thus reducing friction
between them during movements at the joints.

(ii) Hyaline and elastic cartilages provide a supporting framework for the nose, ear, larynx, trachea and bronchi, which allows movement and change in shape.

(ii) Hyaline cartilage forms the basis of endochondral ossification.

Most cartilage is devoid of blood vessels. The exchange of metabolites between chondrocytes and surrounding tissues depends on diffusion through the ground substance and from the surrounding vessels. Few blood vessels contained in canals called cartilage canals are found in some thick cartilages. These are thought to provide nutritive support for the cartilage.

2. Hyaline Cartilage (Figs. 1, 2 and 3)

This is the most common type of cartilage found in the larynx, trachea, at the articular surfaces of bones and at sternal ends of ribs. It has a translucent appearance in its fresh state. It is surrounded by a dense connective tissue covering called the perichondrium and consists of aggregations of chondroblasts and chondrocytes embedded in an amorphous matrix.

The matrix consists of:

(i)   collagen fibres (type II)
(ii) ground substance which is composed of:
    —glycosaminoglycans and proteoglycans (mainly chondroitin sulphate, hyaluronic acid with smaller amounts of ketatan and heparan sulphates)
    —glycoproteins, e.g. chondronectin
    —tissue fluid

In haematoxylin-and-eosin-stained slides, the matrix at the periphery of the cartilage near the perichondrium is eosinophilic, whereas it becomes basophilic in the deeper parts of the cartilage. The matrix surrounding the isogenous groups (described below) is intensely basophilic due to a high content of sulphated glycosaminoglycans and is called territorial or capsular matrix.

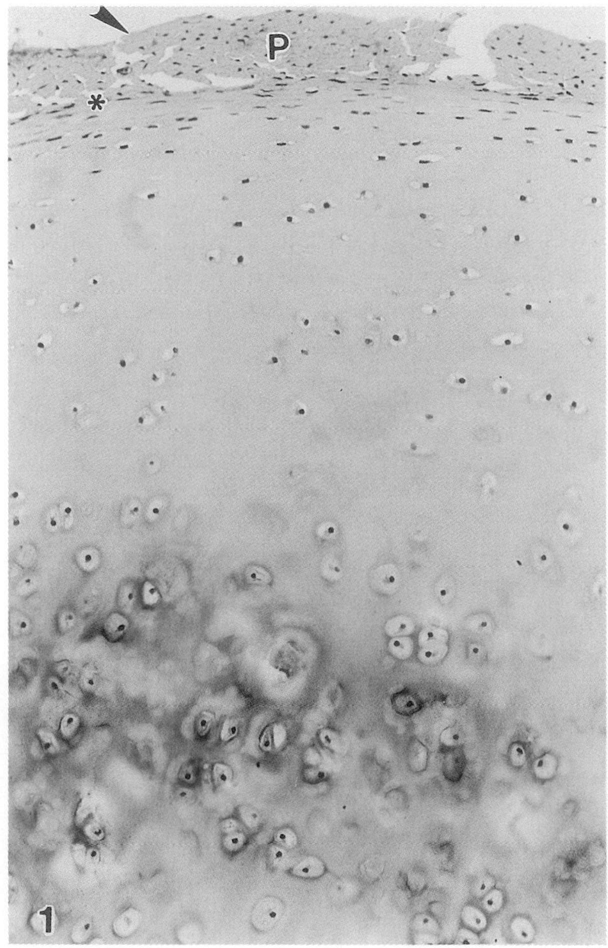

Fig. 1. Transverse section through a costal cartilage. Chondrocytes can be seen in lacunae. The cartilage is surrounded by perichondrium (P) which has an inner chondrogenic layer (*) and an outer fibrous layer (arrowhead). (Magnification 90×)

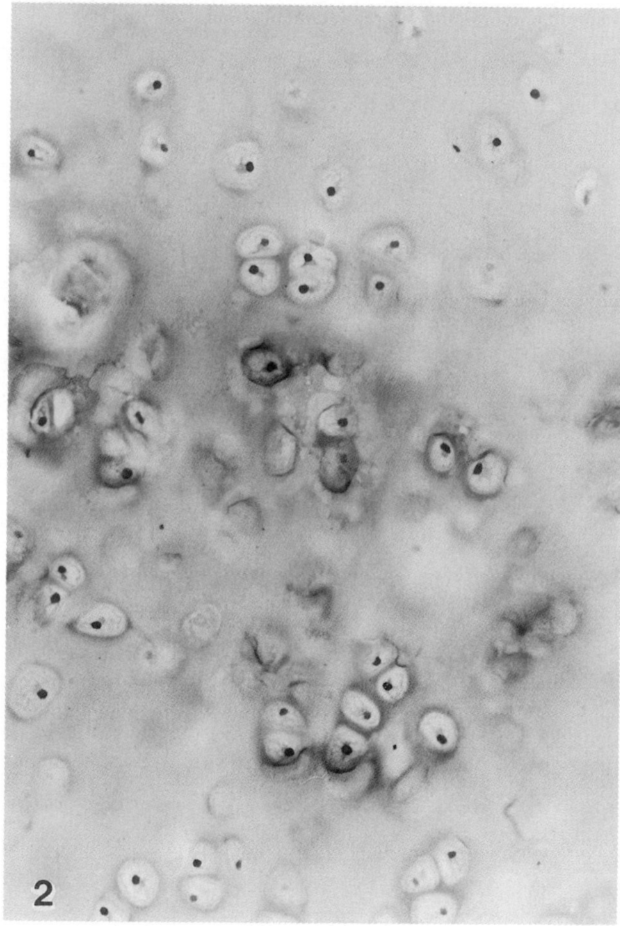

Fig. 2. At high magnification of the costal cartilage, chondrocytes are seen in round lacunae embedded in the matrix. (Magnification 140×)

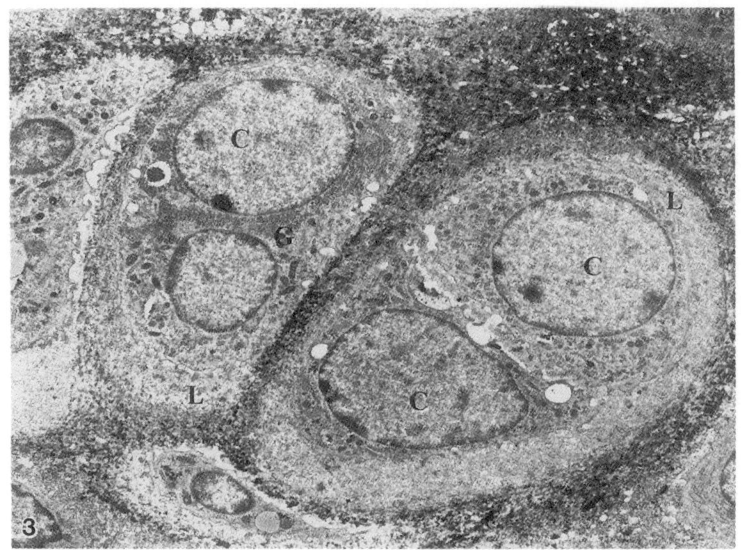

Fig. 3. An electron micrograph of hyaline cartilage from trachea showing chondrocytes (C) occupying lacunae (L). Glycogen particles (G) can be seen in one of the chondrocytes. (Courtesy of Prof. E.A. Ling; magnification 9000×)

3. Cells (Chondrocytes)

Chondrocytes are responsible for synthesising the components of the matrix. At the periphery of the cartilage, chondrocytes are elliptical in shape. Deeper in the cartilage they are round and may appear in clusters of up to eight cells originating from mitotic divisions of a single chondrocyte. These groups are called isogenous groups.

Chondrocytes are contained in spaces in the matrix called lacunae. During life, chondrocytes fill the lacunae but their cytoplasm shrinks during histological preparations.

At the electron microscopic level, chondrocytes show a large amount of rough endoplasmic reticulum and a prominent Golgi apparatus. Lipid droplets and glycogen granules are also present.

4. Perichondrium

Except at the articular surfaces of bones, hyaline cartilage at all other sites is covered by a layer of connective tissue called perichondrium which consists of two layers — inner chondrogenic and outer fibrous.

The outer layer consists of bundles of collagen fibres and fibroblasts. Fibroblasts in the connective tissue of the inner layer have the potential to transform into chondrocytes.

5. Histogenesis

Cartilage develops from the mesenchyme in the embryo. Mesenchymal cells round up, multiply rapidly and form mesenchymal condensations. The rounded cells are now called chondroblasts, which start secreting cartilaginous matrix materials. The deposition of the matrix separates the cells from one another. When completely surrounded by the cartilage matrix, a chondroblast is termed chondrocyte. Peripheral mesenchyme condenses around the developing cartilage mass to form the perichondrium.

6. Growth

The cartilage continues to grow by two processes: (i) interstitial growth, and (ii) appositional growth. Interstitial growth results from the division of existing chondrocytes and gives rise to isogenous groups. Appositional growth results from the differentiation of stem cells in the chondrogenic layer of the perichondrium, first into chondroblasts and then into chondrocytes. It is responsible for continued increase in the thickness of the cartilage.

7. Elastic Cartilage (Fig. 4)

Elastic cartilage is found in the external ear, eustachian tube and epiglottis. It is structurally identical to hyaline cartilage except that its matrix contains a dense network of elastic fibres in addition to

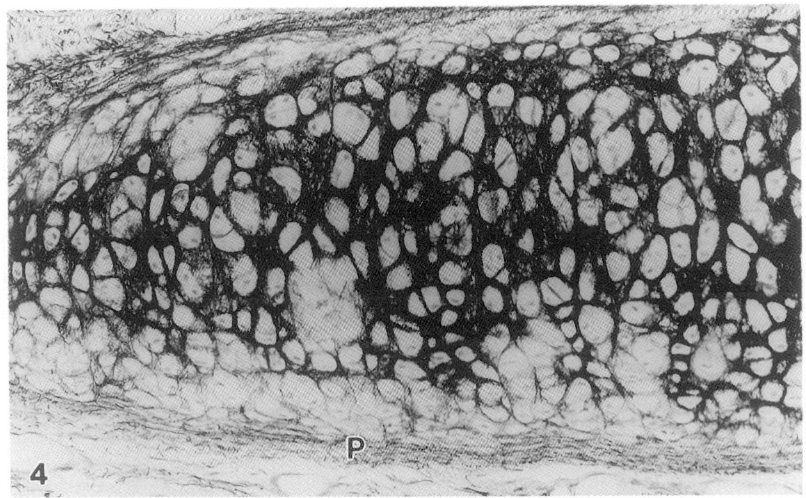

Fig. 4. Section through the epiglottis showing elastic cartilage. Elastic fibres in the matrix are stained black. In between the fibres, lacunae containing the chondrocytes can be seen. Perichondrium (P) surrounds the cartilage. (Magnification 110×)

collagen fibres. The chondrocytes characteristically occur in isogenous groups. A perichondrium surrounds the cartilage. Histogenesis and growth are similar to the hyaline cartilage.

8. Fibrocartilage (Fig. 5)

Fibrocartilage has characteristics intermediate between those of dense connective tissue and hyaline cartilage. It contains chondrocytes similar to hyaline cartilage, either singly or in isogenous groups. Chondrocytes may be arranged in long columns. Numerous collagenous fibres either form irregular bundles between the groups of chondrocytes or are aligned in a parallel arrangement along the columns of chondrocytes. There is no perichondrium in fibrocartilage. Fibrocartilage develops from dense connective tissue by means of differentiation of fibroblasts into chondroblasts and chondrocytes.

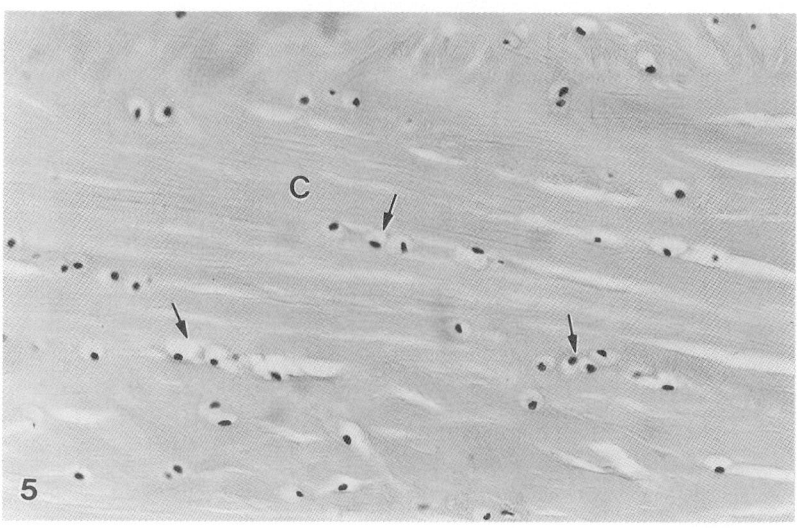

Fig. 5.   Fibrocartilage from an intervertebral disc. Islands of hyaline cartilage (arrows) containing chondrocytes in lacunae can be seen in a dense network of collagen fibres (C). (Magnification 270×)

9. Regeneration of Cartilage

Regeneration of cartilage following injury is poor and always incomplete. When cartilage is injured, the fibroblasts in the perichondrium lay down new connective tissue at the site of injury. Some fibroblasts may transform into chondroblasts and chondrocytes which synthesise cartilage matrix but this process is slow and incomplete.

10. Acknowledgements

The author expresses deep gratitude to Prof. E.A. Ling for his valuable comments during the preparation of this chapter. The technical assistance of Ms. L.S. Ng and Mr. P. Gobalakrishnan and the secretarial help of Mrs. M. Singh are gratefully acknowledged.

Advances in Tissue Banking Vol. 5

9 BASIC ANATOMY AND PHYSIOLOGY OF HUMAN SKIN

JAN KOLLER

Ruzinov General Hospital
Centre for Burns and Reconstructive Surgery
Central Tissue Bank
Ruzinovka 6, 82606 Bratislava
Slovak Republic

1. Introduction

Skin is the largest and most visible organ of the human body. The average adult human skin area is approximately $2\,m^2$ while its average weight is about 5 kg. Skin represents a very unique interface between the organism and its environment with many functions. It is adapted to withstand several physical, chemical and biological stresses. The most important skin functions include barrier function, participation in thermoregulation of the human body, sensory function, excretion, immune function, production of melanin and vitamin D and cosmetic packaging of the individual organism. Damage and/or loss to large areas of the skin, such as in extensive burns or other affections, can cause severe systemic alterations, and even death of the individual.

2. Structure of the Skin

Anatomically, the skin is composed of two major layers: the *epidermis* and *dermis.* The tissue lying deeper to the dermis is called the *hypodermis* (subcutis) (Fig. 1). Both skin layers contain cells and extracellular structures.

In the epidermis, there is a prevalence of cells with very scarce or almost no extracellular matrix. The epidermal cells are permanently renewed from the basal layer. The viability of the cells decreases towards the surface of the epidermis. Dead cells completely filled

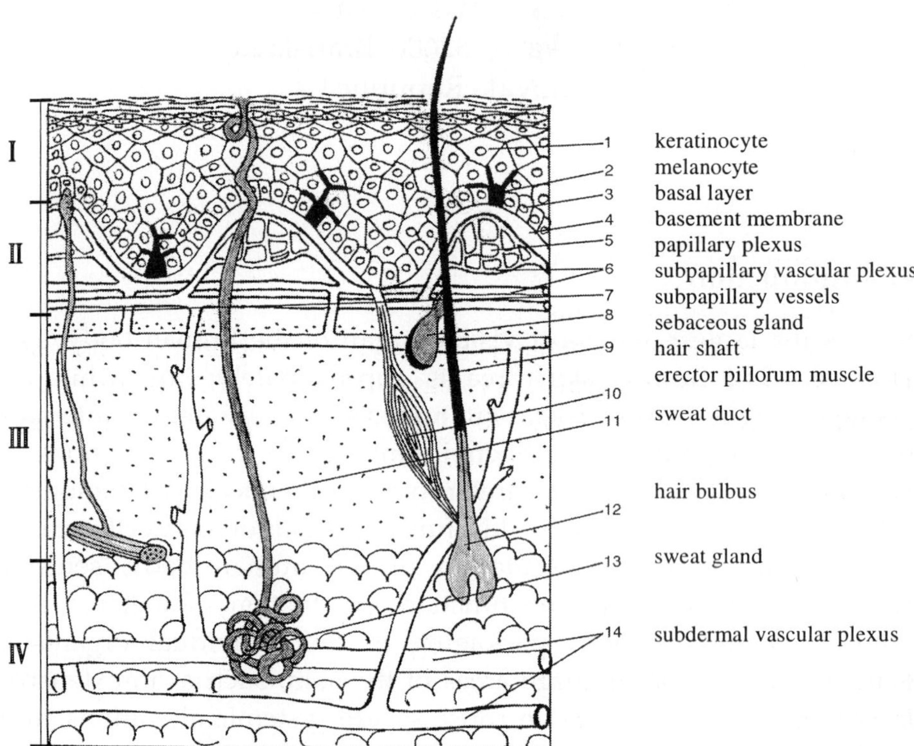

I. Epidermis; II. Papillary dermis; III. Reticular dermis; IV. Subcutis

Fig. 1. Structure of the skin.

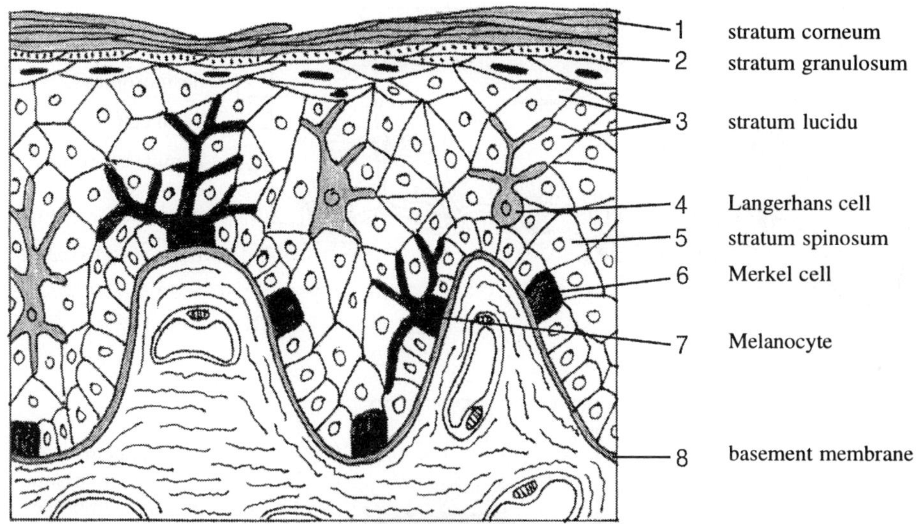

Fig. 2. Layers of epidermis.

by keratohyaline granules are desquamated from the surface of the skin (stratum corneum, Fig. 2).

In the dermis, there are more extracellular components than cells. They include an integrated system of fibrous, filamentous and amorphous connective tissue that facilitates vascular, nerve and cutaneous immune system networks. The organisation of the collagen and elastic tissue of the dermis is a distinctive feature of human skin.

The uppermost part of the dermis adjacent to the epidermis is called the *papillary dermis* because of the dermal papillae interdigitating with the deeper epithelial layers. The junction itself between the epidermis and dermis is represented by the *basement membrane zone system* (Fig. 3).

Deeper layers of the dermis are called the *reticular dermis*, according to the arrangement of the fibres. Blood vessels and nerve fibres are included in the dermis only, whereas the epidermis is avascular. Other structures situated mostly in the dermis are skin appendages, which include the sweat glands and ducts, hair follicles,

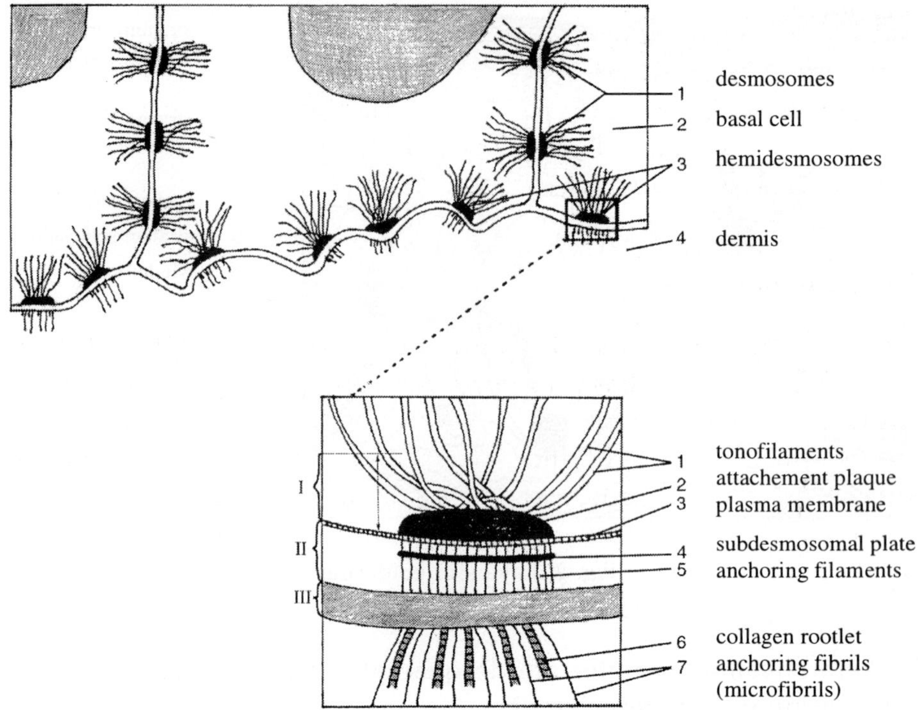

I. Hemidesmosome; II. Lamina lucida; III. Lamina densa

Fig. 3. The basement membrane zone (modified according to Clark, 1988).

sebaceous glands, arrectores pillorum smooth muscle fibres, special nerve receptors, and nail beds with nails.

3. Epidermis

The epidermis is a multilayered sheet of cells with very little extracellular matrix. It is the outermost, continuously renewing part of the skin which is composed of several layers (Fig. 2) and which includes several cell types.

3.1. Epidermal cells

There are at least five cell types in the adult epidermis: keratinocytes, Langerhans cells, melanocytes, Merkel cells and dendritic cells. The last two types are found only occasionally in the epidermis and oral mucosa. The dendritic cells are of the same type as in the dermis.

3.1.1. Kerainocytes

There are the most frequently found principal cells of the epidermis. From the lowermost basal layer to the uppermost shedding cells of stratum corneum, they progressively change their form. Keratinocytes are of ectodermal origin and, in addition to their basic product — keratin, they can produce different fibrous proteins, such as tonofibrils. Keratinocytes act as a mechanical protective barrier to the human body and they also play a major role in the immune functioning of the skin.

3.1.2. Langerhans cells

There constitute about 4% of the nucleated epidermal cells distributed throughout the epidermal layers. In routine light microscopic preparations, they are difficult to see. They originate from a mobile pool of bone-marrow-derived precursor cells playing a major role in immune functions of the skin. Phenotypically, Langerhans cells display a variety of different markers and receptors on their surface, such as CD45, MHC-I, MHC-II, CD54, S100, Vimentin, HLA-D-li, GM-CSF, M-CSF, IL-2 chains, etc. They are extremely potent stimulators of antigen-specific T-cell activation, which initiates protective immune responses against endogenous and exogenous antigens. Other functions of the Langerhans cells include phagocytosis, antigen presentation, participation in cutaneous immune surveillance and involvement in skin allograft rejection. Impairment of these cells can have deleterious consequences for the immunological defence of the host.

3.1.3. Melanocytes

They are pigment-producing cells derived from the neural crest. Melanocytes are evenly distributed in the basal layer of the epidermis with a frequency of one melanocyte for every ten basal keratinocytes. Through their dendrites, one cell can acquire a relation of up to 36 keratinocytes. It is very interesting that the number of melanocytes in the epidermis is the same, regardless of race and skin colour. Racial differences in skin colour are determined by the density and size of the melanosomes.

Melanin — the pigment produced by the melanocytes, is synthesised in a complex organelle called the melanosome. Chemically, there are two basic types of melanin — namely, eumelanin which is brown-black and insoluble, and phenomelanin which is yellow-red and soluble in dilute alkali. Produced melanin granules move from the melanocytes to other cells where they assume a static array. In keratinocytes, they form a supranuclear cap that acts as a shield against UV radiation. It has been shown that exposure to sunlight stimulates the melanocytes to produce larger melanosomes, making the distribution of these proteins to resemble the pattern found in dark-skinned individuals.

3.1.4. Merkel cells

They are mostly found in special regions such as the lips, oral cavity, hair follicles, the glabrous skin of the digits, or as a part of certain tactile discs. They are attached to adjacent keratinocytes by desmosomes (Fig. 3). There are two prevailing hypotheses regarding the origin of the Merkel cells: the neural crest and cutaneous origin hypotheses. The *tactile Merkel cells* are opposed to small nerve plates connected by short, non-myelinated axons to myelinated axons. These complex structures serve as tactile mechanoreceptors (Fig. 4). *Epidermal Merkel cells* seem to stimulate local proliferation and differentiation of keratinocytes.

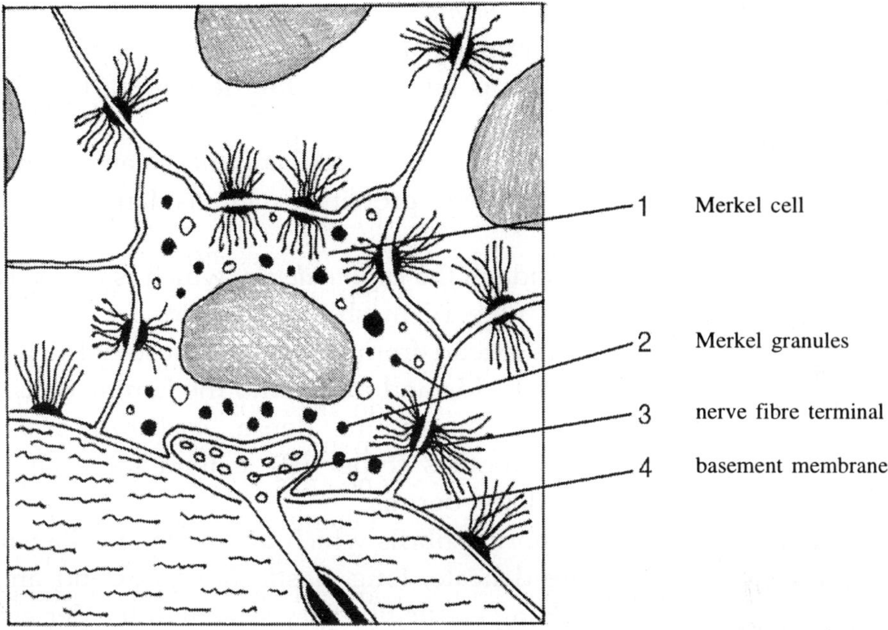

Fig. 4. Merkel cell with nerve fibre terminal (modified according to Clark, 1988).

4. The Basement Membrane Zone System (Fig. 3)

The basement membrane is an important interface which separates the epidermis from the dermis both physically and functionally. All its components except the anchoring fibrils and microfibrils, are synthesised by the basal cells of the epidermis. As the epidermis is a non-vascularised structure, the basement membrane zone helps to regulate proper proliferating and differentiating mechanisms of the epidermis. It is also responsible for epidermal–dermal adherence, probably serves as a selective macromollecular filter, and is also the major site of immune reactant localisation in cutaneous diseases.

The structures of the basement membrane zone include:

(i) The part of the *cell membrane* of the basal cells that faces the dermis and includes a structure called the *hemidesmosome*.

Tiny fibres called *tonofilaments* cross the basal cell cytoplasma and attach to the epidermal part of the hemidesmosome. The *subdesmosomal dense plate* is attached to the dermal part of the hemidesmosome

(ii) Adjacent to the cell membrane is the *lamina lucida* — an electron lucent layer where adherent proteins, such as laminin, are located.

(iii) Next to the lamina lucida is the *lamina densa*, which is basically composed of collagen type IV mesh-like scaffold.

(iv) The *anchoring filaments* extend from the subdesmosomal dense plate across the lamina lucida and insert into the lamina densa.

(v) From the inner face of the lamina densa, *anchoring fibrils*, composed of collagen rootlets (type VII), extend for a short distance into the papillary dermis.

(vi) In addition to the anchoring fibrils which are made of collagen, *microfibrils*, which are delicate, long elastic fibrils, extend and blend with the underlying elastic fibrillary system of the dermis.

5. Dermis

The dermis is composed of cells, extracellular matrix, blood and lymphatic vessels, and skin appendages.

The dermis contributes with its bulk, density, compliance, elasticity and tensile strength to the skin properties. This is due to the presence of dermal matrix containing fibrous and non-fibrous connective tissues. Among the fibrous molecules, the most important are collagen and elastin. Non-fibrous molecules are represented mainly by proteins and glycosaminoglycans (ground substance).

Collagen is the ultimate product of fibroblasts and its presence result in tensile strength of the skin. At least seven types of mature collagen are currently recognised.

Elastic fibers consist of two protein components — the more common *elastin* (amorphous appearance at electron microscopy, around 90%), and the *elastic microfibrils* composed of a specialised glycoprotein.

Elastin is the second major fibrous protein in connective tissue. Elastin contributes to great extent to a the skin elasticity.

In addition to water and electrolytes, *Ground substance* constituents are the glycosaminoglycans (GAGs), glycoproteins, and mucoproteins. Current interest in some ground substance components relates to their hypothetical capacity for *actively directing tissue repair.*

5.1. Other components

Laminin is a large glycoprotein, an *essential component of basement membranes*, adjacent to the cell membranes.

Fibronectin is a ubiquitous, high-molecular weight glycoprotein. It is found in plasma and can be associated with cell surfaces, basement membranes and pericellular matrices. Fibronectin can bind some macromolecules, including collagen, fibrin, heparin and proteoglycans. Its role is important in wound repair as a functional and structural component.

The two main anatomical portions of the dermis are the *papillary dermis* and *reticular dermis*.

The *papillary dermis* is situated immediately deep to the epidermis and basal membrane zone. It is relatively thin and has little structure when viewed with the light microscope. The papillary dermis contains different protein forms with a high proportion of type III collagen. The boundary between the papillary and reticular dermis is defined by a horizontal subpapillary vascular plexus. The papillary dermis is populated more densely by dermal cells than the reticular one.

The *reticular dermis* represents the bulk of the dermis containing the majority of dermal collagen organised into coarse bundles. It is composed primarily of type I collagen. Each collagen bundle is associated with elastic fibres that could be demonstrated microscopically only by special stains.

The blood flow required for the nutrition of the skin is very small. In normal conditions at ordinary skin temperature, the amount of blood flowing through the skin is ten times more than is needed for nutrition.

The dermis is a highly vascularised structure with a special kind of vascular networks (plexuses). The superficial vascular plexus, called *subpapillary plexus,* is situated on the boundary between the papillary and reticular dermis and is composed of arterioles and post-capillary venules. From this plexus, a terminal arteriole extends into each dermal papilla, where an arterial capillary is formed. The arterial capillary makes a U-turn and becomes a venous capillary and a post-capillary venule coming back to the subpapillary plexus. A second, larger and deeper vascular network is situated in the subcutaneous tissue immediately deeper to the dermal layer and is called the *subdermal plexus.* The vascular connections between these two networks are realised by arterioles and venules running perpendicularly to the skin surface through the reticular dermis. This causes, the vascular supply of the reticular dermis to be less abundant than that of the papillary dermis which can play an important role in wound healing, particularly in deep dermal burns. The blood flow through the two plexuses is involved in the regulation of body temperature as well as in the metabolic supply of the whole skin. There are also some direct vascular communications between the arterial and venous plexuses, which are present in some skin areas exposed to maximal cooling, such as the volar surfaces of hands and feet, the lips, nose and ear.

The lymphatics of the skin form a complex and random network beginning as lymphatic capillaries near the epidermis. A superficial lymphatic plexus is formed from which lymphatic channels drain to regional lymph nodes. The lymphatic channels are important for the clearance of fluids, macromolecules and cells from the dermis.

5.2. Dermal cells

The majority of dermal cells are of mesodermal origin, such as fibroblasts, mast cells, macrophages, dendritic cells and T-lymphocytes.

5.2.1. Fibroblasts

Fibroblasts are the most frequent connective tissue cells. In the papillary dermis, they are located mostly in the papillary region and around vessels, in the reticular part in the interstices between collagen fibre bundles. Fibroblasts play an important role in wound healing processes. In newly formed tissue, they can migrate along capillaries and produce matrix components. They produce many different extracellular matrix and structural proteins. Among the extracellular matrix proteins, the most important are all types of collagens, elastin, fibronectin and proteoglycans. The structural proteins include enzymes, enzyme inhibitors, integrins, actin, vimentin and tubuline.

5.2.2. Mast cells

They are derived from the bone marrow. Mast cells are present in all regions of the dermis. They are more frequent in the upper dermis around vessels and epidermal appendages, and in the subcutaneous fat. Dermal mast cells are surrounded by fibronectin which helps them to anchor to the extracellular matrix in inflammatory sites where they proliferate and release different mediators. They are involved in a variety of physiological and pathological events. They store active proteins and respond to a variety of immunologic and non-immunologic stimuli. They release a variety of vasoactive mediators, chemotactic mediators and enzymes.

5.2.3. Macrophages

Macrophages are large, mobile phagocytic cells. They look very similar to neutrophils, from which they differ by an unlobed nucleus and absence of specific granules. They are derived from the bone-marrow precursor cells which differentiate into monocytes in the blood and macrophages in the tissue. They play an active role in cell-mediated immune mechanisms. They are capable of phagocytosis of foreign particles such as cellular debris and bacteria. Their number increases after a local inflammatory stress. Macrophages carry a high number of major histocompatibility complex (MHC) class-II antigens and bear different receptors. They are also active antigen-presenting cells. Macrophages play a key role in wound healing mechanisms.

5.2.4. Dendritic cells

Dermal dendritic cells are located in the perivascular areas. They are different from the epidermal Langerhans cells. Their cytoplasm contains organelles involved in active cellular metabolism. They can also be located in the basal layer of the epidermis. Dermal dendritic cells bear several receptors such as CD36, CD54, etc., and carry large numbers of MHC class-II antigens. Their functional role in the skins immune system is still not clear.

5.2.5. T-lymphocytes

T-lymphocytes migrate from the blood predominantly to the dermis and are located mostly around post-capillary venules and the skin appendages. They contribute to the immune surveillance and homeostasis of the skin.

5.3. Skin appendages

Skin appendages include hair follicles, sebaceous glands, sweat glands with sweat ducts, nails and special nerve receptors.

6. Skin Functions

The most important skin functions include protective and barrier function, participation in thermoregulation of the human body, sensory function, excretion, immune function, production of melanin and vitamin D and cosmetic packaging of the individual organism. The epidermis is continuously renewed from its deepest basal layer.

6.1. Protective and barrier function

The skin acts as a protective barrier of the human body against external environmental stimuli. It is structured to prevent loss of essential body fluids, and to protect the body against the entry of toxic environmental chemicals. It protects the body from mechanical injury, thermal stimuli and microbial invasion. The skin pigment melanin protects the nuclear structures against damage from ultra-violet irradiation.

6.2. Thermoregulation

The skin contributes to a great extent to the body's temperature regulation system, protecting us against hypothermia and hyper-thermia. This is assured by regulation of skin blood circulation, sweat evaporation, and partly by insulation properties of the subcutaneous fat. Exposure to extreme cold reduces the rate of cutaneous blood flow to very low values to prevent the loss of heat. On the other hand, in hot environment, the rate of cutaneous blood flow can increase up to seven times the normal value to ensure maximal heat loss from the body. The loss of heat is further enhanced by sweat excretion and evaporation.

6.3. Immune functions

The skin is part of the innate immunity of the body against invasion of microorganisms. It represents the first barrier to invasion by microorganisms and is the peripheral arm of the immune system. The dryness and constant desquamation of the skin, the normal flora of the skin, the fatty acids of sebum and lactic acid of sweat, all represent natural defence mechanisms. Langerhans cells have an antigen-presenting capacity and also play an important role in immuno-surveillance against viral infections. They interact with neighbouring keratinocytes, which secrete a number of immuno-regulating cytokines, and epidermotropic T-cells forming the skin immune system. The immune mechanisms of the skin intercept and eliminate pathogens and discard cells that have undergone malignant transformation.

6.4. Excretion

The excretory functions of the skin include excretion of sweat and sebum.

Sweating is the normal response to exercise or thermal stress by which the human organism controls its body temperature through evaporative heat loss. Under extreme conditions, the amount of perspiration can reach several litres a day. In addition to the secretion of water and electrolytes, the sweat glands serve as excretory organs for heavy metals, organic compounds and macromolecules. Sweat is composed of 99% water, electrolytes, lactate, urea, ammonia, proteolytic enzymes and other substances.

Sebum has a protective and nutritive effect to the skin and hair. Sebaceous glands are found on all areas of the skin, with the exception of the palms, soles and dorsum of feet. They are holocrine glands, i.e. their secretion is formed by complete destruction of the cells. The sebum is composed of triglycerides and free fatty acids, wax esters, squalene and cholesterol. The sebum controls moisture loss from the epidermis. It also protects against fungal and bacterial infections of the skin due to its contents of free fatty acids.

6.5. Synthesis

Skin cells synthetise some important substances, such as vitamin D (from provitamine mediated by UV irradiation), cholesterol and melanin. Vitamin D_3 is produced in the skin by the action of UV light on dehydrocholesterol. It is then activated in the liver and kidney.

6.6. Sensory functions

The skin is a huge sensory receptor for heat, cold, pain, touch and tickle. It is innervated with around one million afferent nerve fibres.

Sensory endings of the skin are of two main kinds — corpuscular which embrace non-nervous corpuscles, and "free" which do not. The brain receives two types of sensations:

— *superficial sensations* including pain, crude touch and temperature
— *deep sensations*, including sense of position, movement, vibration, muscle sense and fine touch

6.7. Cosmetic packaging and identity functions

Each individual is characterised by a special colour, texture and contours of skin, which are signs of its identity and individuality. Skin is also an organ of emotional expression and a site for the discharge of anxiety. The elevated ridge patterns of the finger pulps (visualised as fingreprints) are unique for each individual and are successfully used for indentification in criminology.

6.8. Epidermal regeneration

The cells in the basal layer (stratum basale) renew by cell division and as they ascend towards the surface, they undergo a process known as keratinisation which involves the synthesis of the fibrous protein — keratin. The cells on the surface of the skin forming the horny layer (stratum corneum) are fully keratinised dead cells which are gradually peeled off. The rate of cell production must be balanced by the rate of cell loss at the surface. The control mechanism of epidermopoiesis consists of a balance of stimulatory and inhibitory signals mediated by diffusible factors, including cytokines and growth factors. Some of them, such as epidermal growth factor, transforming growth factor-alpha, interleukins and basic fibroblast growth factor are stimulating the epidermal cells; others like chalones, transforming growth factor-beta, interferons and tumour necrosis factor have inhibitory action. The epidermis renewal time under normal conditions varies between 50 and 75 days.

In summary, skin is a very special and unique organ of the human body with a characteristic structure and many functions.

This is why extensive damage to the skin due to injuries or diseases can cause deleterious effects on the human organism and must be taken into consideration. If the damage to the skin is superficial, the skin is capable of regeneration and restoration of its functions. Destruction of the whole thickness of the skin on large body surface areas can be fatal, unless the lost skin is replaced temporarily or permanently by skin substitutes and/or skin grafts.

7. References

CHAMPION, R.H., BURTON, J.L. and BURNS, D.A. (eds.) (1998). *Textbook of Dermatology*, 6th edn., Blackwell, Oxford.

CLARK, W.H. (1988). The skin. In: *Pathology*, E. Rubin, J.L. Farber, eds., J.B. Lippincott, Philadelphia, pp. 1194–1211.

FITZPATRICK, T.B., EISEN, A.Z., WOLFF, K., FREEDBERG, I.M. and AUSTEN, K.F. (eds.) (1997). *Dermatology in General Medicine*, 3rd edn., 2 vols, McGraw-Hill, New York.

GANONG, W.F. (1989). *Review of Medical Physiology*, 14th edn., Appleton & Lange, Connecticut.

GRAHAM-BROWN, R. and BURNS, T. (1990). *Lecture Notes on Dermatology*, 6th edn., Blackwell, Oxford.

10 ANATOMY AND EMBRYOLOGY OF HUMAN PLACENTA, AMNION AND CHORION

HASIM MOHAMAD

Department of Surgery, Hospital Kota Bharu
155867 Kota Bharu, Kelantan
Malaysia
and
National Tissue Bank
Hospital University Sains Malaysia
Kubang Kerian, 16150 Kota Bharu, Kelantan
Malaysia

Abstract

Before one can understand the anatomy of the placenta, it is quite important to understand the fate of the human ovum after fertilisation. At the time of fertilisation, the ovum is still lying in the outer one-third of the fallopian tube. After about five to six days, the zygote reaches the uterine cavity from the fallopian tube. During this passage, the zygote is transformed into two cells, four, eight and so on. This process of segmentation results in the formation of the morula, which is about 0.5 mm in diameter. The real mechanism of how this happen is uncertain. However, it is believed that the ciliated

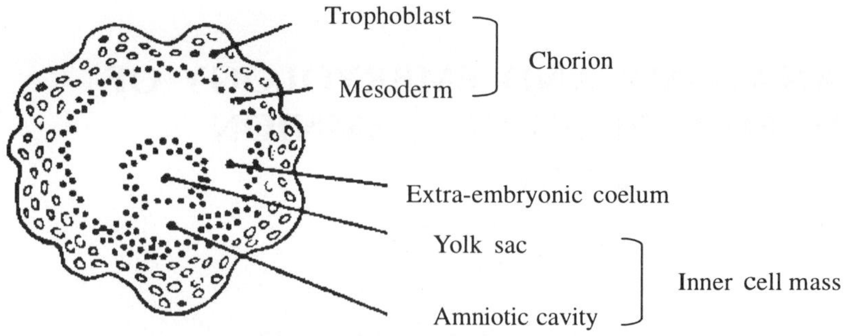

Fig. 1. Blastocyst. Formation of amnion and yolk sac in formative cell mass.

cells in the fallopian tubes help the passage of the ovum through the fallopian tube. The fallopian tubes also show some peristaltic movement but the importance of this movement is less certain. Whatever the mechanism is, the ovum usually reaches the uterine cavity by five to six days after fertilisation.

Before reaching the uterine cavity, the morula developes further into the blastocyst whilst it is still in the fallopian tube. Meanwhile, the outermost cells of the blastocyst (Fig. 1) form the trophoblast, which is capable of eroding and digesting the outer epithelial surface of the uterine decidua.

The embryo develop from the inner cell mass, and the two cavities from the inner cell mass develop into the amniotic cavity and the yolk sac. Ultimately, the embryonic cavity develop into the foetal membrane, which surrounds the embryo and becomes continuous with the embryonic ectoderm at the umbilicus.

1. Early Development of Blastocyst

After segmentation, the zygote begins to divide and forms the morula. The blastocyst forms when a cavity develops in the morula. This development occurs while the morula is in the fallopian tube.

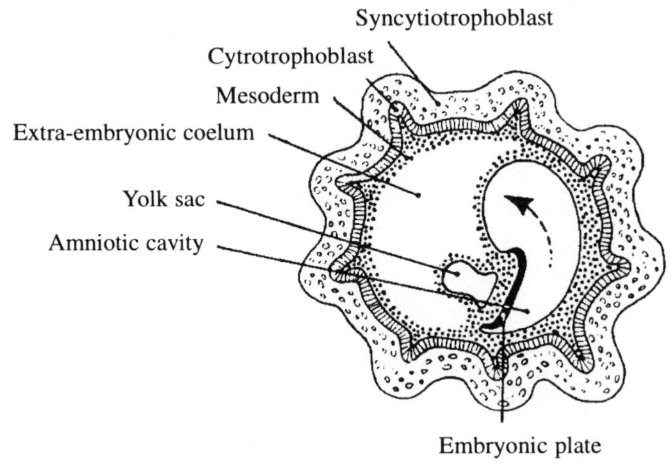

Fig. 2. Extension of amniotic cavity. Early formation of chorionic villi.

The outermost cells of the blastocyst form the trophoblast, which is capable of eroding the surface of the decidua and the fertilised ovum sinks into the inner layer of the decidua, lying in the cavity of the stroma between endometrial glands. The growing zygote enlarges and pushes aside the endometrial glands. The trophoblast cells invade the maternal blood vessels and extravasation of maternal blood occurs around the zygote. The trophoblast becomes differentiated into two layers, a thick outer layer of syncytiotrophoblast and an inner layer of cytotrophoblast. The trophoblast cells therefore form the nutritional organ for the developing embryo.

The combined layer of the mesoderm and the trophoblast is called the chorion and within the chorion is the amniotic membrane that bounds the amniotic cavity (Fig. 2).

The placenta is developed from the extra-embryonic coelom and the chorion. The extra-embryonic mesoderm is continuous with the central tissue of the villi. Therefore, each villus has an outer covering of trophoblast and a central mesodermal core. These projections join together to form primitive blood vessels, extending through both the embryo and the extra-embryonic mesoderm. Hence, the placental circulation is formed and the foetal heart not only pumps blood to the foetus but also to the placenta (Figs. 3 and 4).

The blastocyst contains the inner cell mass which later develops into the foetus. The junction between the trophoblast and the inner cell mass forms the body stalk, which ends as the umbilical cord.

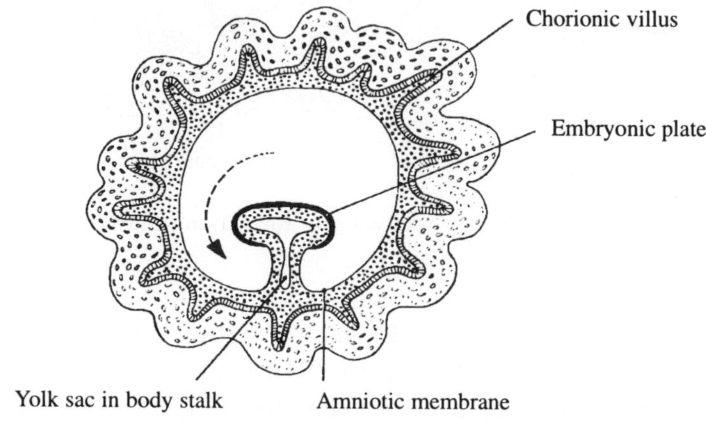

Fig. 3. Chorionic villi and body stalk.

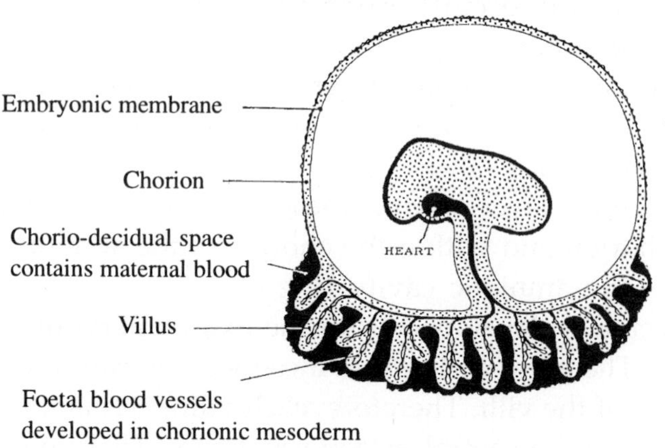

Fig. 4. Formation of the placenta and membranes.

The earliest change in the inner cell mass is the formation of two cavities, each lined with cuboidal epithelium. These cavities are the amniotic, cavity lined by the ectodermal cells, and the yolk sac lined by endodermal cells. Between these cavities lie other cells known as mesodermal cells.

Thus, in the region where the amniotic cavity and the yolk sac come closest together are situated the ectoderm, endoderm and mesoderm cells. Because all the cells necessary for the formation of the foetus are found here, this zone is called the embryonic plate. The skin, hair, nails, nervous system, the lens of the eyes and the enamel of the teeth arise from the *ectoderm*. The alimentary tract, liver, pancreas, lungs and thyroid glands arise from the *endoderm*, while the heart, blood and blood vessels, lymphatics, bones, muscles, kidneys, ovaries and testicles arise from the *mesoderm*.

2. Development of the Placenta

In the early phase of foetal development, the gestational sac is covered by villi formed all over its surface. Between the 12th and 16th weeks, the villi on the capsular surface rapidly degenerate while those on

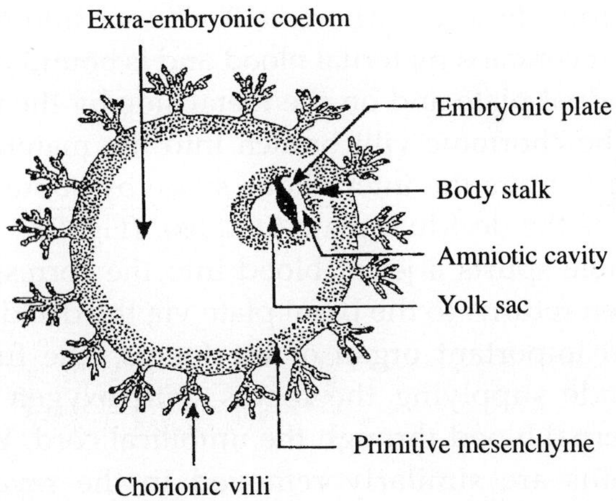

Fig. 5. Development of the placenta, the early changes in the blastocyst.

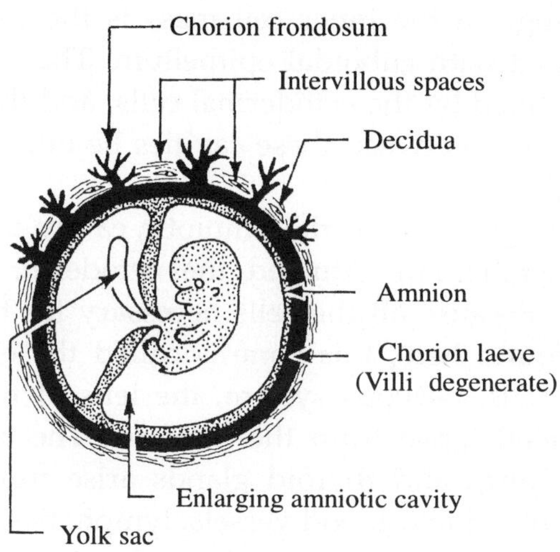

Fig. 6. Formation of the placenta.

the decidua basalis compensate by hypertrophy and become matted to a solid structure called the placenta (Fig. 5).

The placental growth is proportionate with the foetal growth and by term, it is discoid in shape, about 20 cm in diameter and 3 cm in thickness. Usually, it weighs about 500 gm at birth.

The placenta is made up almost entirely of a multitude of chorionic villi, which protrude in an arborescent manner into the intervillous blood spaces. It contains maternal blood and is bound on the maternal side by a decidual plate and on the foetal side by the chorionic plate from which the chorionic villi branch into the maternal blood. The maternal blood enters the intervillous space by about 200 arterioles, which perforate the decidual plate (basalis) (Fig. 7).

Each arteriole spurts a jet of blood into the corresponding foetal lobule and then returns to the basal plate via the decidual veins. The placenta is an important organ of the foetus. The functions of the placenta include supplying the foetus with oxygen and nutrients from the maternal blood through the umbilical cord. Waste products from the foetus are similarly removed in the reverse way. The placenta provides certain amount to protection to the foetus from maternal viral or bacterial infection. However, this protection is not

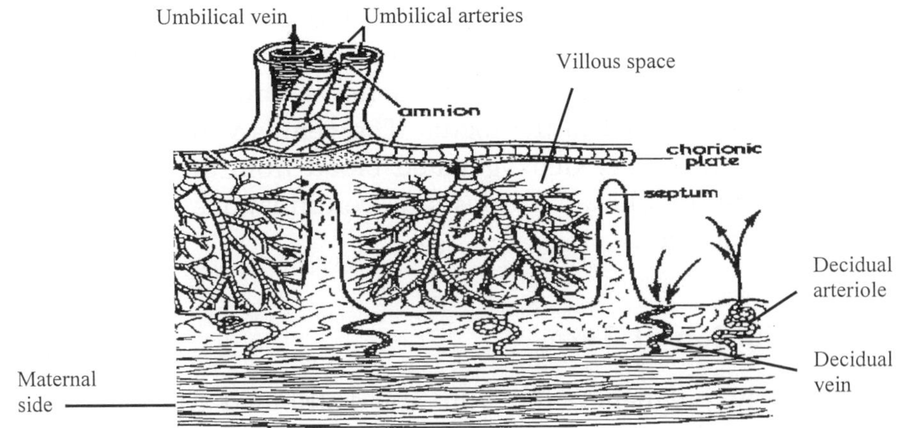

Fig. 7. The placenta.

complete because certain viruses and bacteria can still cross the placenta and infect the foetus. Lastly, the placenta also secretes chorionic gonadotrophin, estrogen, progesterone and other hormones to help maintain the pregnancy.

3. The Placenta at Term

The placenta is circular in shape at term and forms a spongy disc about 20 cm in diameter. It is about 2.5 cm in thickness at the centre and slightly thinner at the edge. The chorion spreads away from the edge of the placenta to form the outer layer, which encloses the foetus and the liquor amnii. The placenta is actually the specialised part of the chorion that serves the foetus.

The placenta has both maternal and foetal surfaces. The maternal surface is rough and spongy and presents a number of polygonal areas called the cotyledons. There are about 15–20 cotyledons in each placenta, which depends on the number of end arteries into which the umbilical arteries divide. The foetal surface is covered by smooth amnion underneath which is loosely attached the chorion. These structures can be stripped off as far as the insertion of the umbilical cord to the placenta.

The umbilical cord usually reaches the placenta at the foetal surface at the centre of the disc. The cord carries with it two arteries and one vein. The oxygenated blood flows through the umbilical vein from the placenta to the foetus. The vein is valveless. The two umbilical arteries carry deoxygenated blood from the foetus to the placenta. The umbilical arteries are continuations of the foetal hypogastric arteries.

4. The Chorion at Term

During early pregnancy, the villi are distributed over the entire surface of the chorionic membrane. The villi that are in contact with the decidual basalis forms the chorion frondosum, which ultimately forms the placenta. Once the definitive placenta is formed, the rest of the chorion atrophies and is denuded of villi (chorionic laeve). This persists only as a thin, friable membrane between the amnion and the decidua. These occurrences are perhaps due to direct pressure or interference of blood supply to the area. At birth, the chorion is seen as an opaque fibrous membrane which is in continuity with the placental edge. It lines the uterine decidua to which it is attached loosely. At term, the thickness of the chorion varies from 0.02 to 0.2 mm, and it has little tensile strength and ruptures easily. Microscopically, it is composed of thin layers of tissues but contains no blood vessels, lymphatics or nerves.

5. The Amnion at Term

As the amnion enlarges, the growing embryo is gradually engulfed into the amniotic cavity. The apposition of the mesoblasts of the chorion and amnion at the end of the first trimester results in the obliteration of the extra-embryonic coelom, hence the attachment of the chorion to the amnion. This attachment is never intimate, even at term, and they can be separated easily at birth.

The amnion is usually about 0.02 to 0.5 mm in thickness and the epithelium consists of a single layer of non-ciliated cuboidal cells.

It is a tough, shiny membrane devoid of blood vessels, lymphatics and nerves. Accordingly, the amnion consists of five layers, i.e. the epithelium, basement membrane, compact layer, fibroblastic layer and spongy layer. The amnion is much stronger than the chorion and is seldom retained in the maternal uterus.

The epithelium is made up of a single layer of non-ciliated epithelial cells. However, under electron microscopy, the apices of the amnion epithelial cells are covered with numerous microvilli while the basal border bears podocytic evaginations. Intercellular canals pass between the lateral aspect of the two membranes of adjacent cells.

The basement membrane is composed of a narrow band of reticulous tissue lying along the base of the epithelial cells to which it is securely adherent by means of fine fibrils and half desmosomes. The basement membrane consists of very fine fibrils adjacent to the epithelial cells. There is a layer of coarse fibrils without periodicity and also coarse collagen fibrils.

The compact layer is a dense, acellular layer immediately subjacent to the basement membrane. This layer shows a marked resistance to leucocytic infiltration so that its boundaries can be easily observed in membranes suffering from a severe inflammatory response.

Fibroblast layer is the most complex layer. It consists of fibroblasts and Hofbauer cells buried in a routine mesh. The thickness of this layer varies considerably in different parts of the amnion and this layer would appear to play quite a considerable part in the transmission of fluid between the foetal and maternal compartment.

The spongy layer is composed of a reticulum of extra-embryonic coelom. It is capable of considerable distention and contains large quantities of mucus. It allows movements of the amnion upon the underlying chorion.

In all the layers in the amnion, there is no identifiable structure of blood vessels, lymphatic vessels or nervous tissues.

6. References

BURNETT, C.W.F. and ANDERSON, M.M. (1979). *The Anatomy and Physiology of Obstetrics*, Faber and Faber.

CLAYTON, S.G., LEWIS, T.L.T. and PINKER, G.D. (1985). *Obstetrics by Ten Teachers*, Edward Arnold.

PHILIPP, E., BARNES, J. and NEWTON, M. (1987). *Scientific Foundations of Obstetrics and Gynaecology*, Heinemann.

PRITCHARD, J.A., MACDONALD, P.C. and GANT, N.F. (1985). *Williams Obstetrics*, Prentice Hall Int.

ZAINOL, J. (1996). *Production and Uses of Laminar Air Dried Amnion in Burns*, Dissertation for Masters in Surgery, University Science Malaysia.

11 ELECTRON MICROSCOPY OF HUMAN AMNIOTIC MEMBRANCE

MAHMOOD FARAZDAGHI

International Federation of Eye Banks
Tissue Banks International
815 Park Avenue, Baltimore, MD 21201
USA

JIRI ADLER

Tissue Bank University Hospital
Brno, Czech Republic

SAMEERA M. FARAZDAGHI

Johns Hopkins University
Johns Hopkins School of Hygiene and Public Health
615 N Wolfe Street, Baltimore, MD 21205
USA

Abstract

Davis reported the first use of foetal membranes for transplantation in 1910. However, in time, the scope of its application increased to a multitude of surgical uses. It has since been used for skin grafting (Davis, 1910; Sabella, 1913;

Tronensegaard-Hansen, 1950; Subramanyam, 1995); treatment of venous ulcers (Stern, 1913; Ward *et al.*, 1989); vaginal reconstruction (Burger, 1937; Dhall, 1984; Nisolle and Donnez, 1992; Georgy and Aziz, 1996); peripheral vascular disease (Tronensegaard-Hansen, 1956); burns (Kirschbaum and Hernandez, 1963; Quinby *et al.*, 1982), as a physiological wound dressing (Colocho *et al.*, 1974; Gruss *et al.*, 1978); for leg ulcers (Trelford and Trelford-Sauder, 1979; Faulk *et al.*, 1980; Ward *et al.*, 1984); otolaryngologic, head and neck surgery (Zohar *et al.*, 1987; Talmi *et al.*, 1990); pelvic surgery (Rennekamff *et al.*, 1994; Gharib *et al.*, 1996), etc.

Amniotic membranes have been widely used in the field of ophthalmology as well. The first use was reported in 1940 for repair of conjunctival defects (de Rotth, 1940) and thereafter for treatment of caustic burns of the eye (Lavery, 1946; Sorsby *et al.*, 1946). However, since conjunctival epithelial cells transdifferentiate into cornea-like cells (Tseng *et al.*, 1984; 1987), utilisation of amniotic membrane as a carrier has received renewed interest. Recently, amniotic membrane has been used to treat conditions such as Stevens-Johnsons disease (Prasad *et al.*, 1986; Tsubota *et al.*, 1996); ocular surface disorders (Lee and Tseng, 1997; Rodriguez-Ares, 1999); chemical and thermal burns (Kim and Tseng, 1995; Shimazaki, 1997); deep corneal ulcers (Kruse *et al.*, 1999); pterygium (Prabhasawat *et al.*, 1997); bullous keratopathy (Pires *et al.*, 1999); removal of tumour, scar or adhesion (Tseng *et al.*, 1997); etc.

Surgical application of amnion for treatment of a wide variety of pathological conditions is due to its unique characteristics and properties. Immunologically, amniotic membrane is a suitable transplant material since it does not express HLA-A, B, or DR antigens and therefore rejection does not occur (Akle *et al.*, 1981; Adinofli *et al.*, 1982; Houlihan *et al.*, 1995). Its anti-adhesive effect (Shimazaki *et al.*, 1998), ability to inhibit neovascularisation (Trelford and Trelford-Sauder, 1979; Kim and Tseng, 1995) and prevent local inflammatory response (Choi *et al.*, 1998) are uncommon qualities among transplantable tissues. Its antimicrobial properties reduce risk of post-operative infection (Talmi *et al.*, 1991). It is reported to reduce pain decrease electrolyte, fluid, and protein loss and promote epithelialisation (Trelford and Trelford-Sauder, 1979). It has also been observed to decrease corneal haze (Choi *et al.*, 1998). The transplanted membrane may perform as a structural barrier to impede proliferation of fibrous tissue and thus decrease scarring (Shimazaki *et al.*, 1998; Tseng *et al.*, 1999).

The membrane consists of proteins, carbohydrates and lipids along with a variety of different growth factors, protease inhibitors, etc., all of which are assumed to play an important role in the effectiveness of the tissue for transplantation. Studies demonstrate that amniotic membrane supports suppression of transforming growth factors (Tseng, 1998) and is therefore superior to collagen shields or plastic for its anti-scarring effect. However, the mechanism of its action is not yet understood and more research is required.

Amniotic membrane is approximately 1,500 cm^2, of which the reflected amnion is 1,200 cm^2. Depending on the application, a large number of grafts of various sizes may be prepared from a single placenta, thus decreasing processing costs. In addition, in countries where cadaveric tissue donation is not in accord with traditional beliefs, skin banks are limited and tissue is scarce. However, obtaining amnion is not a difficult task.

Ideally, placenta should be obtained following elective Caesarean section rather than delivery per vias naturales to avoid structural defects associated with stretching of the membrane during labour and delivery as well as to prevent contamination by vaginal normal flora, or herpes, chlamydia, etc. The membrane should be processed within 12 hours of retrieval to prevent degeneration of cells and detachment of basement membrane from the compact layer. For safety, the donor should be screened for medical contraindications and serologically tested before, and six months after delivery, during which the tissue should be quarantined. Recommended serological tests are for HIV-1 and -2 antibodies, HTLV-1 and -2 antibodies, HbsAg, Hepatitis B core IgG/IgM, HCV, HIV-1 P_{24} antigen and syphilis, to comply with the American Association of Tissue Banks (AATB) standards.

Among grafts of different preservation methods, i.e. fresh, frozen, tissue-culture-maintained and lyophilised membranes, the latter has been demonstrated to have a higher graft take (Ward *et al.*, 1989). In addition, lyophilised membranes have a longer shelf life, are easier to store and safer, due to gamma irradiation. For membranes processed under good laboratory procedures and practices, 1.8 Mrad (18 kGy) is proved to be an effective dose for sterilisation, while collagen structure remains intact (Farazdaghi *et al.*, 2000). Figure 1 demonstrates the explant of a single conjunctival cell growing on freeze-dried amnion.

Also of interest is the attempt by Tseng *et al.* (1999) and our own studies (Farazdaghi and Adler, unpublished data) to demonstrate that cells will grow on the fibroblast layer of amnion. We have also been able to demonstrate that even epithelium-denuded membranes facilitate epithelialisation.

To have a better perspective in processing and utilisation of amniotic membrane, it is necessary to understand the structure, function and composition of the tissue. This is a brief overview of the morphology and characteristics of the amniotic membrane. However, aetiology pathological conditions and diseases as well as processing and preservation methods are beyond the scope of this article.

The amnion is an avascular membrane consisting of five layers — the epithelium, basement membrane, compact layer, fibroblast layer and spongy layer.

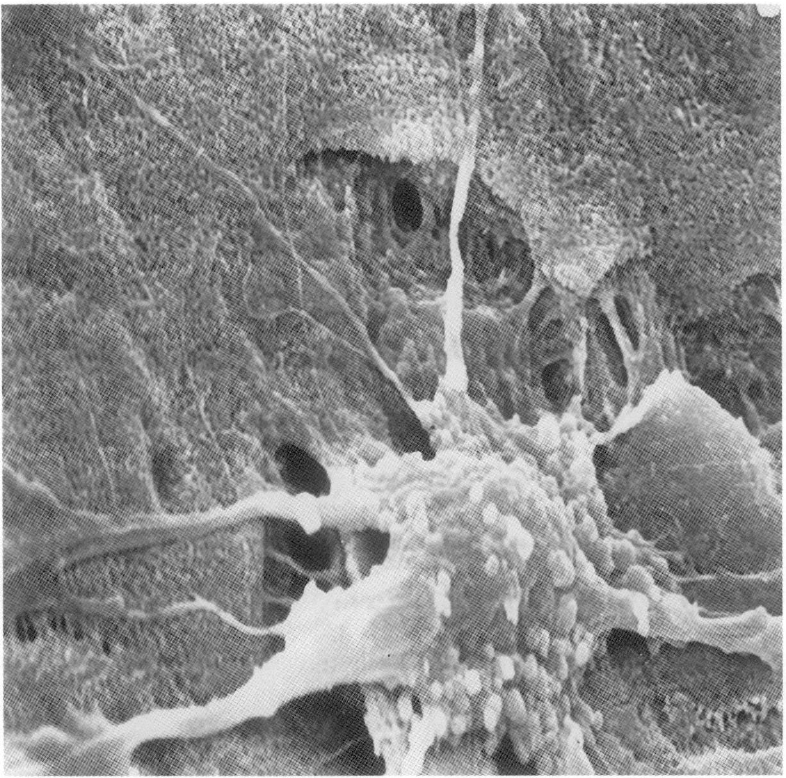

Fig. 1. Single conjunctival cell explant growing on freeze-dried irradiated amniotic membrane (SEM, magnification 3,000×).

1. Epithelium

Electron microscopy of reflected amnion demonstrates a single-layered epithelium of cuboidal to polygonal cells with rounded corners and a convex top surface (Fig. 2). The height of these cells varies from 4–15 μm. Whereas cells of the placental amnion are exclusively cuboidal with a height of 15–22 μm epithelium of the cord amnion may consist of as many as five layers of flattened cells with a height of 2–5 μm (Hempel, 1972) (Fig. 3).

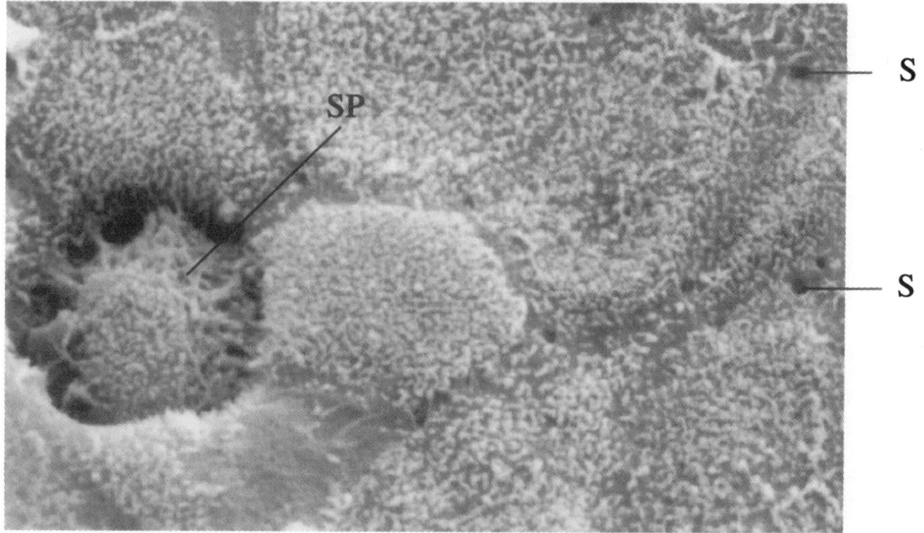

Fig. 2. Polygonal epithelial cells with rounded corners and convex roof. Rough surface of cells demonstrates presence of microvilli. Stoma (S) at multicellular junctions. "Spider cell" (SP) as a precursor to epithelial cell degeneration (SEM magnification 3,000×).

Transmission electron microscopy (TEM) and scanning electron microscopy (SEM) reveal numerous microvilli as plump and club-shaped protrusions of 1.5–3 µm (Schmidt, 1992) extending from the free surface of the epithelial cells into the amniotic fluid (Fig. 4). They are generally single, though occasionally appear as a group arising from a common base or as branched formations. There are canal-like elements consisting of numerous fine rods which extend 0.25–0.5 µm into the cytoplasm (Bourne, 1962), thus making the cytoplasm appear more dense adjacent to the microvilli when observed under lower magnification (Fig. 6).

The cytoplasm is fairly uniform, dense, granular and weakly basophilic. Filaments of 5–10 nm parallel to the apical surface are extended to the desmosomes of lateral cell wall. These filaments contain actin, cytokeratin and vimentin, and contribute to the tensile strength (Wolf *et al.*, 1991). TEM shows numerous vacuoles and

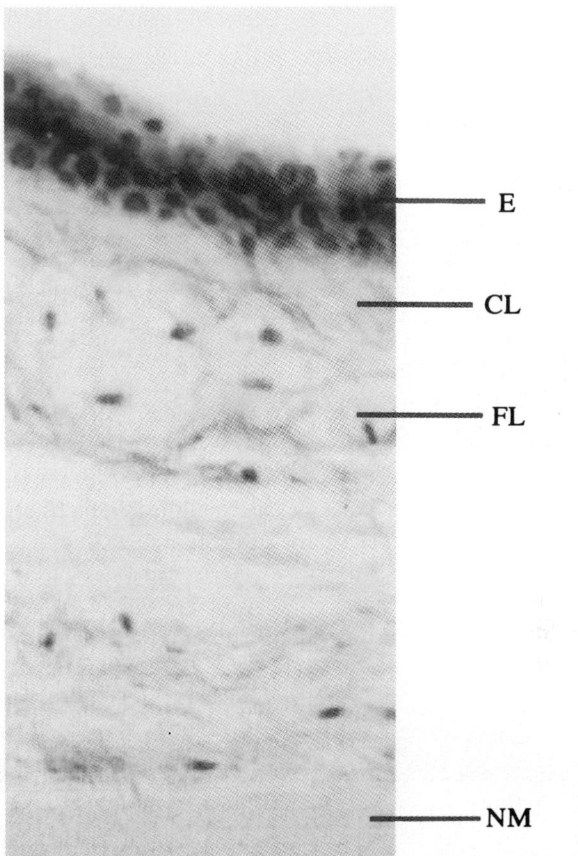

Fig. 3. H & E near cord: Multilayered epithelium (E), accellular compact layer (CL) and fibroblast layer with a loose network of fibres. The amnion is attached to a nitrocellulose carrier membrane (NM). (Magnification 100×)

vesicles of varying size in the cytoplasm. Vesicles may be empty and demonstrate themselves as membrane-bounded vacuoles or filled with an amorphous material of low electron density (Figs. 5 and 6). About 20–55 lipid droplets of 1–5 μm diameter are usually situated around the nucleus in a rosette-like pattern (Fig. 5). Lipid droplets appear in early stages of development and are an integral part of amniotic epithelial cells unless cells are in a

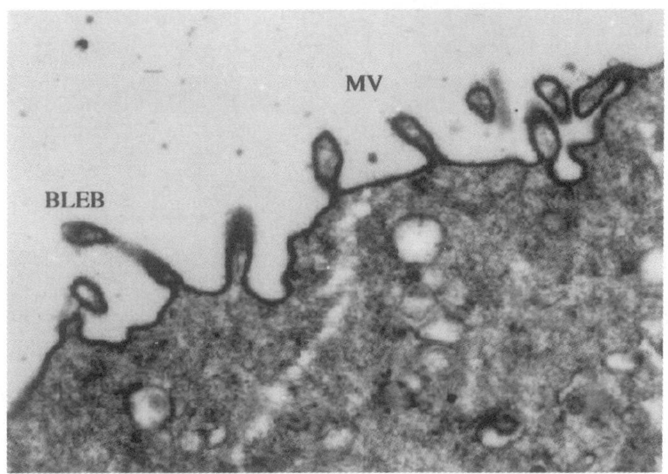

Fig. 4. Apical border of epithelial cells: microvilli (MV), blebs and small vacuoles in the cytoplasm are observed. (TEM, magnification 16,000×)

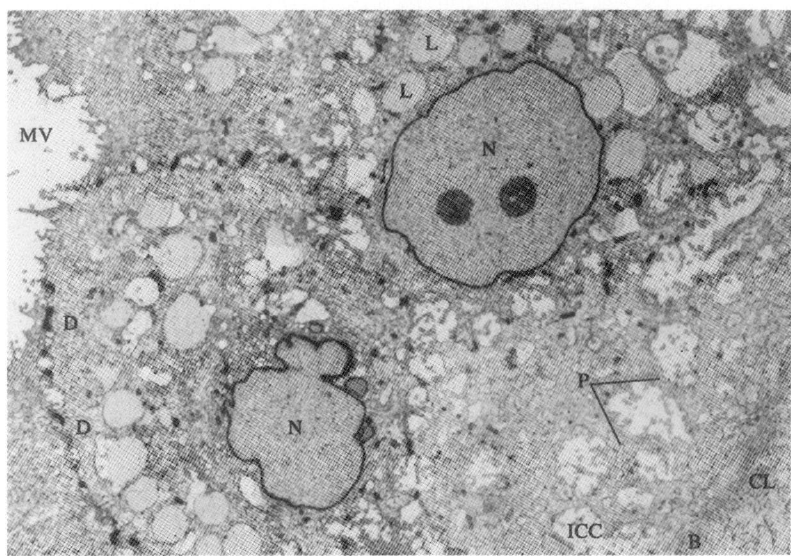

Fig. 5. Epithelial cells with microvilli (MV), a large irregular nucleus (N) with two nucleoli, lipid inclusions (L) in a rosette formation around the nucleus, desmosomes (D) at cell junctions, vacuoles (V), intercellular canals (ICC), basal processes (P), basement membrane (B) and compact layer (CL). (TEM, magnification 3,300×)

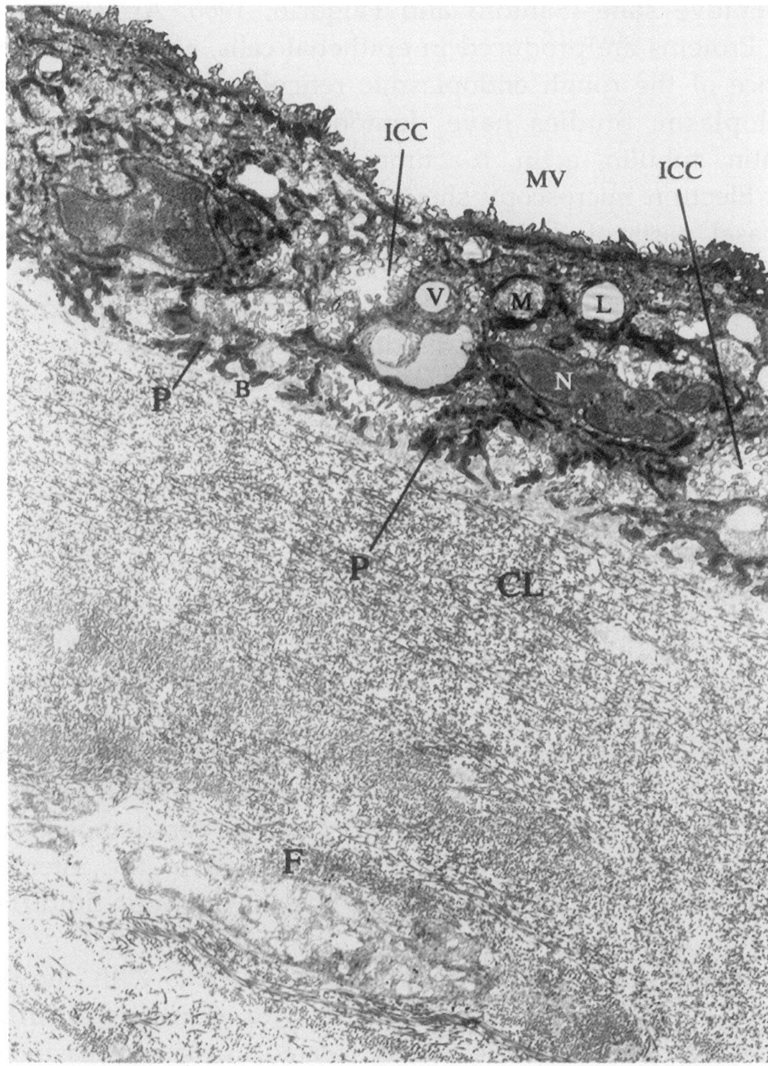

Fig. 6. Reflected amnion: Apical border reveals numerous microvilli (MV); cytoplasm immediately adjacent to the microvilli appears slightly dense. The large, dense nucleus (N) is surrounded by lipid inclusions (L) and vacuoles (V). Meconium (M) appears as material of moderate electron density. Basal processes (P) are protruding into the basement membrane (B), intercellular canals (ICC) are seen between the cells. Compact layer (CL), fibroblast layer (FL) along with a fusiform fibroblast (F) are also observed. (TEM, magnification 2,400×)

degenerative state (Santoro and Falgorio, 1966; Armstrong *et al.*, 1968). Proteins are produced in epithelial cells, as evidenced by the presence of the rough endoplasmic reticulum (rER) and abundant reticuloplasm. Studies have demonstrated presence of keratin, vimentin, tubulin, actin, α-actinin, ezrin and fodrin (Wolf *et al.*, 1991). Electron microscopy shows presence of keratin in the apical and basal parts of the cell. While tubulin is found in the entire cytoplasm with concentration in the base and basal processes, actin is seen as a band in the apical part, extending to the microvilli and lateral protrusions. Fodrin is distributed along the entire cell surface and desmoplakin is limited to desmosomes and hemidesmosomes (Schmidt, 1992).

Narrow bands of condensed cytoplasmic filaments connect two adjacent cells and desmosomes form button-like points of intercellular contact (Fig. 5). Series of irregular shaped lateral vacuoles are joined by narrow channels between adjacent cells to form intercellular canals (Figs. 5 and 6). Although lateral vacuoles and intercellular canals contain microvilli, their presence is less than those of the apical surface of the epithelium (Figs. 5 and 6). Stoma (opening) often occurs at multicellular junctions (Figs. 2 and 7). Together with the stoma, intercellular canals are an important factor in transport and exchange between membrane and amniotic fluids (Bourne, 1962). Experimentally, methylene blue or trypan blue can demonstrate this function. Presence of tracers can be detected in the intercellular space shortly after their introduction into the amniotic fluid (Franke and Estel, 1978).

Epithelial cells generally have a single nucleus with one or two nucleoli (Fig. 5). The nucleus is round with an irregular outline. It is rather large, dense and centrally located in the cytoplasm with a volume of 113 to 290 μm³ (Diegritz, 1949). About 5–7% cells may have more than one nucleus (Schwarzacher, 1959; Schwarzacher and Klinger, 1963). Polynucleosis is a result of amitotic division and is supported by the fact that the total DNA content of a polynuclear cell corresponds to the DNA content of a mononuclear cell (Schwarzacher and Klinger, 1963; Schmidt, 1992). A study by Schwarzacher and Klinger (1962) reveals that cells with one nucleus

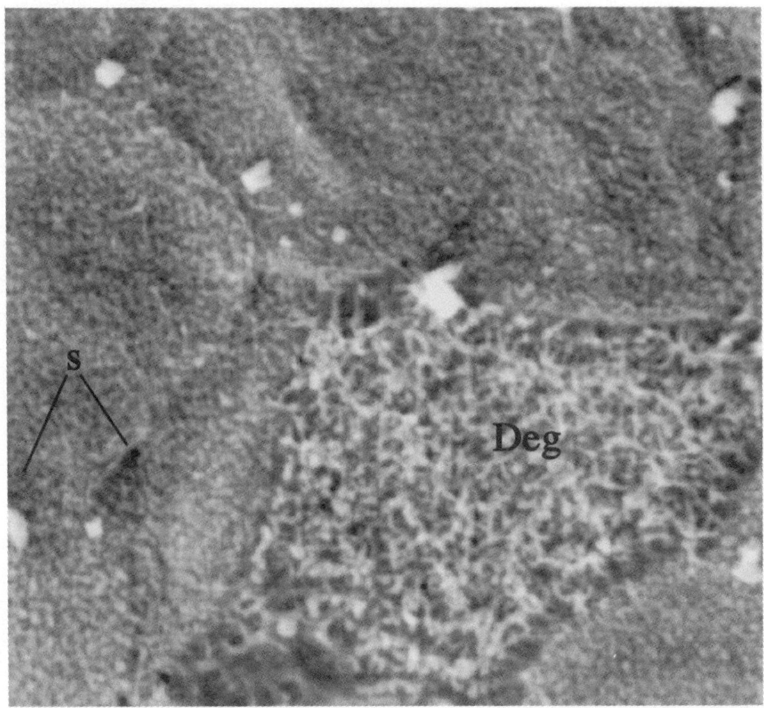

Fig. 7. Epithelial surface: Polygonal cells with rounded corners; stoma (S) at cell junctions; a degenerating cell (Deg); and microvilli as rough, uneven surface. (SEM, magnification 2,400×)

are primarily diploid (2n set of chromosomes), however, higher ploidy, i.e. tetra- (4n), octo- (8n) and even decaploidy have been observed.

The basal region of the epithelium is deeply attached by irregularly-shaped basal processes or pedicles to the basement membrane (Figs. 5, 6 and 8). Although they infiltrate the membrane, they do not extend beyond it. These processes appear as a "narrow layer of granular material", and depending on their functional state, they may be long and narrow or short and plump. Occasionally, they may be connected to one another by autodesmosomes (Petry, 1980). Basal processes are found to be more complex in the region

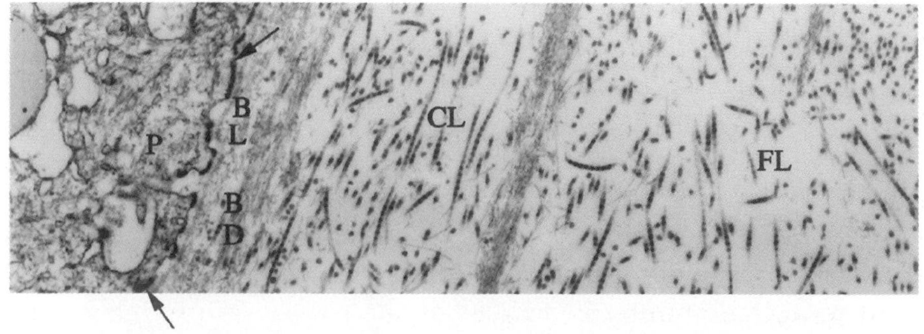

Fig. 8. Semidesmosomal plates where the lamina lucida is firly adherent to the epithelial layer (SP↑); basal processes (P); basement membrane with lamina lucida (BL) and lamina densa (BD); compact layer (CL) and fibroblast layer (FL) (TEM, magnification 20,000×)

of intercellular canals. Material of moderate density, similar to the basement membrane, fills the space between the basal processes and occasionally extends into the epithelial cells and intercellular spaces (Fig. 8).

Amniotic epithelial cells are specially adapted to perform three major functions as a covering epithelium secretory epithelium and for intercellular and transcellular transport (van Herendael et al., 1978). "Light", Golgi-type (Thomas, 1965) or Type I (Schmidt, 1992) are epithelial cells containing remarkably well-developed rER large Golgi apparatus which comprises dictyosomes and abundant elongated mitochondria. Lysosomes and multi-vesicular bodies are present in the cytoplasm. As a result of these characteristics, they are assumed to be secretory in function. Dense amniotic epithelial cells consolidate to form large mosaic-like areas. Optical density is due to high tubulin content and particular profusion of cytoskeletal components. These cells have been classified as Type II (Schmidt, 1992), "dark" or "fibrillary type" (Thomas, 1965) and their function is assumed to be absorption. Microfilaments are abundantly present in the cytoplasm the endoplasmic reticulum is narrow and dense the Golgi apparatus is not well developed and the nucleus contains large amounts of heterochromatin and small rounded mitochondria (Franke and Estel, 1978; Schmidt, 1992). "Light" cells are known to be remarkably less frequent than "dark" cells with a ratio of 1:2 to 1:8. Organ culture of term amnion reveals that after five days of incubation, the apparent differences between "light" (Golgi or Type I) and "dark" (fibrillary or Type II) cells disappear and the above-mentioned differences are due to adaptation of epithelial cells to a specific function (Schmidt, 1992).

At term, the amnion is a tissue at the end of its productive life. Generally, epithelial cell loss is always present with degenerating (spider) cells losing their nuclei (Figs. 2 and 7). However, occasionally, large areas of degenerating epithelial cells may be present in the form of "roads", where strips of epithelium with a few cell width may have lost their nuclei. The cause of this necrosis, which resembles foetal scratching, is unknown.

2. Basement Membrane

The basement membrane is a thin acellular structure of reticular tissue adhered to the base of the amniotic epithelium. It is PAS positive and in haematoxylin and eosin (H & E) stain, it appears eosinophilic. The thickness varies from the placenta to reflected amnion. The basement membrane contains collagens of type III, type IV and type V (Azzarelli and Lafuze, 1987) fibronectin and laminin (Klima and Schmidt, 1988).

It consists of two distinct layers. The lamina lucida is deeply adherent to the base of epithelial cells, forms the basal cristae and extends itself to epithelial cells and intercellular space (Fig. 8). The lamina densa is interposed between the lamina lucida and compact layer from its deeper aspect (Verbeek *et al.*, 1967). Adherence of the basement membrane to the compact layer is firm and separation of the two layers is not easily achieved. However, if epithelial cells are dead or diseased, or if membrane preparation is delayed for several hours after delivery, the basement membrane will separate from the underlying compact layer but remain adherent to the epithelial layer (Bourne, 1962).

3. Compact Layer

The compact layer is a thin, acellular structure, uniform in depth and density. It is comprises a network of reticular fibres and is interposed between the basement membrane and the underlying fibroblast layer (Figs. 8 and 9). Bundles of reticular fibres construct a uniform woven mesh throughout the structure and spaces formed by the meshwork are filled with mucus. This special structure provides a remarkable tensile strength to the entire amniotic membrane. Tension on the amniotic membrane changes the shape of the mucus-filled mesh, "rather like a piece of expanding wooden lattice-work". The compact layer mainly comprises collagen type I, type III and type V. Though the membrane has a low affinity for

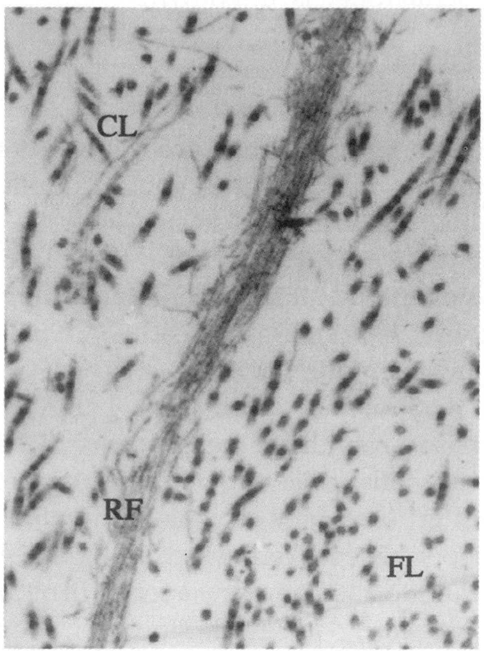

Fig. 9. Compact (CL) and fibroblast (FL) layers: Bundles of reticular fibres are visible (RF). Fibres in fibroblast layer are loosely packed in contrast to compact layer. (TEM, magnification 20,000×)

stain, it is relatively dense and is seen as weakly eosinophilic when stained with H & E. This acellular membrane has the ability to resist infiltration of maternal leukocytes, except in cases of severe chorio-amnionitis. (Bourne, 1962).

4. Fibroblast layer

The fibroblast layer is the fourth layer of the amnion. With a thickness of 0.05 to 0.5 mm, it is responsible for the main thickness and variation in diameter of the amnion. It is difficult to stain due to its high mucin content. It stains weakly eosinophilic. However, its affinity to stain depends upon the thickness of the layer. A more condensed and thinner layer appears as a strip-containing spindle-shaped nuclei, but when sparse, it is less recognisable. This layer is composed of a reticular mesh interspersed with a loose fibroblast network. The fibroblasts are usually stellate or fusiform in shape (Fig. 6) containing a dense, oval, disc-shaped nucleus and two to ten cellular processes. They vary in size depending upon their age and physiological state. Some have a diameter of 50 or 60 μm, containing three or four nuclei with five to ten cellular processes, while others may be mononuclear with a diameter of 10–20 μm and two or four cellular processes. Long axes of the cells are approximately parallel to the basement membrane. Cellular processes which may vary in length and shape form short and blunt to long protuberances extending for many millimetres to form the fibroblast network. In response to stress, cellular processes alter their shape by elongation and narrowing to align themselves parallel to the applied force. This response is similar to that of the reticular network. The disc-shaped nucleus of fibroblasts lies along its longitudinal axis and parallel to the epithelial surface of the amnion. Therefore, its shape is not easily appreciated in cross-sections. The cytoplasm is weakly basophilic. It contains a considerable number of small dense glycogen granules and lipid droplets well-developed rER, relatively small Golgi apparatus and limited mitochondria (Bourne, 1962).

The fibroblast layer also contains Hofbauer cells/histiocytes which are morphologically similar to fibroblasts as well as macrophages. They are oval in shape with small pseudopodia-like processes and stain denser than fibroblasts. The cytoplasm contains glycogen granules, lipid droplets and large vacuoles. Some cells contain meconium in the form of a yellowish-brown granular material. Meconium released in amniotic fluid passes through the intercellular space and intercellular canals of epithelium. When it reaches the connective tissue, it is absorbed into the cells by phagocytosis (Schmidt, 1992).

5. Spongy Layer

The spongy layer is the fifth and last layer of the amnion. It is compressed between the chorion and developing amniotic sac and is therefore also called "stratum intermedium" or "in-between layer". Although it adheres to both membranes, its adhesion to amnion is stronger, especially over the reflected membranes. It consists of a complex network of fine fibrils surrounded by mucus. The fibrils appear as straight or wavy. They are composed of reticulin, collagen type I and type III (Klima and Schmidt, 1988). The spongy layer contains two types of cells, i.e. fibroblasts and Hofbauer cells that are similar to those in the fibroblast layer. Hofbauer cells are usually observed in groups of six or more cells. Fibroblasts are mostly mononuclear, fusiform or stellate cells with 20–40 μm diameter. Bundles of wavy or straight fibres originate from the cellular processes of these cells and are scattered throughout the layer. The spongy layer acts as a visco-elastic pad between the two membranes, thus enabling amnion to move over the chorion, which is attached to the uterine wall. This important function protects the amnion against trauma and rupture during dilation of the cervix in labour. When tension is increased and results in rupture of the chorion, the amnion can glide freely and prevent direct tension on the amniotic sac. The spongy layer is remarkably hygroscopic and thickness can increase from 5 μm to as much as 10 mm in the event of oedema (Bourne, 1962).

6. Acknowledgements

We would like to thank Prof. Drahoslav Horky, Medical Faculty of the Masryk University, for providing invaluable cooperation, and Ms. Jana Komarkova, Tissue Bank University Hospital, for her excellent technical assistance.

7. References

ADINOFLI, M., AKLE, C.A. and McCOLL, I. (1982). Expression of HLA antigens β_2-microglobulin and enzymes by human amniotic membrane. *Nature* **295**, 325–327.

AKLE, C.A., ADINOFLI, M., WELSH, K.I., LEIBOWITZ, S. and McCOLL, I. (1981). Immunogenecity of human amniotic epithelial cells after transplantation into volunteers. *Lancet* **2**, 1003–1005.

ARMSTRONG, W.D., WILT, J.C. and PITCHARD, E.T. (1968). Vacuolisation of human amnion. Cell studies by time-lapse photography and electron microscopy. *Am. J. Obstet. Gynecol.* **102**, 932–948.

AZZARELLI, B. and KAFUZE, J. (1987). Amniotic basement membrane: A barrier of neutrophil invasion. *Am. J. Obstet. Gynecol.* **156**, 1130–1136.

BOURNE, G.L. (1962). In *The Human Amnion and Chorion*. Lyold-Luke, London.

BURGER, K. (1937). Artificial vaginal reconstruction with the help of amnios. *Zentralblatt Fur Gynakol.* 2437–2440.

CHOI, Y.S., KIM, J.Y., WEE, W.R. and LEE, J.H. (1998). Effect of application of human amniotic membrane on rabbit corneal wound healing after excimer laser photorefractive keratectomy. *Cornea* **7**, 389–395.

COLOCHO, G., GRAHAM, W.P., GREEN, A.E., MATHESON, D.W. and LYNCH, D. (1974). Human amniotic membrane as a physiologic wound dressing. *Arch. Surg.* **109**, 370–373.

DAVIS, J.W. (1910). Skin transplantation with a review of 550 cases at the Johns Hopkins Hospital. *Johns Hopkins Med. J.* **15**, 307.

DE ROTTH, A. (1940). Plastic repair of conjunctival defects with fetal membranes. *Arch. Ophthalmol.* **23**, 522–525.

DHALL, K. (1984). Amnion graft for treatment of congenital absence of the vagina. *Br. J. Obstet. Gynaecol.* **91**, 279–282.

DIEGRITZ (1949). Über die Kern-Plasmrealation der Amnionzelle. *Z. Anat.* **114**, 283–308.

FARAZDAGHI, M., ADLER, J., KOMARKOVA, J. and HORKY, D. (2000). Preserved human amniotic membrane grafts: An evaluation of morphology, elasticity and biocompatibility. *Proc. European Eye Bank Association 12th Conference*, January.

FAULK, W.P., MATTHEWS, R.N., STEVENS, P.J., BENNETT, J.P., BURGO, H. and HSI, B.L. (1980). Human amnion as a adjunct in wound healing. *Lancet*, 1158.

FRANKE, H. and ESTEL, C. (1978). Untersuchungen über die Ultrastuktur und Permeabilitat des Amnions unter besonderer Berücksichtigung mikrofilamentarer and microtubularer Strukturen. *Arch. Gynaekol.* **225**, 319–338.

GEORGY, M.S. and AZIZ, N.L. (1996). Vaginoplasty using amnion graft new surgical technique using laproscopic transillumination light. *J. Gynaecol. Surg.* **16**, 262–264.

GHARIB, M., URE, B.M. and KLOSE, M. (1996). Use of amniotic grafts in the repair of gastrochisis. *Pediatr. Surg.* **11**, 96–99.

GRUSS, J.S. and JIRSCH, D.W. (1978). Human amniotic membrane a versatile dressing. *J. Can. Med. Assoc.* **118**, 1237–1246.

HEMPEL, E. (1972). Die ultrastrukturelle Differenzierung des menschlichen Amnionepithels unter besonderer Berücksichtigung des Nabelstranges. *Anat. Anz.* **132**, 356–370.

HOULIHAN, J.M., BIRO, P.A., HARPER, H.M., JENKINSON, H.J. and HOLMES, C. (1995). The human amniotic membrane is a site of MHC class 1b: Evidence for the expression of HLA-E and HLA-G. *J. Immuno.* **154**, 565–574.

KIM, J.C. and TSENG, S.C.G. (1995). Transplantation of preserved human amniotic membrane for surface reconstruction in severely damaged rabbit corneas. *Cornea* **14**, 473–484.

KIRSCHBAUM, S.M. and HERNANDEZ, H. (1963). Use of amnion in extensive burns. *Proc. Third Int. Cong. Plastic Surg.* Excerpta Medica, Amsterdam.

KLIMA, G. and SCHMIDT, W. (1988). Immunhistochemische Untersuchungen über die Natur der Bindegewebsfibrillen in den Fruchthüllen. *Acta Histochem. (Jena)* **84**, 195–203.

KRUSE, F.E., ROHRSCHNEIDER, K. and VÖLCKER, H.E. (1999). Multilayer amniotic membrane transplantation for reconstruction of deep corneal ulcers. *Ophthalmol.* **106**, 1504–1511.

LAVERY, F.S. (1946). Lime burn of conjunctiva and cornea treated with amnioplastin graft. *Trans. Ophthalmol. Soc. UK* **66**, 668.

LEE, S. and TSENG, S.C.G. (1997). Amniotic membrane transplantation for persistent epithelial defects with ulceration. *Am. J. Ophthalmol.* **123**, 303–312.

NISOLLE, M. and DONNEZ, J. (1992). Vaginoplasty using amniotic membranes in cases of vaginal agenesis or after vaginectomy. *J. Gynecol. Surg.* **8**, 25–30.

PETRY, G. (1980). "Autodesmosomen", desmosomale Kontakte von Teilen derselben Zelle im menschlichen Chorion laeve and Amnion. *Eur. J. Cell. Biol.* **23**, 129–134.

PIRES, R.T.F., TSENG, S.C.G., PRABHASAWAT, P., PUANGRICHARERN, V., MASKIN, S.L. and KIM, J.C. (1999). Amniotic membrane transplantation for symptomatic bullous keratopathy. *Arch. Ophthalmol.* **117**, 1291–1297.

PRABHASAWAT, P., BARTON, K., BURKETT, G. and TSENG, S.C.G. (1997). Comparison of conjuctival autografts, amniotic membrane grafts and primary closure for pterygium excision. *Ophthalmol.* **104**, 974–985.

PRASAD, J.K, FELLER, I. and THOMPSON, P.D. (1986). Use of amnion for the treatment of Stevens-Johnsons syndrome. *J. Trauma.* **26**, 945–946.

QUINBY, W.C. Jr., HOOVER, H.C., SCHEFLAN, M., PHILEMON, T.W., SUMNER, A.S. and CONRADO, C.B. (1982). Clinical trials of amniotic membranes in burn wound care. *Plastic Reconstructive Surg.* **70**, 711–716.

RENNEKAMPFF, H.-O., DOHRMAN, P., FORY, R. and FANDRICH, F. (1994). Evaluation of amniotic membrane as adhesion prophylaxis in a novel surgical gastrochisis model. *Invest. Surg.* **7**, 187–193.

RODRIGUEZ-ARES, M.T., TOURINO, R., CAPEANS, C. and SANCHEZ-SALORIO, M. (1999). Repair of scleral perforation with preserved scleral and amniotic membrane in Marfan's syndrome. *Ophthalmic. Surg. Lasers* **30**, 485–487.

SABELLA, N. (1913). Use of fetal membranes in skin grafting. *Med. Records NY* **83**, 478–480.

SANTORO, A. and FALAGARIO, M. (1966). Sulla fine strutturadelle cellule epithiali dell'amnion umano a termine di gestatione. *Attual. Ostet. Ginecol.* **12**, 933–938.

SCHMIDT, W. (1992). The amniotic fluid compartment: The fetal habitat. *Adv. Anat. Embryol. Cell. Biol.* **127**, 1–98.

SCHWARZACHER, H.G. (1959). Zur Frage der Zellvermehrung im wachsenden menschlichenAmnion. *Verh. Anat. Ges. Jena.* (Suppl. to *Anat. Anz.* **105**, 156–159).

SCHWARZACHER, H.G. and KLINGER, H.P. (1962). Deoxyribonukleinsaure-(DNS)-Gehalt und Geschlechtschromatin mehrkerniger Amnioneoithelzellen des Menschen.*Verh. Anat. Ges. Jena.* (Suppl to *Anat. Anz.* **111**, pp. 94–102).

SCHWARZACHER, H.G. and KLINGER, H.P. (1963). Die Entstehung mehrherniger Zelln durch Amitose im Amnionepithel des Menschen und die Aufteilung des chromosoamlen Materials auf deren einzelne Zellkerne. *Z. Zellforcsh.* **60**, 741–754.

SHIMAZAKI, J., SHINOZAKI, N. and TSUBATO, K. (1998). Transplantation of amniotic membrane and limbal autograft for patients with recurrent pterygium associated with symblepharon. *Br. J. Ophthalmol.* **82**, 235–240.

SHIMAZAKI, J., YANG, H.-Y. and TSUBATO, K. (1997). Amniotic membrane transplantation for ocular surface reconstruction in-patients with chemical and thermal burns. *Ophthalmol.* **104**, 2068–2076.

SORSBY, A. and SYMMONS, H.M. (1946). Amniotic membrane grafts in caustic burns of the eye (burns of second degree). *Br. J. Ophthalmol.* **30**, 337–345.

STERN, W. (1913). The grafting of preserved amniotic membrane to burned and ulcerated skin surfaces substituting skin grafts. *JAMA* **13**, 973–974.

SUBRAHMANYAM, M. (1995). Amniotic membrane as a cover for microskin grafts. *Br. J. Plastic Surg.* **48**, 477–478.

TALMI, Y.P., FINKELSTEIN, Y. and ZOHAR, Y. (1990). Use of human amniotic membrane as a biologic dressing. *Euro. J. Plastic Surg.* **13**, 160–162.

TALMI, Y.P., SIGLER, L., and INGE, E. (1991). Antibacterial properties of human amniotic membranes. *Placenta* **12**, 285–288.

THOMAS, C.E. (1965). The ultrastructure of human amnion epithelium. *J. Ultrastruct. Res.* **13**, 65–84.

TRELFORD, J.D. and TRELFORD-SAUDER, M. (1979). The amnion in surgery, past and present. *Am. J. Obstet. Gynecol.* **134**, 833–845.

TROENSAGAARD-HANSEN, E. (1950). Amniotic grafts in chronic ulceration. *Lancet* **1**, 859–860.

TROENSEGAARD-HANSEN, E. (1956). Amnion implantation in peripheral vascular disease. *Br. Med. J.* **2**, 262.

TSENG, S.C.G., LI, D.-Q. and MA, X. (1999). Suppression of transforming growth factor bets isoforms, TGF-ß receptor type II, and myofibroblast differentiation in cultured human corneal and limbal fibroblasts by amniotic membrane matrix. *J. Cell. Physiol.* **179**, 325–335.

TSENG, S.C.G., FARAZDAGHI, M. and RIDER, A.A. (1987). Conjunctival transdifferentiation induced by systemic vitamin A deficiency in vascularized rabbit corneas. *Invest. Ophthalmol. Vis. Sci.* **28**, 1497–1504.

TSENG, S.C.G., HIRST, L.W., FARAZDAGHI, M. and GREEN, W.R. (1984). Goblet cell density and vascularization during conjunctival transdifferentiation. *Invest. Ophthalmol. Vis. Sci.* **25**, 1168–1176.

TSENG, S.C.G., PRABHASAWAT, P. and LEE, S.-H. (1997). Amniotic membrane transplantation for conjunctival surface reconstruction. *Am. J. Ophthalmol.* **124**, 765–774.

TSENG, S.C.G., PRABHASAWAT, P., BARTON, K., GRAY, T. and MELLER, D. (1998). Amniotic membrane transplantation with or without limbal allografts for corneal surface reconstruction in-patients with limbal cell deficiency. *Arch. Ophthalmol.* **116**, 431–441.

TSUBOTA, K., YOSHIYUKI, S., OHYAMA, M., TODA, I. TAKANO, Y., OHO, M., SHINOZAKI, N. and SHIMAZAKI, J. (1996). Surgical reconstruction of the ocular surface in advanced ocular cicatricial pemphigoid and Stevens-Johnsons syndrome. *Am. J. Ophthalmol.* **122**, 38–52.

VAN HERENDAEL, B.J., OBERTI, C. and BROSENS, I. (1978). Microanatomy of the human amniotic membranes: A light microscopic, transmission and electron microscopic study. *Am. J. Obstet. Gynecol.* **131**, 872–880.

VERBEEK, J.H., ROBERTSON, E.M. and DARIA HAUST, M. (1967). Basement membranes (amniotic, trophoblastic, capillary) and adjacent tissue in term placenta, an electron microscopic study. *Am. J. Obstet. Gynecol.* **99**, 1136–1146.

WARD, D.J. and BENNETT, J. P. (1984). The long term results of the use of human amnion in the treatment of leg ulcers. *Br. J. Plastic Surg.* **37**, 191–193.

WARD, D.J., BENNETT, J. P., BURGOS, H. and FABRE, J. (1989). The healing of chronic venous leg ulcers with prepared human amnion. *Br. J. Plastic Surg.* **42**, 463–467.

WOLF, H.J., SCHMIDT, W. and DRENCKHAHN, D. (1991). Immunocytochemical analysis of the cytoskeleton of the amniotic epithelial cell. *Cell Tissue Res.* **266**, 385–389.

ZOHAR, Y., TALMI, Y.P., FINKELSTEIN, Y., SHVILI, Y., SADOV, R. and LAURIAN, N. (1987). Use of human amniotic membrane in otolaryngologic practice. *Laryngoscope* **97**, 978–980.

SECTION III:

MICROBIOLOGY

12 INTRODUCTION TO MEDICAL MICROBIOLOGY

GAMINI KUMARASINGHE

Division of Microbiology
Department of Laboratory Medicine
National University Hospital
5 Lower Kent Ridge Road
Singapore 119074

Abstract

Antonie van Leeuwenhoek, in 1674, first saw what he called "ammalcules" — bacteria and protozoa — in biological samples, including those taken from his own body. Many important developments related to clinical microbiology took place during the latter part of the 19th century. In 1875, F.J. Cohn published an early classification of bacteria, using the genus name *Bacillus* for the first time. Robert Koch described anthrax in 1876, the culture plate technique in 1881 and the aetiology of tuberculosis in 1884. He was awarded the Nobel Prize for his contributions to medicine in 1905. Joseph Lister demonstrated the isolation of bacteria in pure culture, Louis Pasteur introduced the concept of vaccination with attenuated microorganisms and Paul Ehrlich demonstrated the formation of antibodies, all during the 19th century. Since then, medical microbiology has evolved at an explosive rate (ASM, 1999). A wide variety of emerging pathogens continue to be described as various advances are made in medicine (CDC, webpage). During the last two decades, molecular diagnostic techniques have led to a revolution in our abilities to identify, classify and understand microorganisms. Increasing numbers of diagnostic tests, including those commercially available, are based on molecular techniques. Some enthusiasts predict that they may replace culture as the routine laboratory method of investigation.

Microbiology is the science concerned with studying all microorganisms. Medical microbiology restricts this to the microbes that live on the human surface, and those there or elsewhere that may invade human tissues or otherwise cause infectious disease. In a nutshell, medical microbiology involves the diagnosis, treatment and control of human infection.

Clinical microbiology has matured into a wide-ranging science, not just a service to process specimens and provide results but also to advise on the collection of specimens, the interpretation of results and management of patients, the selection of antimicrobial agents and in the control of hospital-acquired infections.

Conventional pathogens are capable of causing infections in previously healthy people. The organisms isolated from clinical specimens may derive from bacteria and fungi that are permanently living on body surfaces (commensals) or from the environment. Opportunistic pathogens are those that usually do not cause disease in normal people, but may cause serious infections in immunocompromised patients. Hence, the significance of laboratory findings will depend on how the specimen was collected and needs to be assessed in the context of the clinical situation. Serious nosocomial infections are often caused by commensals and environmental organisms. A clear distinction between a primary pathogen, a commensal and a contaminant is not always clear-cut. This situation is frequently encountered in immunologically compromised patients. As a result, the liaison between the medical microbiologist and the clinician is of paramount importance to ensure a sensible interpretation of laboratory findings.

1. Biological Background

We live in a germ-filled world. Microbes can be found everywhere in the environment, including the air, the soil, the water, and the food we eat. Microbes of almost infinite variety and complexity colonise our body surfaces and orifices. The chemical reactions produced by microorganisms help to make the soil fertile, and to decompose organic material piling up in the environment. They help to improve the quality of certain types of food and synthesise vitamins. The microbial flora resident on our body surface protects us from less desirable microbes, which is referred to as colonisation resistance.

The general perception about microbes is that they are invisible creatures that cause disease, whereas the beneficial aspects are often ignored. A few can be harmful by causing disease, a few can spoil food, a few can destroy valuable materials. When something undesirable happens, we become aware of microbes, and may not realise the important contributions that are being made by them and the fact that living without them is impossible. Both mitochondria and chloroplasts essential to animal and plant life are probably evolved from endosymbiont bacteria (Alberts *et al.*, 1994).

2. Infectious Diseases

Infectious diseases cause problems in all specialities of medicine. Any system may be affected. An adequate knowledge of infectious diseases is desirable in any practising clinician. Infectious disease is the world's major cause of illness (**morbidity**) and death (**mortality**). Classical infectious diseases are caused by primary pathogens that affect healthy individuals. Some are more commonly seen in developing areas of the world, e.g. typhoid, tuberculosis and malaria. Others, such as *Escherichia coli*, *Staphylococcus aureus* and *Streptococcus* *pneumoniae*, are common worldwide. Opportunist infections affect patients whose defence mechanisms are damaged. They are more commonly encountered where medical services are more advanced, e.g. in places where there are advanced techniques in medicine and surgery that render the patient more susceptible to infection, e.g. immunosuppressive agents, prosthetic devices and intensive care.

3. Epidemiology of Infectious Disease

Epidemiology is the study of the nature, distribution, causation, mode of transfer, prevention and control of infection. Most studies concentrate on factors that influence acquisition and spread because this knowledge is essential for prevention and control. Infectious diseases can be categorised on the basis of how often they occur. If a disease, such as the common cold, is constantly present in a community, it is said to be **endemic**. An **epidemic** is present when the occurrence of a disease exceeds expected levels. When an epidemic of a disease becomes worldwide, it is considered to be **pandemic**. The occurrence of infectious diseases is affected by geography, climate, poverty, politics, wars and human behaviour. The patient's history regarding job, pastimes, sexual proclivities, travel, etc., will give clues as to the cause of the illness.

4. Pathogenesis

Pathogenicity is defined as the ability of a microorganism to cause disease. Virulence refers to the extent of pathogenicity, so it is a measure of the damage an organism is capable of causing to the host. There are many mechanisms that contribute to virulence. Bacteria that possess **capsules** are more virulent because the capsule inhibits phagocytosis, e.g. *Neisseria meningitidis*. The presence of **fimbriae** may endow a bacterium with the power to adhere to the host's cells. Some bacteria produce **exotoxins** that permit them to cause a wide range of diseases, e.g. diphtheria, tetanus, gas gangrene and food poisoning. The infectivity of an organism depends on two main factors: (i) the minimum number of cells required to colonise or cause an infection, and (ii) its ability to invade the susceptible site. Shigellae are capable of causing infections with a dose as small as 10^1–10^2 organisms, whereas salmonellae requires about 10^5–10^6 organisms to establish an infection (Duerden, 1987). The mode of transmission varies according to the ability of the organism to invade tissues. Hepatitis A virus is capable of penetrating intestinal mucosa, whereas Hepatitis B virus cannot penetrate the skin or mucosa (Volk, 1996).

5. Basic Features of Bacteria

The rigid **cell wall** of a bacterium determines the shape of the cell. Without it, the cell would swell and burst due to the high concentration of intracellular solutes. The strength of the cell wall is imparted by mucopeptide (peptidoglycan), which can be damaged by certain antibiotics, e.g. penicillins. Partially-treated infections may result in organisms with inhibited cell walls known as **protoplasts**, **spheroplasts** and **L-forms**. These resemble mycoplasmas — bacteria that are inherently deficient in peptidoglycan. Such organisms may play a role in the pathogenesis of chronic and recurrent infections because they can survive host defence mechanisms that target cell walls (Butler and Blakey, 1975). The result of the Gram stain varies according to the composition of the cell wall. Gram-positive organisms are blue-staining and Gram-negatives are red-staining. The principal differences being a far greater amount of mucopeptide in Gram-positives and the presence of an outer cell membrane of lipopolysaccharides in the Gram-negatives' cell wall. Lipopoly-saccharides liberated during the disintegration of cells are responsible for the clinical situation of Gram-negative sepsis, a cause of systemic immune response syndrome — SIRS (Nystrom, 1998).

The **cytoplasm** and the peripherally-bound membrane form the protoplasm. This consists of a watery sap packed with large numbers of tiny granules called ribosomes. These are the sites of protein synthesis and differ from those found in human cells in size and composition. These differences explain the selective action of several antibiotics that inhibit bacterial more than human protein synthesis.

The **chromosome/nuclear body** is the area in the cytoplasm where DNA is located and has little resemblance to the human cell nucleus. There is no nuclear membrane in prokaryotes.

Plasmids are DNA molecules that exist independently from the bacterial chromosomes. They may carry genes that confer properties of medical importance, such as antibiotic resistance. They are often possessed by multiresistant bacteria found in hospitals.

Transposons are pieces of DNA, nicknamed "jumping genes" because of their ability to move between chromosomes, plasmids and bacteriophages.

Bacteriophages are specialised viruses — the smallest infectious agents — which infect only bacteria. Plasmids, transposons and phages provide bacteria with a system for genetic mixing that may be advantageous for rapid adaptation to unfavourable circumstances. Although these genes are dispensable to the bacterium, they may persist within the progeny over long periods of time (Mercer *et al.*, 1984).

Capsules are possessed by some bacteria and help to evade certain human defence mechanisms, such as phagocytosis. Capsular antigens are used in the identification of organisms and in the synthesis of vaccines.

Flagellae are fine whip-like organelles of locomotion that move bacteria towards food and other attractants. Only some bacteria have flagellae. They play a role in the pathogenesis of some infections, e.g. urinary tract infections, by aiding bacteria to move upstream from the urethra to the bladder.

Fimbriae or **pili** are shorter hair-like protrusions and are organelles of adhesion that help bacteria to attach to a host cell. Specialised fimbriae play an additional role in the attachment of donor to recipient bacteria during conjugation. In this process, bacteria exchange genetic information. In uropathogenic strains of

Escherichia coli, fimbriae have been established as a virulence factor prompting colonisation and invasion (Hull *et al.*, 1981).

Spores are possessed by certain species of bacteria. They possess thick, highly resistant cell walls. Spores can withstand adverse conditions, including extraordinary high and low temperatures. Boiling cannot destroy spores, so autoclaving is essential to achieve a complete sterilisation process (Levinson and Jawetz, 1994).

Antimicrobial agents used in the treatment of infections target various sites such as the cell wall, cell membrane, ribosomes, nucleic acids and folate synthesis (O'Grady *et al.*, 1997). There are structural and functional differences between these cellular targets and the human equivalents. This enables us to design drugs which damage bacterial systems while causing less or no harm to human ones.

6. Reproduction

Bacteria reproduce by binary fission, some as quickly as every 20 minutes; others are much slower (Levinson and Jawetz, 1994). Fast growers may contaminate specimens and result in high counts, leading to the misinterpretation of results. In the case of slow growers like *Mycobacterium tuberculosis*, cell division requires 12–20 hours. They may take several weeks to produce a visible growth on culture media. The clinician may have to wait 8–12 weeks for reports of laboratory investigations (Volk, 1996).

7. Classification of Microorganisms

Bacteria are grouped into several categories according to their shape. Cocci are spherical, bacilli are rod-shaped, and spirochaetes appear as corkscrew-like spirals. Organisms such as actinomycetes and *Nocardia* are filamentous and branching. Mycobacteria cannot be stained well by Gram's method, but can be stained by acid-fast stains as in the **Ziehl–Neelson method**. However, it is not possible to distinguish between *Mycobacterium tuberculosis* and other mycobacterial species merely by examining a stained preparation. The cell-wall-deficient forms described earlier cannot be Gram-stained either. Morphological characteristics are extremely helpful during the preliminary stages of laboratory investigations. A presumptive identification of a pathogen may be made based on the Gram stain and the clinical picture. Such information will help the clinician to embark on empirical antimicrobial therapy on a rational basis. The results of the stain also guide the laboratory in performing further investigations. A brief statement on relevant clinical findings provided on the request forms accompanying specimens will also facilitate this service.

Rickettsiae, *Coxiella burneti* and chlamydiae are bacteria that have some characteristics of viruses. They are obligate intracellular parasites capable of causing a variety of infections in humans and animals. They cannot be cultured on agar, but can be grown in living cells.

In the past, no standard classification of bacteria was universally accepted and applied, although Bergy's Manual of Systemic Bacteriology was (Bergy's Manual, 1989) widely used as an authoritative source. The traditional method of identifying organisms is based on characteristic features such as cell shape, Gram reactions, nutritional requirements, chemical tests and pathogenicity. This system suffers from the weakness that decisions taken about the relative importance of different characters are often arbitrary.

A novel method of classifying bacteria is based on the genetic constitution of organisms, as well as phenotypic, biochemical and antigenic properties (Woese, 1990). By measuring the guanine and cytosine $(G+C)$ contents of bacteria, it can be shown that although there is a very wide range in the $G+C$ component of DNA, it is relatively fixed for any one species. This provides the basis for a much more accurate and consistent classification of microorganisms. The International Committee for Systematic Bacteriology reviews regularly the vocabulary of microbiology. The proposed changes and names of newly described bacterial genera and species are published in the *International Journal of Systematic Bacteriology* (ICSB, 1995).

Viruses, in contrast to bacteria, fungi and parasites, are not "living cells". They do not possess nuclei or organelles and cannot reproduce independently. They replicate within host cells. They are too small to be seen with a light microscope but some virus particles can be detected and characterised by their size and morphology by means of an electron microscope. The infectious particle is known as the virion, which consists of nucleic acid and a protein coat called the capsid. Because viruses replicate only in living cells, and because many viruses are inactivated at room temperature, it is important to transport specimens in a suitable medium on ice and to put them into cell cultures as soon as possible.

Fungi (yeasts and moulds) are eukaryotes and differ from bacteria in several practical aspects. The fungal cell wall consists primarily of chitin, and is thus resistant to antibacterial drugs. The cell membrane contains ergosterol in contrast to cholesterol in human cells. The most effective antifungal drugs exploit this difference to achieve selective action.

Parasites live on or in higher forms of life, and they include protozoa and helminths (worms). They have complex life cycles. There is a whole host of fungi and parasites that have recently become important, especially because of the increasing number of immunologically-compromised patients.

Prions are infectious protein particles with no nucleic acid, and have been implicated as the cause of certain "slow" diseases, such as Creutzfeldt–Jacob disease in humans and scrapie in sheep, and more recently, bovine spongiform encephalopathy (BSE) — "mad cow disease". Prions are much more resistant to inactivation by ultraviolet light, heat and formaldehyde. However, they are inactivated by higher concentrations of hypochlorite, sodium hydroxide and by autoclaving for a prolonged period of time at high temperature (Steelman, 1994). They are not well understood and there is no treatment available.

8. Physiology of Bacteria

Bacteria differ widely in their physiological properties and metabolic needs. Based on the oxygen requirements of bacteria, four groups have been described:

(i) **Obligate (or strict) aerobes**, such as mycobacteria, pseudomonad, etc., require oxygen for growth.

(ii) **Facultative anaerobes**, including enteric bacteria and staphylococci, are capable of growth in the presence or absence of oxygen.

(iii) **Microaerophilic organisms**, like certain streptococci and campylobacters, grow best at low oxygen tensions.

(iv) **Obligate anaerobes** grow only in the absence of oxygen but vary considerably in their sensitivity to it. Many obligate anaerobes are extremely sensitive to the presence of oxygen and are rapidly killed by exposure to air. As a result, special precautions must be taken for their isolation and study.

Transport media should be used to provide appropriate conditions for the survival of organisms. According to clinical information available, the laboratory will be able to provide an ideal environment suitable for a suspected pathogen.

Carbon dioxide is often necessary in small amount, such as is present in the atmosphere. A higher concentration, 5–10%, is necessary for some organisms, e.g. *Neisseria gonorrhoeae*, *Brucella* spp. and some streptococci.

The optimal temperature for growth is species dependent. Growth may be inhibited above or below this optimum. The largest group of bacteria are the **mesophiles**, in which optimal growth occurs between 20°C and 40°C. Nearly all of the human pathogens are best suited to temperatures around 37°C. **Psychrophiles** are cold loving organisms that can grow effectively in a refrigerator, e.g. *Listeria monocytogenes* grows in soft cheeses and certain species of pseudomonads in banked blood stored at 4°C. **Thermophiles** can be found growing in hot springs, oceanic thermal vents and in rotting vegetable matter. The thermostable enzymes of these bacteria have become useful for repeated thermal cycling of polymerase chain reactions carried out at high temperatures (Saiki *et al.*, 1998).

The pH is one of the major factors that limit the growth of bacterial cultures. Most medically important bacteria grow best at a neutral or slightly alkaline pH. *Vibrio cholerae* grows well above pH 8. However most medically important fungi grow well at a lower pH than that of bacteriological agars.

The physiological requirements of microorganisms should be taken into consideration and can be exploited when attempting to isolate them. This can be done only with the cooperation of the clinicians who can provide relevant information to the laboratory.

9. Metabolic Products

There are several by-products of bacteria that are of medical importance. Many bacteria, mostly Gram-positive organisms release potent exotoxins into their environment, e.g. *Clostridium tetani* and *Corynebacterium diphtheriae*. Exotoxins are proteins. **Endotoxin** is a lipopolysaccharide. It is derived from the outer membrane of Gram-negative bacteria and is liberated on cell death. The presence of endotoxin in the bloodstream can result in fever, inflammation and frequently, shock. Sepsis is one of causes of SIRS, also referred to as septic shock. In severe cases, this shock becomes irreversible and death follows. There are many extracellular enzymes of medical importance, such as **hyaluronidases** (help in the spread of the organisms), **coagulase** (helps to form a fibrin barrier typical of an abscess to wall off the hosts' defence mechanisms), **collagenase** (helps the spread by breaking down collagen, which is the ground substance of bone, skin and cartilage), and **streptokinase** (helps the spread of the organism by dissolution of blood clots).

Some bacteria are capable of producing **pigments** that can be seen macroscopically. As a result, phenomena, such as the red colouration of food items, the simulation of blood in sputa and babies' napkins have been described (Collier, 1998).

There are numerous other harmful bacterial products such as haemolysins, leucocidins, neurotoxins, pyrogens, etc. On the other hand, some products such as vitamins, are beneficial to humans.

10. Normal Microbial Population on the Human Body

All of us carry millions of microorganisms on the skin and lining surfaces (mucous membranes) of internal organs — mouth, respiratory, gastrointestinal and urogenital tracts. Under normal circumstances, these organisms are commensals, living in partnership with the host. The other areas of the human body are normally sterile. If the opportunity arises, these colonisers may invade these sterile sites and cause disease. Some sterile sites, such as the lungs, gall bladder, urinary bladder and uterus, are in communication with colonised sites. The entry of organisms is prevented by various physiological mechanisms. Under favourable circumstances, any organism can cause harm and behave as a pathogen. These categories of symbionts, commensals and opportunists are useful only in describing the usual role of the organism in relation to the host (Volk, 1996). Any organism coming from the environment will have to compete with the flora already colonising the human body. The protective effect of the normal flora is called colonisation resistance. Many pathogens, in contrast to commensals, have the capacity to invade normal defence barriers and to cause disease.

10.1. The skin

The superficial skin surface is colonised by some bacteria and yeasts, but the majority are found in deeper structures, such as hair follicles, the most common being *Staphylococcus epidermidis*. *Staphylococcus aureus* is present to a much lesser extent. Propionibacteria and other anaerobic organisms are commonly found in deeper structures of the skin.

10.2. The eye

The bacterial counts on the conjunctival surface are kept to a minimum by the mechanical washing action of the eyelids and the tears. The tears contain a bactericidal enzyme called lysozyme. The organisms commonly found are *Staphylococcus epidermidis* and *Corynebacterium* species.

10.3. The respiratory tract

Many bacterial species normally colonise the upper respiratory tract of healthy people. "Viridans streptococci", *Neisseria* spp., *Corynebacterium* spp. and anaerobes are carried by the majority of people. There are asymptomatic carriers of recognised pathogens, such as *Streptococcus pyogenes* (2–5%), *Streptococcus pneumoniae*, *Haemophilus influenzae* and *Corynebacterium diphtheriae* (less than 0.1%). Transient colonisation may occur with organisms such as *Klebsiella* spp., *Escherichia coli, Pseudomonas* spp. *and Candida albicans* following antibiotic therapy (Shanson, 1999). However, sites below the larynx normally remain sterile.

10.4. The digestive tract

The mouth has a large variety of organisms, including certain species of spirochaetes. Because of the difficulties in isolation, many organisms have not been identified. The acid content of the gastric juice prevents any organism from colonising the gastric mucosa. One bacterium (*Helicobacter pylori*) can do this, but this is regarded as a harmful infection, not colonisation. Large numbers of bacteria begin to appear at the lower end of the ileum with a wide variety of organisms in the large intestine, the majority being anaerobes. The potentially pathogenic anaerobic organisms such as *Bacteroides fragilis* and *Clostridium perfrigens* can normally be found in the intestine. The other organisms usually found include aerobes such as *Escherichia coli, Klebsiella* spp. and *Enterococcus faecalis*.

10.5. The genito-urinary tract

The distal urethra is colonised by skin organisms and sometimes by mycoplasmas and ureaplasma. *Mycobacterium smegmatis* is normally found in the smegma — the material that collects under the foreskin of the penis.

10.6. The blood

The bloodstream is sterile except for the transient presence of microorganisms without any signs and symptoms of an infection (bacteraemia) that occurs during day-to-day activities, such as brushing one's teeth. These organisms are promptly removed by the immune system (Volk, 1996).

11. Transmission of Pathogens

Some pathogens originate from the human normal flora and others are derived from animals, e.g. *Brucella* species and *Yersinia pestis*. The routes by which microorganisms are disseminated are as follows:

11.1. Contact

This is either direct (inadequate hand-washing, sexual activity) or indirect (inanimate objects — "fomites" — like inadequately sterilised instruments, door handles, telephone hand sets, etc.; and insect vectors, such as flies and cockroaches).

11.2. Inoculation

Organisms that cannot directly invade the skin gain access as a result of penetrating wounds (e.g. tetanus), needle stick injuries (e.g. hepatitis B), biting insects and other arthropods — malaria, dengue and many others.

11.3. Ingestion

Microorganisms disseminated via this route are *Salmonella typhi,
Shigella* spp., *Hepatitis A* and *E*, and *Giardia intestinalis.*

11.4. Aerial spread

Microorganisms disseminated by inhalation are, for example, TB,
chickenpox, mumps and measles. The dispersal of staphylococci
via skin scales is of especial importance in operating theatres, as
each person can emit about 10,000 bacteria per minute at rest,
increasing to 50,000 per minute during activity as the friction of
clothing against the skin releases more skin scales or squames
(Howarth, 1985).

11.5. Vertical transmission

The acronym TORCH was devised to highlight organisms infecting
the foetus *in utero* — *Toxoplasma gondii*, rubella virus, cytomegalovirus and herpes simplex virus (Nehmias, 1971). This acronym is
now obsolete because of its inability to cover all agents now known
to cause vertical transmission. An alternative, PoRTHaTCH, minus
the vowels (parvovirus B19, rubella, *Toxoplasma gondii*, HIV, *Treponema
pallidum*, cytomegalovirus and herpes simplex virus) would encom-
pass most of them (Inglis, 1996).

11.6. Endogenous infections

Organisms previously colonising the body surfaces may invade
sterile areas and cause disease (e.g. intestinal organisms causing
post-operative wound infections in large bowel surgery).

12. Diagnostic Techniques

The following techniques are commonly used in clinical microbiology
laboratories.

12.1. Microscopy

The observation of bacteria by means of staining procedures is an important initial step in the identification and presumptive diagnosis of an infecting agent. Of all the staining methods, the most important by far is the stain developed by Christian Gram in 1883. In this procedure, a heat-fixed smear on a glass slide is stained with crystal violet followed by iodine. It is briefly decolourised with acetone and counter-stained with, e.g. safranin. Gram-positive bacteria are those that retain the initial dye to stain blue, whereas Gram-negatives lose the original colour and are counter-stained to appear red. This reflects the differences in the two types of cell walls. The Gram-positive cell wall retains stain because of its thick, multilayered peptidoglycan, which account for 40% of the mass of the Gram-positive cell. Unstained preparations and wet mounts are useful for demonstrating certain constituents, e.g. fungal hyphae, in body fluid (e.g. urine, CSF) and to enumerate cells. Special stains, e.g. the Ziehl–Neelson method are useful for demonstrating *Mycobacterium tuberculosis* and other mycobacteria. Long-chain fatty acids in the cell wall render the organism resistant to the decolourising agent, a mixture of acid and alcohol, hence, they are referred to as "acid-fast". Parasites in blood films are demonstrated by the Giemsa stain and electron microscopy is valuable for the rapid diagnosis of viral infections.

12.2. Culture

To confirm the findings of microscopic examination, it is necessary to isolate bacteria in cultures for full identification and to test for antimicrobial susceptibilities. Culture is also more sensitive than microscopy, which is sometimes negative when small numbers of a pathogen are present initially. The selection of appropriate culture media depends on the type of specimen processed and the type of organism expected as the nutritional requirements of microorganisms are variable. Some will grow on simple nutrient agar and others may require media enriched with more nutrients, such as blood agar and chocolate agar. Special culture media are used for the selection of certain organisms from a mixture, e.g. MacConkey's agar with bile salts for intestinal organisms, and potassium tellurite to detect *Corynebacterium diphtheriae*. Whether the organism requires aerobic or anaerobic conditions, and the optimum temperature for growth are important considerations. Liquid media, e.g. blood culture bottles are used to recover small numbers of organisms from specimens. Living cells are necessary to isolate viruses.

12.3. Antimicrobial susceptibility testing

Antibiotic resistance is a worldwide problem and the patterns of resistance vary from place to place. In certain clinical situations, effective antimicrobial therapy can be predicted empirically, but laboratory confirmation is essential to determine the exact situation. Because of *in vitro* and *in vivo* differences in antimicrobial activity with regard to certain organisms for certain antibiotics, the identification of bacteria is essential to guide the selection of appropriate drugs, e.g. *Salmonella typhi* show marked *in vivo* and *in vitro* differences against aminoglycosides; *Stenotrophomonas maltophilia* against aminoglycosides and quinolones (Garrison *et al.*, 1996). Generally, it takes about 48 hours from the time the specimen is received in the laboratory to produce these results. Most laboratories perform the disc diffusion test by seeding agar plates with the test organism and placing antibiotic-impregnated discs over the inoculated plate. A dilution method to determine the lowest concentration of an antimicrobial agent inhibiting a visible growth (the minimum inhibitory concentration) *in vivo* is more laborious, but useful in the treatment of more serious infections and more difficult organisms. Susceptibility testing of slow growing organisms such as *M. tuberculosis* usually takes several weeks to produce results. Antifungal and antiviral susceptibility testing techniques are available only in reference laboratories.

12.4. Immunological methods

Antigens are molecules that react with antibodies. Various components of microorganisms are antigenic and capable of inducing specific globulin proteins or immunoglobulins, called antibodies in humans. Immunological methods employed during investigations can be set up to detect either the antigen or antibody. The antibody detection tests are most widely used. The common methods used in clinical microbiology work include agglutination: a visible reaction in the presence of homologous antigen and antibody; haemagglutination: antigens attached to red blood cells act as bridges linking and producing visible reaction; enzyme immunoassay: antigen–antibody reaction is detected with a labelled enzyme to initiate a colour reaction; immunofluorescence: the presence of bound antibody is detected using a second anti-human immunoglobulin labelled with fluorescein and visualised by ultraviolet light microscopy.

12.5. Molecular techniques

There are several techniques to detect genes or components of organisms, of which the polymerase chain reaction (PCR) and gene probes are the most popular. These tests are based on the principle that any microorganism will have unique DNA sequences that are not found in any other agent. In PCR, this target sequence can be amplified more than a million fold within a few hours, and then detected by various methods. In the case of gene probes, a target sequence can be identified by means of a hybridisation reaction with a specific labelled DNA probe. The molecular techniques have been successfully used in the detection of antibiotic resistance genes, microbial typing and in the identification of a variety of bacteria, viruses, and parasites, including those not cultivable using present techniques (Pitt, 1997).

13. Sterilisation and Disinfection

Sterilisation refers to the destruction of all infectious agents. Disinfection has a less precise meaning and generally refers to the removal of harmful microorganisms to a level below that required to cause infection, the difference being that bacterial spores are usually not destroyed. Physical cleaning is the cheapest and most important method of disinfection, which involves the removal of dirt, dust, blood clots, body fluids, microbial contaminants or the "**bioburden**", etc. found on an item. After thorough washing, the low bioburden presents a relatively low challenge to sterilisation and disinfection systems (Chu *et al.*, 1999). Washing is an essential initial step to ensure proper sterilisation or disinfection. Failure to physically clean equipment is the commonest reason for the failure to disinfect or sterilise it. Sterilisation is essential for equipment that come into contact with a break in the skin or mucous membranes, e.g. needles, scalpel blades, artery forceps, etc. Disinfection is adequate for items used on the intact skin and mucous membrane, e.g. face masks. A high-level disinfection is necessary for items such as bronchoscopes because of the risk of tuberculosis, and proctoscopes and sigmoidoscopes because of cryptosporidiosis. It is recommended these items be immersed in 2% gluteraldehyde for at least 20 minutes and rinsed with sterile water before using on another patient (APIC, 1996). Heat is cheap, reliable and easy to control. It is the best form of sterilisation or disinfection. Whereever possible, heat should be used instead of chemicals. Certain materials like plastics, fibre-optic endoscopes and optical instruments cannot stand high temperatures, so chemical methods become desirable.

Sterilising methods used in hospitals include autoclaving, hot air at 160°C, and ethylene oxide. Ionising radiation is used by industry to sterilise heat-sensitive disposable items like plastic syringes and rubber gloves. Bone allograft banks commonly sterilise frozen bone by irradiation. Recently, it has been found that gamma irradiation is not a significant virus inactivation method for bone allografts

(Campbell, 1999). Because organs, cells and most tissue grafts cannot be subjected to sterilisation steps, the risk of infectious disease transmission remains and thorough donor screening and testing are especially important (Eastlund, 1995). Methods of disinfection include boiling at 100°C for 5 mins, pasteurisation at 65°C for 30 minutes, low-temperature steam and washing with a wide variety of chemicals. There is no perfect disinfectant. They vary in their ability to destroy different types of organisms. A mixture of low-temperature steam and formaldehyde is useful for situations where a high degree of disinfection is essential. There are many factors that may render a disinfectant ineffective: freshly prepared solutions of correct strengths are extremely important for optimal activity. For example, different strengths of hypochlorite solutions have been recommended for different purposes: for blood spillage 10,000 ppm, laboratory jars 2,500 ppm, general environment 1,000 ppm and 125 ppm available chlorine for infant feeding utensils (Shanson, 1999). Organic matter like faeces or blood inactivates disinfectants ("quenching") — some are more vulnerable than others.

The types of chemical disinfectants used in hospitals include alcohols, aldehydes, diguanides, halogens, phenolics, quaternary ammonium compounds. Paracetic acid has been recently recommended as an alternative to glutaraldehyde for the decontamination of endoscopes. The choice of a disinfectant must be made by assessing the properties of the disinfectant and the situation in which it is used. Examples of various commercial products of disinfectants are given in Table 1 and the properties of these agents are compared in Table 2, to help in the selection of an appropriate compound on a rational basis.

The Central Sterile Supply Department (CSSD) and Theatre Sterile Supply Units (TSSU) in busy hospitals are designed to provide an efficient faster service under supervision of trained personnel.

Table 1. Commercial products of disinfectants.

Types of Disinfectant	Commercial Products		
Aldehydes	Cidex		
	Formalin		
	Aldecyde		
Halogens	Choros	Multichlor	Presept
	Domestos	Vim	
	Sterite	Ajax	
	Milton	Countdown	
	Septonite	Betadine	
	Diversol BX	Disadine	
Phenolics	Stericol	Lzal	
	Hycolin	Amphyl	
	Clearsol	Lysol	
	Dettol		
	Ibcol		
	Jeyes fluid		
Diguanides	Chlorhexidine		
	Hibiscrub		
	Savlon		
	Hibisol		
	Hibidi		
Alcohol	Ethanol		
	Isopropyl		
Quarternary	Roccal		
Ammonium	Zephiran		
Compounds	Marinol		
	Cetavlon		

Table 2. Properties of disinfectants.

Type of Disinfectants	Vegetative Bacterial	Bacterial Spores	TB	Viruses	Fungi	Comments
Aldehydes	√	√	√	√	√	A good alternative for equipment that cannot be heat sterilised.
Halogens	√	√	d	√	√	First choice where viruses are present. Corrodes metal & damage plastic and fabrics. Cannot use on dirty surfaces.
Phenolics	√	d	√	d	√	Cheap & useful for environmental disinfection. Can use on dirty surfaces
Alcohol	√	d	d	d	√	Disinfection of surfaces and for skin prior to injections.
Diguanides	good activities against gram-positives	–	–	d	√	4% chlorhexidine has good activity against Gram-negative bacilli and viruses as well. Useful skin and mucour membrane disinfectant. Compatible with alcohol.
Quarternary Ammonium compounds	some activity against gram-positives	–	–	d	√	Good detergents. Cannot use as disinfectants.

√   good activity
d   poor activity
–   no activity

14. References

ALBERTS, B., BRAY, D., LEWIS, J., RAFF, M., ROBERT, K. and WATSON, J.D. (1994). *Molecular Biology of the Cell*. Garland Publishing Inc. New York & London.

APIC (Association for Professional in Infection Control and Epidemiology, Inc.) (1996). Guidelines for infection, prevention and control in flexible endoscopy. *Am. J. Infect. Control* **22**, 19–38.

ASM (1999). Microbiology's fifty most significant events during the past 125 years. A poster supplement to *ASM News* **65**, 5.

BERGEY'S MANUAL OF SYSTEMATIC BACTERIOLOGY VOLS. 1 and 2 (1989). Krieg, N.R. and Holt, J.G., eds., Williams and Wilkins, Baltimore, London.

BUTLER, H.M. and BLAKEY, J.L. (1975). A review of bacteria in L-phase and their possible clinical significance, *Med. J. Aust.* **20**, 463–467.

CAMPBELL, D.G. and LI, P. (1999). Sterilization of HIV with irradiation: Relevance to infected bone allografts. *Aust. NZ J. Surg.* **69**, 517–521.

CDC: NATIONAL CENTRE FOR INFECTIOUS DISEASES. *Emerging Infectious Diseases*. Atlanta, GA 30333, USA, Webpage: http://www.cdc.gov/ncidod/eid/index.htm

CHU, N.S., CHAN-MYERS, H., GHAZANFARI, N. and AUTONOPOLO, S.P. (1999). Levels of naturally occurring micro-organisms on surgical instruments after clinical use and after washing. *Am. J. Infect. Control* **27**, 315–319.

COLLIER, L., BALOWS and SUSSMANAN, M. (1998). Systematic bacteriology. In: *Topley and Wilson's Microbiology and Microbial Infections*, Arnold, Great Britain. Vol. 2. pp. 69, 1016.

DUERDEN, B.I., REID, T.M.S, JEWSBURY, J.M. and TURK, D.C. (1987). *A New Short Textbook of Microbial and Parasitic Infection*. Hodder and Stoughton. London, Sydney, Auckland, Toronto, pp. 31–36.

EASTLUND, T. (1995). Infectious disease transmission through cell, tissue, and organ transplantation: Reducing the risk through donor selection, *Cell Transplant* **4**, 455–477.

GARRISON, M.W., ANDERSON, D.E., CAMBELL, D.M., CARROLL, K.C., MALONE, C.L. and ANDERSON, J.D. (1996). *Stenotrophomonas maltophilia*: Emergence of multidrug resistant strains during therapy and in an *in vitro* pharmodynamic chamber mode. *Antimicrob. Agents Chemother.* **40**, 2859–2804.

O'GRADY, F., LAMBERT, H.P., FINCH, R.G. and GREENWOOD, D. (1997). Modes of action. In: *Antibiotic and Chemotherapy*, Churchill Livingstone, London, pp. 10–22.

HOWARTH, F.H. (1985). Prevention of airborne infection during surgery. *Lancet* **16**, 386–388.

HULL, R.A., GILL, R.E., HSU, P., MANSHEW, B.H. and FALKOW, S. (1981). Construction and expression of recombinant plasmids encoding type 1 or D-mannose-resistant pili from a urinary tract infection. *Escherichia coli* KI isolate. *Infect. Immun.* **33**, 933–938.

INGLIS, T.J.J. (1996). Congenital and neonatal infections. In: *Microbiology and Infection*. Churchill Livingstone, New York, Edinburgh, London, Madrid, Melbourne, San Francisco and Tokyo, pp. 137–143.

ICSB (Subcommittee on the Taxonomy of Mollicutes) (1995). Revised minimal standards for description of new species of the class millicutes. *Int. J. Syst. Bacteriol.* **45**, 605–612.

LEVINSON, W. and JAWETZ, E. (1994). (a) Structure of bacterial cells (b) Growth. In: *Medical Microbiology and Immunology*, Appleton & Lange, USA. pp. 3–13; pp. 13–14.

MERCER, A.A., MORELLI, G., HEUZENROEDER, M., KAMKE, M., and ACHTMAN, M. (1984). Conservation of plasmids among *Escherichia coli* K1 isolates of diverse origins. *Infect. Immun.* **46**, 649–657.

NEHMIAS, A.J., JOSEY, W.E., NAIB, Z.M., FREEMAN, M.G., FERNANDEZ, R.J. and WHEELER, J.H. (1971). Perinatal risk associated with maternal genital *Herpes simplex* virus infection. *Am. J. Obstet. Gynecol.* **110**, 825–837.

NYSTROM, P.O. (1998). The systemic inflammatory response syndrome: Definitions and aetiology. *J. Antimicrob. Chemother.* **41** Suppl A, 1–7.

PITT, T.L. (1997). Classification and identification of microorganism. In: *Medical Microbiology*. D. Greenwood, R.L.B. Slack and J.F. Peutherer, eds., Churchill Livingstone, UK, pp. 25–35.

SAIKI, R.K., GELFAND, D.H. STOFFEL, S., SCHARF, S.J., HIGUCHI, R., HORN, G.T., MULLIS, K.B. and ERLICH, H.A. (1988). Primer-directed enzymatic amplification of DNA with a thermostable DNA polymerase. *Science* **239**, 487–491.

SHANSON, D.C. (1999). (a) ENT and eye infections. (b) Disinfectant and sterilization. In: *Microbiology in Clinical Practice*. Butterworth-Heinemann, Great Britain, pp. 210–212; pp. 459–470.

STEELMAN, V.M. (1994). Creutzfeld-Jacob disease: Recommendations for infection control. *Am. J. Infect. Control* **22**, 312.

VOLK, W.A., GEBHARDT, B.M., HAMMASKJOLD, M.-L. and KADNER, R.J. (1996). (a) Microbial cells and their function: A review of cell biology. (b) *Mycobacterium*, (c) & (d) Normal flora, infections, and bacterial invasiveness. In: *Essentials of Medical Microbiology*. Lippincott-Revan, Philadelphia, PA, pp. 3–13; pp. 429–439; pp. 315–328.

WOESE, C.R., KANDLER, D. and WHEELS, M.L. (1990). Towards a natural system of organisms: Proposal for the domains Archea, Bacteria, and Eucarya, *Proc. Natl. Acad. Sci.* USA, **87**, 4576–4579.

Advances in Tissue Banking Vol. 5
© 2001 by World Scientific Publishing Co. Pte. Ltd.

13 BIOBURDEN ESTIMATION IN RELATION TO STERILISATION

NORIMAH YUSOF

Tissue Bank, Malaysian Institute for
Nuclear Technology Research (MINT)
Bangi, 43000 Kajang, Selangor
Malaysia

1. Introduction

According to the International Standard ISO 11137 (ISO, 1995a), bioburden is defined as the population of viable microorganisms on a product. In the context of sterilisation, bioburden is the total count of viable microorganisms on a product determined immediately prior to the sterilisation process. It is therefore the initial or pre-sterilisation count, reflecting the degree of microbiological contamination of the product. Bioburden represents the sum of contamination contributed from a number of sources, including the microbiological status of raw materials (tissue itself, packaging materials, etc.), the environment in which the product is processed (the room, laminar flow cabinet, washing solutions, etc.), the personnel who handle it (during washing, cleaning, drying, packaging, storing, etc.) and the equipment or tools which are in direct contact with tissues (freeze-dryer, bandsaw, autoclave, scissors, forceps, glassware, etc.). The International Standards for sterilisation of healthcare products require that adventitious microbiological contamination of a healthcare product from all sources be minimised to the lowest degree possible. Even though the product has been processed or produced under standard manufacturing practices, prior to sterilisation, the processed product still has microorganisms on it, albeit in low numbers. Such a product is non-sterile and must be subjected to sterilisation. The purpose of sterilisation is therefore to inactive or kill the microbiological contaminants and thereby transform the non-sterile product into a sterile one.

The inactivation of a pure culture of microorganisms by any physical and/or chemical agents for sterilisation often follows an exponential relationship (Yusof, 1999). It means that there is always a finite probability that a microorganism may survive regardless of the extent of treatment applied. For a given treatment, the probability of survival/killing is determined by the number and resistance of microorganisms and by the environment in which the organisms exist during treatment. Inevitably, the sterility of any one-product item from a batch of products subjected to sterilisation treatment cannot be guaranteed. The sterility of the treated batch of product items has to be defined in terms of the probability of the existence of a non-sterile item in that batch. The ISO 9000 series of International Standards designated sterilisation as a special process because process efficiency cannot be verified by inspection and testing of the product (ISO, 1994). For this reason, any sterilisation process selected to sterilise a product has to be validated before use. The performance of each step of the process has to be monitored routinely and the equipment properly maintained. It is equally important to validate the microbiological challenge in terms of the number and types of microorganisms presented for treatment.

2. Bioburden

In practice, bioburden or the investigation of microbiological contamination level is determined using a defined technique.

According to the International Standard ISO 111737-1 (ISO, 1995b), bioburden estimate is the value established for the number of microorganisms comprising the bioburden by applying to a viable count or pre-sterilisation count a factor compensating for the recovery efficiency. The standard specifies the general criteria to be applied for the estimation of bioburden. The annexes of the standard provide additional guidance and methods which may be used for validating the technique. Bioburden estimations are performed to validate and revalidate a sterilisation process for which the extent of exposure to the sterilisation treatment is to be directly related to the bioburden estimate or for which a general knowledge of bioburden is required. Bioburden is also conducted as a routine control of the manufacturing process, as an overall environmental monitoring programme, as the assessment of the efficiency of a cleaning process in removing microorganisms and as the monitoring of raw materials, components or packaging. The bioburden estimation of a healthcare product generally consists of four distinct stages:

- Removal of microorganisms from the medical product;
- Transfer of these isolated microorganisms to culture conditions;
- Enumeration of the microorganisms with subsequent characterisation; and
- Application of the correction factors(s) determined during bioburden recovery studies in order to calculate the bioburden estimate for the pre-sterilisation count.

Bioburden estimation is expressed as total count per unit product (either as one product item, or in unit weight or unit volume).

3. Methodologies

It is not possible to define a single technique to be used in any microbiological count analysis because of the wide variety of materials and the varied design of healthcare products. Furthermore, the selection of a technique is influenced by the level and types of contaminants in and on top of the product. It is necessary to validate the technique before employing it for routine use. The ISO 11737-1 (ISO, 1995b) document provides guidance on selection of a technique and outline method(s), which may be used to validate the technique selected. However, ISO 11737-1 is not applicable for the enumeration or identification of viral contamination.

It is important that bioburden estimations are conducted under controlled conditions. The laboratory facilities used for the estimations, whether as a part of a tissue bank or located in another organisation, should be managed and operated in accordance with a documented quality system. If bioburden estimations are performed in a laboratory under the direct management of the tissue banking set-up the operation of the laboratory should be within the tissue bank's quality system. If an external laboratory is used, such a laboratory is recommended to be formally certified against appropriate ISO documents, such as the ISO/IEC Guide 25 (ISO, 1990).

Tools that are in direct contact with product, microbiological media and eluents, should be sterile. Working area must be kept clean and disinfected before and after use. Personnel must be well trained and be aware of all safety procedures.

Ideally, bioburden should be estimated for each production batch on a regular basis. However, this may not always be practicable in tissue banking. Tissues processed are often in small batches and the number of tissue items produced per batch is usually small. In such circumstances, tissue products may be grouped on the basis of tissue type and equivalence of processing environment, and raw materials used. The frequency of conducting bioburden estimation is very high during the initial production of a new tissue type, and later, the frequency can be reduced when the bioburden data is consistently low and all production parameters are maintained.

The sequence of the technique for bioburden estimations is summarised as follows:

Product sampling

↓

Treatment

↓

Transfer to culture medium

↓

Incubation
(Bacteria at 30–35°C, yeast and mould at 20–25°C)

↓

Enumeration

↓

Identification/ characterisation (if necessary)

↓

Interpretation of data

Product sampling is done at random in its standard packaging immediately before sterilisation. If the choice is limited, a product that is not suitable for clinical use or is rejected can be selected. However, the product must have undergone all essential stages of processing, including cleaning and packaging, preferably in the same processing batch, using the same batch of washing solutions and chemicals (if any) and carried out by the same tissue-bank operator. The selected product should reflect as closely as possible the product ready for sterilisation. The bioburden estimation should utilise the whole product. If this is not practicable due to size, a portion of the product is allowed, but it must be carefully selected so that the bioburden of this portion is a good representative portion for the whole product.

Treatment is required to remove microorganisms from a product. The degree of adhesion of microorganisms to tissue surfaces varies with the nature of tissues and the types of microorganisms. Treatments employed may consist of rinsing together with physical force (such as using shaker, vortex mixer, stomacher, ultrasonicator). Addition of surfactant such as Tween 80 (at concentration between 0.01 and 0.1%) in rinsing solution can enhance removal. Careful selection of the surfactant concentration is necessary in order to avoid foaming. Any treatments used should be reproducible and not affect the viability of microorganisms. Swabbing can be used for irregularly shaped product, relatively inaccessible areas and when a

Table 1. Examples of eluents and diluents (ISO, 1995b).

Solution	Concentration in Water	Applications
Ringer	¼ strength	General
Peptone water	0.1%–1.0%	General
Buffered peptone water	0.067M phosphate 0.43% sodium chloride 0.1% peptone	General
Phosphate-buffered saline	0.02M phosphate 0.9% sodium chloride	General
Sodium chloride	0.25%–0.9%	General
Calgon Ringer	¼ strength	Dissolution of calcium alginate swabs
Thiosulfate Ringer	¼ strength	Neutralisation of residual chlorine
Water		Dilution of aqueous samples; preparation of isotonic solutions of soluble materials prior to counting

Note: This list is not exhaustive.

large area has to be sampled. However, the method is prone to errors as the way the swab swabbing is done cannot be controlled, and not all microorganisms are likely to be collected, or if collected, they might be trapped in the swab matrix and therefore cannot be detected.

Rinsing solutions or eluents and diluents commonly used in bioburden estimation as listed in ISO 11737-1 (ISO, 1995b) are shown in Table 1.

The transfer to culture medium is carried out after dilution in which the microorganisms are well separated into single-cell suspension. There are several methods for growing the microorganisms. For the enumeration method using colony counts, each viable microorganism should be able to express itself as a visible colony. Plating on medium agar is the best choice where one of these three common methods is used:

3.1. Membrane filtration

Membrane filters having pore size 0.45 μm are generally used to remove microorganisms from the eluent, which is poured through them. The membrane filter is washed by passing sterile water through and then placed either on an agar surface or on an absorbent pad soaked in nutrient medium. After incubation, colonies grown on the surface of the membrane filter can be counted and isolated for identification/characterisation. The membrane filtration method is particularly useful for products of low bioburden.

3.2. Pour plating

A certain volume or aliquot of suspension (eluent) is mixed with molten agar that has been cooled to 45°C. The contents are mixed by gently swirling the plate to disperse the microorganisms throughout the medium and allowing it to solidify. Colonies grow within the medium as well as on its surface. Pour plating is chosen for products of high bioburden after serial dilution, and only a small volume of eluent is used.

3.3. Spread plates

A certain volume or aliquot of suspension (eluent) is spread on the surface of a solid medium using a spreader. The aliquot, usually in small quantity, has to be absorbed into medium so that discrete colonies can grow.

Some examples of commonly used media and incubation conditions as listed by ISO 11737-1 (ISO, 1995b) are shown in Table 2.

Incubation period as recommended in ISO 11737-1 (ISO, 1995b) varies from two to seven days (refer to Table 2). The agar plates are incubated invertedly at 30–35°C for bacteria and at 20–25°C for yeast and mould.

Enumeration of microbial colonies grown on plates is the sum of the total bacterial colonies (both aerobic and anaerobic) and total colonies of yeast and mould. The bioburden estimation of a product is the total count per unit product. If unit weight or unit volume is used in the analysis, a correction factor should be applied for the final estimation. A factor compensating for the recovery efficiency of the colonies as described in ISO 11737-1 (ISO, 1995b) should also be included. Bioburden estimations are always likely to be underestimated because no single culture medium or incubation conditions will enable the growth all types of micro-organism (Gardner and Peel, 1986).

Identification characterisation: it is not necessary to isolate and identify each type of natural contaminant. It is sufficient just to identify the most commonly found contaminants and the most resistant ones for the selected sterilisation treatment.

4. Facility

All items of equipment should be calibrated and subjected to regular maintenance. Table 3 lists some of the basic equipment, tools and other items required for conducting bioburden estimation. Any microbiological laboratory must be able to accommodate these equipment without causing any cross-contamination. Entrance to the laboratory should be restricted especially during working.

Table 2. Examples of media and incubation conditions (ISO, 1995b).

Types of Microorganisms	Solid Media	Liquid Media	Incubation Conditions[a]
Non-selective aerobic bacteria	(Soybean casein digest agar) Tryptone soya agar Nutrient agar Blood agar Glucose tryptone agar	(Soybean casein digest broth) Tryptone soya broth Nutrient broth	30°C to 35°C for 2 days to 5 days
Yeast and moulds	Sabouraud dextrose agar Malt extract agar Rose Bengal Chloramphenicol agar (Soybean casein digest agar) Tryptone soya agar	Sabouraud dextrose broth Malt extract broth (Soybean casein digest broth) Tryptone soya broth	20°C to 25°C for 2 days to 5 days
Anaerobic bacteria	Reinforced clostridial agar[b] Schaedler agar[b] Prereduced blood agar[b] Fastidious anaerobe agar[b] Wilken-Chalgren agar[b]	Robertson's cooked meat broth Fluid thiglycollate broth	30°C to 35°C for 2 days to 5 days

Note: This list is not exhaustive.

[a] The incubation conditions listed are those which are commonly used for the types of microorganisms listed.

[b] Cultured under anaerobic conditions.

Table 3. Laboratory equipment and tools for bioburden estimation work.

Equipment	Tool	Others
Laminar airflow cabinet	Membrane filtration system and pumps	Surgical gloves
Incubators	Anaerobic jars	Head covers
Autoclave	Forceps	Shoe covers
Water purification system	Scissors	Laboratory coats
Water bath	Spreaders	Face masks
Microscopes	Inoculating loops	Disinfectants
Dry steriliser (Oven)	Thermometers	Hand soaps and creams
Refrigerators	Petridishes	Staining kit
Vortex mixer	Glass slides and covers	Media
Magnetic stirrer hotplates	Glassware (bottles, beakers, flasks, test tubes, pipettes etc)	Chemicals
Ultrasonic cleaner	Automatic pipettes and tips	Identification kit
Sealing machine	Bunsen burner and gas tank	
Electronic balances		
pH meter		

Note: This list is not exhaustive.

5. Discussion

Bioburden estimation as the initial contamination level of a product prior to sterilisation can be one of the quality control parameters for a tissue production. The level is also essential in determining the extent of sterilisation treatment in meeting the requirement for sterility assurance. In the case of radiation sterilisation, bacterial spores and viruses are generally most resistant to radiation. From bioburden estimation, the most resistant type of natural bacterial contaminants can be further isolated into pure culture. The radioresistancy or D_{10} value of the identified bacteria can be obtained from literature. If not available, a dose response curve of the bacteria can be conducted by exposing a bacterial spore population at a concentration of 10^7 or 10^8 counts per ml to incremental doses of radiation ranging from 0 to 12 kGy. The survival fraction is plotted on a semi-logarithmic scale against the radiation doses. From the dose response curve, the linear gradient or dose required to reduce one log cycle, D_{10} value, can be determined (Yusof, 1999). The radiation dose for sterilisation can be determined based on bioburden (assuming that all the contaminants have the maximum resistance level although the identified bacterial spores may constitute only a small percentage of the whole contaminant population) and D_{10} value, in order to achieve high sterility assurance level of 10^{-6} (the probability of getting one product non-sterile among one million products). Bioburden estimation therefore warrants the validation and revalidation of the sterilisation treatment.

6. References

GARDNER, J.F. and PEEL, M.M. (1986). *Introduction to Sterilization and Disinfection*. Churchill Livingstone, Edinburgh, pp. 183.

INTERNATIONAL STANDARD (ISO) (1990). *General Requirements for the Competence of Calibration and Testing Laboratories*. ISO/IEC Guide 25:1990, Geneva.

INTERNATIONAL STANDARD (ISO) (1994). *Quality Systems — Model for Quality Assurance in Production, Installation and Servicing*. ISO 9002:1994, Geneva.

INTERNATIONAL STANDARD (ISO) (1995a). *Sterilization of Health Care Products — Requirement for Validation and Routine Control — Radiation Sterilization*. ISO 11137:1995(E), Geneva.

INTERNATIONAL STANDARD (ISO) (1995b). *Sterilization of Medical Devices — Microbiological Methods — Part 1: Estimation of Population of Microorganisms on Products*. ISO 11737-1:1995(E). Geneva.

VOLK, W.A. and WHEELER, M.F. (1988). *Basic Microbiology*. Harper & Row, New York, pp. 687.

YUSOF, N. (1999). Quality system for the radiation sterilisation of tissues allografts. In: *Advances in Tissue Banking*, Vol. 3, G.O. Phillips, R. von Versen, D.M. Strong and A. Nather, eds. World Scientific, Singapore, pp. 257–281.

14 TRANSMISSIBLE DISEASES OF PARTICULAR IMPORTANCE IN THE IMMUNOCOMPROMISED AND TRANSPLANT RECIPIENTS

GAMINI KUMARASINGHE

Division of Microbiology
Department of Laboratory Medicine
National University Hospital
5 Lower Kent Ridge Road
Singapore 119074

Abstract

Transmissible diseases are caused by microorganisms such as bacteria, viruses, fungi and parasites. They are caused by living microorganisms. Hence, with adequate measures, diseases may be prevented or even eradicated, e.g. smallpox. Infection is a common problem shared by all medical specialities. Although the incidence of many communicable diseases in developed countries has fallen to very low levels, in developing countries, infections continue to cause considerable morbidity and mortality. On the other hand, infections associated with recent advances in medicine cause new problems particularly in developed countries. The salient features of a few selected organisms that cause infections in immunocompromised and transplant recipients are discussed in this chapter.

1. Hepatitis Viruses

There are several viral causes of inflammation of the liver: hepatitis A, B, C, D, E, G and TT virus, Epstein-Barr virus, cytomegalovirus and yellow fever (a flavivirus).

Hepatitis A and E are enterically transmitted agents, as opposed to B, C, D and TT, which are spread by the parenteral route. The clinical presentations of both viruses are virtually the same, usually mild with fever, nausea and vomiting during the acute period of the illness. Many infections are asymptomatic and resolve spontaneously. Demonstration of IgM and a rising IgG titre is helpful in the diagnosis of HAV, but no routine diagnostic tests are available for HEV. The mainstay of prevention is controlling faeco-oral spread by providing clean drinking water. Active immunisation is available for HAV but not for HEV.

Hepatitis B and C viruses (HBV and HCV) behave similarly, with regard to epidemiology and clinical presentation. Blood and body fluids are infectious. Both viruses are common in intravenous drug abusers. The sexual route is far more efficient for HBV than HCV. HBV is common among sex workers and homosexual men. HBV is transmitted to newborn babies of infectious mothers. Nosocomial infections among healthcare workers due to sharps injuries is a serious problem. HBV infection is one of the major hazards to healthcare workers (Shapiro, 1995). Infections may be followed by spontaneous complete recovery, an asymptomatic carrier state, chronic liver disease or very rarely hepatoma. Relapses of HBV infections are common among patients undergoing liver transplants. HCV is the most common cause of cirrhosis requiring liver transplantation (Detre, 1996) The laboratory diagnosis is by serological testing. Interferon has been used in the treatment of chronic liver disease. There is a genetically-engineered vaccine for active immunisation against Hepatitis B. Hyperimmune anti-hepatitis B immunoglobulin is available for passive immunisation of non-immune persons, e.g. hospital staff who sustain inoculation injuries. There is no vaccine against Hepatitis C yet.

Hepatitis D (Delta agent) is a defective virus. It can only replicate in cells also infected with hepatitis B virus by using its surface antigen as its coat. The transmission is by the same means as HBV and when there is a coinfection with the two viruses, the disease is more severe than with HBV alone. The diagnosis is by serology and alpha-interferon is used to mitigate effects of chronic hepatitis. There is no vaccine against HDV, but those who are immune to HBV will not be infected with HDV.

Hepatitis G is a blood-borne virus. The exact aetiological role in hepatitis has not been clearly demonstrated yet.

TT virus is a novel hepatitis virus discovered in Japan (Nishizawa *et al.*, 1997). The details of its epidemiology and role in liver disease remain to be explored.

2. Herpes Virus Family

The family contains eight viruses which cause a wide range of human infections. All are structurally similar, notorious for causing latent infections with occasional reactivations when exposed to an inciting agent or during immunosuppression. The list of viruses so far described have been classified, on the basis of their biological properties and host ranges, into three broad groups:

(a) α-herpesviruses, e.g. herpes simplex virus (HSV) and varicella-zoster virus (VZV), rapid growth, latency in sensory ganglia.
(b) β-herpesviruses, e.g. cytomegalovirus (CMV), human herpes virus 6 (HHV6) and human herpes virus 7 (HHV7), slow growth, restricted host range.
(c) γ-herpesviruses, e.g. Epstein-Barr virus (EBV), human herpes virus 8 (HHV8), growth in lymphoblastoid cells.

Serology of herpes viruses as a diagnostic tool is usually not helpful except in primary infections. Immunofluorescence to detect the antigen from clinical material and culture to isolate the virus are helpful in clinical practice.

Herpes simplex viruses 1 and 2 are probably the commonest human virus infections. Although type 1 infections are commoner in oral and central nervous system lesions, and type 2 mainly affects the genital tract, the pattern is not clear-cut. Type 1 infections are usually acquired early in childhood by the sharing of toys, cutlery, etc., at home or in nurseries and often present as herpes labialis, "cold sores". Type 2 infections are commoner after adolescence, usually present as herpes genitalis and is one of the commonest sexually transmitted diseases. There was thought to be an association between HSV2 and carcinoma of the cervix but this was discredited and papillomaviruses are now implicated. Recurrent severe herpes infections are a serious problem especially in the immunosuppressed group of patients.

2.1. Varicella-zoster virus (VZV)

This virus causes a highly contagious disease which is transmitted by respiratory droplets. Primary infections with VZV are referred to as chicken pox and the recurrences as shingles or herpes zoster. The diagnosis is almost always made on the basis of the clinical picture. Shingles is a disease of adults, its frequency increasing with advancing age as a consequence of waning immunity. The lesions are usually restricted to the area of the skin and mucous membranes supplied by the sensory nerves of a single dorsal root ganglion. Serious disseminated infections may occur in immunocompromised patients, where antiviral therapy with acyclovir is used. A live attenuated vaccine that is effective in preventing varicella is available, but zoster can still occur because the vaccine does not eliminate the virus in those who had latent infections (Na, 1997). Varicella-zoster immunoglobulin (VZIG) is used for post-exposure prophylaxis when serious complications are expected, such as during the early or late stages of pregnancy. The newborn baby is vulnerable if the mother has not developed antibodies which are passed to the neonate.

VZIG should also be given to immunocompromised patients with no vaicella-zoster antibodies (HMSO, 1996).

2.2. Cytomegalovirus (CMV)

The name derives from the characteristic appearance found in infected cells; marked cellular enlargement and formation of typical intranuclear "owl's eye" inclusions. Primary infection, which usually occurs in childhood, may be asymptomatic and persists for life. The virus is excreted in body fluids, such as urine, saliva, semen, breast milk and cervical fluid. The organism is transmitted by contact with body fluids, sexual activity, transfusion of blood products and transplanted tissues. Respiratory precautions are unnecessary. Nosocomial transmission is preventable by proper disposal of contaminated items and by hand washing after every contact (Faix, 1989).

Infections in normal individuals are usually mild and self-limiting with fever and a mild hepatitis. Infectious mononucleosis syndrome (resembling EBV infections) may occur with atypical lymphocytes, seen in peripheral blood but with a negative Paul-Bunnell reaction. Serious infections are commoner in patients whose cell-mediated immunity is depressed, e.g. transplant recipients and leukaemia patients receiving immunosuppressive drugs. CMV is the commonest infectious disease affecting transplant patients. During pregnancy, CMV may be transmitted transplacentally, more often during delivery or post-natally from breast milk butif causes most damage with earlier infection. Overall, the CMV infection rate *in utero* is 0.3–2% (Ahlfors *et al.*, 1984). Most cases of congenital disease result from primary infections, the commonest manifestations being hepatosplenomegaly and a petechial rash due to thrombocytopaenia (Stagno, 1990).

The demonstration of the mere presence of the virus in surface secretions is not diagnostic of an infection. The conventional cultures require 2–3 weeks for isolation of the virus. CMV early antigen test detects antigen generated by cell culture after incubation for

24 hours (DEAFF test). Serology is generally not helpful in clinical decision-making. Histological evidence in a biopsy of a diseased tissue is helpful in making a definitive diagnosis. PCR is regarded as the diagnostic test of choice to demonstrate viraemia during antiviral therapy with a very high sensitivity and specificity (Rubin, 1994).

2.3. Epstein-Barr virus (EBV)

EBV is one among many viruses that cause a sore throat and where glandular fever is a common manifestation. Transmission of the virus is by saliva and the infection is widespread, with most people infected from early in life, everywhere in the world.

Infectious mononucleosis (glandular fever) may present with exudative pharyngitis suggestive of a bacterial infection and may be treated with antibiotics with no improvement. A florid rash usually develops if patient is given ampicillin.

EBV is associated with Burkitt's lymphoma in Africa and na-sopharyngeal carcinoma in South-east Asia and China. Several other lympho-proliferative conditions have been observed in children with primary immunodeficiencies, in transplant and immuno-suppressed patients (Volk *et al.*, 1995). Active EBV replication is seen in > 80% of organ transplant recipients during anti-lymphocyte antibody therapy. The most serious manifestation of EBV in this type of patient is post-transplant liver disease (Basgoz and Preiksaitis, 1995).

2.4. Human herpes viruses 6 and 7

In 1989, HHV6 was isolated from the blood of patients with lympho-proliferative disorders and HHV7 in 1990 under similar circum-stances. Both viruses infect T-lymphocytes. HHV6 is the cause of a common disease in infancy known as roseola infantum or sixth disease. Although infections due to HHV7 are widespread among young children, the virus has so far not been implicated in any disease. Infections with HHV6 are very common, the seroprevalence approaches 100%, although a country-to-country variation has been noticed (Ranger *et al.*, 1991). After the primary infection, the virus multiplies in salivary glands and is excreted in the saliva. It remains latent in lymphocytes and monocytes and does not cause problems to normal people. It is a major cause of opportunistic viral infections in the immunosuppressed, typically in AIDS patients and transplant recipients, resulting in rejection of transplant organs and death (Campadelli-Fiume, 1999). The most serious clinical manifestations of reactivation are due to disseminated infections of organs, such as the brain, lungs and retina, which may contribute to death (Knox *et al.*, 1994). Similarly, HHV7 can also reactivate in transplant recipients (Osman *et al.*, 1996). A possible associated pathogenic role of HHV6 in the pathogenesis of multiple sclerosis has also been described (Friedman, 1999). The virus can be isolated from saliva by culture and detection is possible by PCR.

2.5. Human herpes virus 8

HHV8 was first identified in 1994 from tissues of Kaposi's sarcoma patients with AIDS (Moore and Chang, 1995). Recent studies have shown evidence of both sexual and non-sexual modes of transmission as well as spread via renal allografts (Martin *et al.*, 1999). Current research on this virus is being concentrated on the role played by the virus in the pathogenesis of Kaposi's sarcoma and body-cavity B-cell lymphoma (Bergstrom, 1999). PCR can detect the virus from clinical material, and it can be isolated in B-cell lymphoma cell lines.

3. Mycobacterial Infections

The increasing incidence of mycobacterial infections has affected both the developing and the developed world. Most illnesses and deaths are due to tuberculosis, although non-tuberculous mycobacteria have contributed to morbidity and mortality in both developing and industrialised countries (Falkinham, 1996). The major pathogens of the *Mycobacterium* species include the *Mycobacterium* complex, which includes four closely related mycobacteria: *M. tuberculosis, M. bovis, M. microti* and *M. africanum*, and *M. leprae.* Other members of the genus are referred to as atypical mycobacteria or mycobacteria other than tuberculosis (MOTT). Unlike *M. tuberculosis*, atypical mycobacteria are widespread in the environment and frequently colonise humans. However, because of their low virulence, overt disease is very uncommon except in those who are profoundly immunodeficient.

3.1. Tuberculosis

In spite of all of the advances that have been made in medicine, mycobacterial diseases remain a major problem resulting in considerable morbidity and mortality throughout the world.

The commonest primary site of tuberculosis is in the lungs and is caused by inhalation of infectious material discharged into the air by coughing or by other means. The primary lesion, the infected lung together with its draining lymph nodes, is referred to as a Ghon complex. Infections can rarely be acquired through the skin or by way of the gastrointestinal tract.

Bacteria may spread via the bloodstream or lymphatics to any part of the body and may cause lesions in any organ. After about ten days, specific T-cell clones which react to mycobacterial antigens expand and infiltrate the infected lesions. A group of activated macrophages surround foci of infection "epithelioid cells" and some fuse together to form "giant cells". The result is a granuloma. The centre of this becomes necrotic, and the cheesy material often formed is described as caseous — this is unique to tuberculosis. This process is usually sufficient to contain and control the primary infection and many patients do not become clinically unwell at this stage. However, the mycobacteria are not killed, merely walled off within granulomas which become surrounded by fibrotic tissue that may calcify. In a minority of patients, the infection is not controlled and any of the following may occur: progression of the primary lesion, spread to the pleural cavity with effusion, spread via the bloodstream to various organs and enlargement of infected lymph nodes, especially in the neck. Miliary tuberculosis refers to the appearance of the chest X-ray in a patient with blood-borne spread. Reactivation of tuberculosis may occur many years after the primary infection. Sometimes, there is a precipitating factor like old age, diabetes mellitus, HIV infection or administration of immunosuppressive drugs. Reactivation may also lead to dissemination.

The bacterium can be demonstrated in clinical material by performing a Ziehl–Neelsen stain. Mycobacteria are stained poorly by the dyes used in Gram stain. The term "acid-fast" refers to the organism's ability to retain the carbol fuchsin stain despite subsequent treatment with an ethanol-hydrochloric-acid mixture. The high lipid content (approximately 60%) of the cell wall makes mycobacteria acid-fast. However, a positive result only shows that a *Mycobacterium* species is present and a culture is necessary to identify whether the organism seen under microscopy is *M. tuberculosis* or a MOTT. On the other hand, the polymerase chain reaction (PCR) is a useful method to quickly differentiate *M. tuberculosis* from MOTT. **A negative microscopy and PCR result do not exclude TB.** The culture method still remains the gold standard. A culture is also necessary to perform antimicrobial susceptibility tests, which have become an essential procedure because of the emerging problem of antituberculous drug resistance (Jereb, 1995).

Automated commercial broth-based systems give faster results than traditional culture techniques. Rapid diagnosis of tuberculous meningitis is important and ZN stains on CSF samples are often negative — molecular methods including PCR are coming into use.

There is no reliable way to diagnose TB serologically. However, the patient's immune status can be assessed by injecting an extract of the tubercle bacillus called purified protein derivative (PPD) intradermally, e.g. Mantoux test. Positive results may be due to previous infection or BCG immunisation. Hence, in a population where BCG is given routinely, the Mantoux test is not useful as a diagnostic tool. A false negative reaction may occur in overwhelming infections and in immunocompromised patients.

Several drugs must be given concurrently or resistance emerges during therapy. All of the drugs have potential, severe side-effects. The initial combination will depend on the level of suspicion that the patient has acquired a resistant strain. The length of therapy depends on the site of infection and the immune status of the patient. Corticosteroids may be indicated: e.g. tuberculous meningitis, pericardial and renal diseases.

Bacille Calmette-Guerin (BCG) is a live attenuated strain of *M. bovis*. There is much debate about just how effective it is. It seems clear that it protects infants and young children from the most devastating forms of meningitis infection, and it is given at birth in areas with higher levels of TB in the population. BCG also protects against leprosy infection.

3.2. "Atypical mycobacteria"

There are many species of saprophytic environmental mycobacteria that normally live in soil and water: they have been detected in 86% of soil samples collected from several locations (Wolinsky, 1968). Human beings are being constantly exposed to these bacteria which may be normally found among the normal flora of the intestine. They may also cause confusion due to contaminated specimen containers and staining reagents used in laboratories.

Some species occasionally cause infections in the immuno-compromised patients. A recent increase in the incidence of infections even in people with normal immunity has been observed (Horsburgh, 1996). *M. kansasii* most often causes lesions resembling TB in the lungs, but also causes infections in the lymph nodes and other places. *Mycobacterium avium-intracellulare* (MAI, or avium complex — MAC) and *Mycobacterium scrofulaceum* more often cause mycobacterial lymphadenitis, but do infect the lungs on rare occasions. There has been a recent increase in the incidence of organisms causing necrotising skin diseases. *M. ulcerans*, *M. marinum* and *M. haemophilum* have affected both healthy and immuno-compromised patients in the last decade (Dobos, 1999). Outbreaks of post-injection abscesses caused by *M. abscessus* have been reported following various procedures due to contamination of multidose vials that served as a common source (Gail *et al.*, 1999). The diagnosis of the lesions caused by atypical mycobacteria may not be established quickly and appropriate treatment may be delayed for long periods or not be given at all. Special culture conditions are required to isolate these organisms. If the organism is clinically suspected, the clinician must liaise with the clinical microbiologist.

Resistance to standard antituberculous drugs is common. Isolation, identification and susceptibility testing are important to guide the appropriate treatment.

4. Human Immunodeficiency Virus Infection

The epidemic due to HIV was first discovered in 1981, following the appearance of clusters of cases of rare opportunistic infections in previously healthy people. However, the existence of the virus long before it was discovered has been demonstrated by recent serological tests done on previously collected blood samples. Now, HIV is one of the leading causes of death in young individuals. The World Health Organisation predicted a cumulative total of 1,025,073 cases of AIDS and 20–40 million cases of HIV by the year 2000 (WHO, 1995).

HIV infects and kills CD4 T-lymphocytes. Other cells that contain CD4 proteins on their surface, e.g. macrophages and monocytes, can also be infected. The resulting loss of cell-mediated immunity makes the infected individual more likely to develop opportunistic infections. The natural infection occurs in humans but certain primates can be infected in the laboratory. The mystery of the origin and the original source of HIV remains unsolved. A similar virus, HIV2, was first isolated in 1986 (Clavel *et al.*, 1986).

The common modes of transmission are by sexual contact and by infected blood products, including, from mother to child during the perinatal period. Infected individuals can be shown to have been exposed to one of the recognised routes of transmission and there is clear evidence that the virus is not spread by casual contact, contamination of intact skin or by inhalation or insect bites. Although a small number of virus can be demonstrated in the saliva, tears and urine, there is little epidemiological evidence that infection can be acquired from these sources. Although the pattern of transmission follows that of hepatitis B virus, the infective dose required to cause an infection is much higher with HIV: 0.1 ml HIV-infected blood compared to 0.001 ml of "e" antigen positive hepatitis B carries blood (Shanson, 1999). Occupational exposure among healthcare workers is a serious potential problem. However, the incidence of occupationally acquired HIV is extremely low. The major risk factor is contaminated needle stick injuries, especially with large bore needles. The risk of transmission is about 0.3% following such an injury (Tokars *et al.*, 1993).

During the acute stage of infection, which usually begins 2–4 weeks later, patients may develop "flu"-like symptoms; these may be associated with generalised lymphadenopathy. Although antibodies may not appear until two months or much later, it may be possible to demonstrate the presence of p24 antigen four weeks after the infection. The patient may remain free of signs and symptoms for long periods measured in years and the viraemia may be low or absent, but the lymph nodes will continue to produce HIV during this latent state. During the late stages, there is a gradual reduction in CD4 cells. These lymphocytes play a central role in the immune response to foreign antigens. When the HIV viral load is high in the advanced stages and the CD4 count falls below $200/\text{mm}^3$, the infected individuals become more susceptible to opportunistic infections, the most characteristic being *Pneumocystis carinii*, *Toxoplasma gondii* and *Candida* species. Cancerous conditions may be precipitated by opportunistic infections: e.g. Kaposi's sarcoma and HHV8, lympho-proliferative disorders and HHV6 (Luppi *et al.*, 1998). Various opportunistic infections seen in AIDS patients include viral infections, such as disseminated herpes simplex, herpes zoster and cytomegalovirus fungal infections caused by *Candida albicans, Cryptococcus neoformans* and dimorphic fungi common in endemic areas, e.g. *Histoplasma capsulatum;* protozoal infections caused by *Toxoplasma gondii, Cryptosporidium parvum, Isospora belli* and *Microsporidia,* and bacterial infections caused by *Mycobacterium tuberculosis,* MOTT, particularly MAI and *Salmonella* species.

Laboratory diagnosis of HIV is initially made by screening samples using an EIA test. Recombinant or synthetic antigens now used in this test have helped to overcome the problem of false-positive reactions that occurred with the original antigen prepared from T-lymphocyte cultures. It is important that a positive result is confirmed by Western blot analysis, where viral proteins are separated by a gel electrophoresis technique before reaction with the patient's serum. In certain situations, especially during the first two months after infection, when antibodies cannot be demonstrated, detection of p24 antigen may be helpful. The virus can be grown in the laboratory, but this facility is available only in a few research centres.

Antiviral therapy prolongs survival and reduces the number of opportunistic infections by inhibiting replication of the virus. The virus is not eliminated from infected cells. Antiviral treatment may be associated with severe haematological complications. Modern therapy with multidrug regimens is highly effective at reducing viral load and improving the health of patient.

Prevention can be achieved in healthcare workers by taking measures known as "Universal Precautions", to avoid exposure to blood and body fluids (CDC, 1991). It is mandatory to regard blood and body fluids of any person as hazardous. All hospitals should enforce these precautions. The vaccines developed so far are directed at viral envelope proteins, and have produced good immune responses in vaccine trials. However, due to the presence of variants with vastly different envelope proteins the protection offered by these vaccines is not expected to be satisfactory. Vaccines targeted against various other components of the virus are under development.

5. Creutzfeldt-Jakob Disease (CJD)

CJD is a poorly understood condition caused by an agent with an incubation period that may last for years. The agent causing CJD behaves similarly to the organisms causing slow virus infections, such as measles causing subacute sclerosing panencephalitis, Kuru, scrapie and bovine spongiform encephalopathy (BSE).

CJD is a pre-senile condition with associated dementia. It is a chronic progressive and ultimately a fatal neurological disease, probably caused by a class of agents referred to as "prions". These are small protein particles resistant to inactivation by sterilisation procedures adopted in routine practice. Hence, additional precautions have been recommended when decontaminating equipment and instruments used for these patients (see Chapter 12).

Diagnosis can be established by a brain biopsy. Isolation precautions similar to those used for patients with HBV and HIV have been advised (Greenlee, 1982). Experiments have clearly demonstrated that prions are transmissible by successfully transmitting the agent to primates and other species. There are also reports of human-to-human transmission of CJD via human dura mater grafts, following corneal transplantation (as with rabies), via intracerebral electrodes and as a result of injecting growth hormone derived from pituitary glands (Fradkin *et al.*, 1991).

5.1. A new variant of CJD (nvCJD)

In the UK, a similar illness rapidly spreading among cattle, bovine spongiform encephalopathy (BSE), first appeared in 1984 (Wells, 1987) which affected 1% of all adult cattle by 1992. The epidemic was attributed to oral ingestion of the infectious agent via cattle food prepared from contaminated cattle and sheep carcasses. The disease is also transmissible to domestic cats and to large cats living in zoos via contaminated feed. In light of the new epidemic spreading among domestic animals, the concern arose that the disease may be transmitted to humans as well. A new variant form of CJD was first identified in 1996 from 14 patients in the UK and one in France.

There is epidemiological, clinical and histopathological evidence to support a possible link between the nvCJD and BSE (Will, 1996). The confirmation of a clinical diagnosis is by the characteristic features demonstrable in a brain biopsy.

6. Fungal Infections

Fungi are ubiquitous, living mostly in the soil and on decaying vegetation. They exist as moulds (filaments) or yeasts (single-celled forms). Dimorphic fungi are able to exist in both forms and change in morphology according to growth conditions.

Infections of the skin (ringworm), hair and nails are caused by mould fungi called dermatophytes. Yeasts, e.g. *Candida albicans*, affect the skin, nail and mucous membranes, but in smaller numbers, are often part of the normal flora at these sites.

Sporothrix schenckii causes subcutaneous infections that spread along lymphatic channels, and sometimes disseminated infection.

Dimorphic fungi may cause deep-seated infections in healthy people. They are coccidioidmycosis, paracoccidioidomycosis, blastomycosis, histoplasmosis and paracoccidiosis. These infections are seen in certain parts of the USA and in many other temperate and tropical areas.

Almost any fungus may cause invasive disease in the severely immunocompromised. The fungi commonly isolated from such patients include *Aspergillus* species, *Trichosporon beigelii*, *Fusarium* species and *Pseudallescheria boydii*. *Penicillium marneffei* causes serious disease in South-East asian AIDS patients. Yeast infections may become disseminated in many unwell patients, including those on antibiotics after a major surgery, as well as those with more defined forms of immunocompromise like neutropaenia.

Cryptococcus neoformans is found in bird excreta and causes central nervous system and respiratory tract infections.

The laboratory diagnosis of fungal infections depends on direct microscopy of tissues, histological examination and culture. Serological tests lack sensitivity or specificity and are not helpful as a diagnostic tool, except in the case of cryptococcosis and histoplasmosis. Most substances that affect fungi are toxic to human cells, because both are eukaryotic. As a result only a few antifungal drugs are available for therapeutic use.

Pneumocystis carinii is an important cause of pneumonia in any condition associated with severe immunosuppression, and is particularly closely associated with AIDS. The organism, previously thought to be a parasite, has been reclassified as a fungus by molecular taxonomic studies. The organism has been demonstrated in many species of animals and is distributed worldwide. However, it is believed that human infection results from exposure to strains found in man. There is no direct invasion of tissues, although dissemination outside the lung does occur particularly in AIDS patients. Following presumed inhalation of cysts, the resulting inflammatory response in alveoli blocks oxygen exchange. The chest X-ray may show characteristic appearance of an interstitial pneumonia. Examination of spontaneously expectorated sputum by Gram staining microscopy seldom reveals the presence of the organism. Silver staining of broncho-alveolar lavage or lung biopsy is a method used to demonstrate cysts. Immunofluorescence is also commonly used to diagnose the infection.

7. References

AHLFORS, K., IVARSSON, S.A., HARRIS, S., SVANBERG, L., HOLMGVIST, R., LERNMARK, B. and THEANDER, G. (1984). Congenital cytomegalovirus infection and disease in Sweden and the relative importance of primary and secondary maternal infections. Preliminary findings from a prospective study. *Scand. J. Infect. Dis.* **16**, 129–137.

BASGOZ, N. and PREIKSAITIS, J.K. (1995). Post-transplant lymphoproliferative disorder. *Infect. Dis. Clin. N. Am.* **9**, 901–923.

BERGSTROM, T. (1999). HHV 6,7 and 8. Recently discovered herpesviruses explain the etiology of well-known diseases. *Lakartidningen* **96**, 3161–3165.

CAMPADELLI-FIUME, G., MIRANDOLA, P. and MENOTTI, L. (1999). Human herpesvirus 6: An emerging pathogen. *Emerg. Infect. Dis.* **3**, 353–366.

CDC: BULL. AM. COLL. SURG. (1991). Recommendation for preventing transmission of human immunodeficiency and hepatitis B virus to patients during exposure-prone invasive procedures. *Centre Dis. Cont. Bull. Am. Coll. Surg.* **76**, 29–37.

CLAVEL, F., GUETARD, D., BRUN-VEZINET, F., CHAMARET, S., REY, M.A., SANTOS-FERREIRA, M.O., LAURENT, A.G., DAUGUET, C., KATLAMA, C. and ROUZIOUX, C. (1986). Isolation of a new human retrovirus from West African patients with AIDS. *Science* **233**, 343–346.

DETRE, K.M., BELLE, S.H. and LOMBARDERO, M. (1996). Liver transplantation for chronic viral hepatitis. *Viral Hepatitis Rev.* **2**, 219–228.

DOBOS, K.M., QUINN, F.D., ASHFORD, D.A., HORSBURGH, C.R. and KING, C.H. (1999). Emergence of a unique group of necrotizing mycobacterial diseases. *Emerg. Infect. Dis.* **5**, 367–378.

FAIX, R.G. (1989). Lack of aerosol dispersal of cytomegalovirus during mechanical ventilation. *Pediatric Infect. Dis. J.* **8**, 330–332.

FALKINHAM, J.O. (1996). Epidemiology of infection by nontuberculosis mycobacteria. *Clin. Microbiol. Rev.* **9**, 177–215.

FRADKIN, J.E., SCHONBERGER, L.B., MILLS, J.L., GUNN, W.J., PIPER, J.M., WYSOWSKI, D.K., THOMSON, R., DURAKE, S. and BROWN, P. (1991). Creutzfeldt-Jacob Disease in pituitary growth hormone recipients in the United States. *JAMA* **265**, 880–884.

FRIEDMAN, J.E., LYONS, M.J., CU, G., ABLASH, D.V., WHITMAN, J.E., EDGAR, M., KOSKINIEMI, M., VAHERI, A., ZABRISKIE, J.E. (1999). The association of the human herpesvirus 6 and MS. *Mult. Scler.* **5**(5), pp. 355–362.

GAIL, K, MILLER, L.A., YAKRUS, M.A., WALLACE, R.J. Jr, MOSLEY, D.G., ENGLAND, B., HUITT, G., McNEILL, M.M. and PERKINS, B.A. (1999). Abscesses due to Mycobacterium abscessus linked to injection of unapproved alternative medication. *CDC* **5**, 5.

GREENLEE, J.E. (1982). Containment precautions in hospitals for cases of Creutzfeldt-Jacob Disease. *Infect. Cont.* **3**, 222.

HORSBURGH, C.R Jr. (1996). Epidemiology of diseases caused by nontuberculosis bacteria. *Semin. Respir. Infect.* **11**, 244–254.

JENNER, E. (1996). Immunisation against infectious disease. Bicentenary Edition HMSO. In: *Varicella.* pp. 251–261.

JEREB, J.A., KLEVENS, R.M., PRIVETT, T.D., SMITH, P.J., CRAWFORD, J.T., SHARP, V.L., DAVIS, W.R. and DOOLEY, S.W. (1995). Tuberculosis in health care workers at a hospital with an outbreak of multidrug-resistant *Mycobacterium tuberculosis. Arch. Intern. Med.* **155**, 854–859.

KNOX, K.K. and CARRIGAN, D.R. (1994). Disseminated active HHV6 infections in patients with AIDS. *Lancet* **343**, 577–578.

LUPPI, M., BAROZZI, P., MORRIS, C.M., MERELLI, E. and TORELLI, G. (1998). Interaction of human herpes virus 6 genome in human chromosomes. *Lancet* **352**, 1707–1708.

MARTIN, J.N. and OSMOND, D.H. (1999). Kaposi's sarcoma — associated herpesvirus and sexual transmission of cancer risk. *Curr. Opin. Oncol.* **11**, 508–515.

MOORE, P.S. and CHANG, Y. (1995). Detection of herpesvirus-like DNA sequences in Kaposi's sarcoma in patients with and without HIV infection. *N. Engl. J. Med.* **332**, 1181–5.

NA, G.Y. (1997). Herpes zoster in three healthy children immunized with varicella vaccine (Oka/Biken); the causative virus differed from vaccine strain on PCR analysis of the IV variable region (R5) and of a *Pstl*-site region. *Br. J. Dermatol.* **137**, 255–258.

NISHIZAWA, T., OKAMTO, H., KONISH, K., YOSHIZAWA, H., MIYAKAWA, Y. and MAYUMI, M. (1997). A novel DNA virus (TTV) associated with elevated transaminase levels in post-transfusion hepatitis of unknown etiology. *Biochem. Biophys. Res. Commun.* **241**, 92–99.

OSMAN, H.K., PEIRIS, J.S., TAYLOR, C.E., WARWICKER, P., JARRETT R.F., MADELEY, C.R. (1996) Cytomegalovirus disease in renal allograft recipients: is human herpesvirus 7 a co-factor for disease progression? *J. Med. Virol.* **48**, 295–301.

RANGER, S., PATILLAUD, S., DENIS, F., HIMMICH, A., SANGARE, A., M'BOUP, S., ITOUA-N'GAPORO, A., PRINCE-DAVID, M., CHOUT, R. and CEVALLOS, R. (1991). Seroepidemiology of HHV-6 in pregnant women from different parts of the world. *J. Med. Virol.* **34**, 194–198.

RUBIN, R.H. (1994). Infection in the organ transplant recipient. In: *Clinical Approach to Infection in the Compromised Host*, eds. R.H. Rubin and L.S. Young, Plenum Press, New York, 629–705.

SALISBURY, D.M. and BEGG, N.T. (1996). Immunisation against infectious disease, Edward Jenner Bicentenary Edition, London HMSO, 251–261.

SHANSON, D.C. (1999). *AIDS and Other Diseases Caused by Retroviruses. Microbiology in Clinical Practice.* Butterworth-Heinemann, Great Britain, 357–382.

SHAPIRO, C.N. (1995). Occupational risk of infection with hepatitis B and hepatitis C virus. *Surg. Clin. North. Am.* **75**, 1047–1056.

STAGNO, S. (1990). Cytomegalovirus. In: *Infectious Disease of the Fetus and Newborn Infant*, eds. J.S. Remington and J.O. Klein, W.B. Saunders, Philadelphia, pp. 41–281.

TOKARS, J.I., MARCUS, R., CULVER, D.H., SCHABLE, C.A., McKIBBEN, P.S., BANDEA, C.I. and BELL, D.M. (1993). Surveillance of HIV infection and Zidovudine use among health care workers after occupational exposure to HIV-infected blood. *Ann. Intern. Med.* **118**, 913–919.

VOLK, W.A. *et al.* (1996). Herpesviridae. In: *Essentials of Medical Microbiology*. Lippincott-Raven Publishers, Philadelphia, pp. 545–556.

WELLS, G.A.H., SCOTT, A.C. and JOHNSON, C.T., *et al.* (1987). A novel progressive spongiform encephalopathy in cattle. *Vte. Rec.* **121**, 419–420.

WILL, R.G., IRONSIDE, J.W., ZEIDLER, M. COUSEN, S.N., ESTIBEIROK, K., ALPEROVITCH, A., POSER, S., POCCHIARI, M., HOFMAN, A. and SMITH, P.G. (1996). A new variant of Creutzfeldt-Jakob Disease in the UK. *Lancet* **347**, 921–925.

WOLINSKY, E. and RYNEARSON, T.K. (1968). Mycobacteria in soil and their relation to disease-associated strains. *Am. Rev. Respirat. Dis.* **97**, 1032–1037.

WORLD HEALTH ORGANIZATION (1995). AIDS — Global data, *Wkly. Epidemiol. Rec.* **70**, 5–7.

SECTION IV:

STERILE TECHNIQUES

Advances in Tissue Banking Vol. 5
© 2001 by World Scientific Publishing Co. Pte. Ltd.

15 PRINCIPLES OF STERILE TECHNIQUE

S.Z. MORDIFFI

Major Operating Theatre Suite
Nursing Department, National University Hospital
5 Lower Kent Ridge Road, Singapore 119074

A. NATHER

NUH Tissue Bank, National University Hospital
5 Lower Kent Ridge Road, Singapore 119074

1. Introduction

All tissue-bank operators must be trained on aseptic technique in order to perform sterile procurement of tissues from living and deceased donors. It is vital that each new technologist be attached to the operating room for at least two or three months to learn and practise hands-on all principles of sterile technique. The technologist must learn not only how to scrub and gown in a sterile fashion. He or she must also learn how to maintain sterility in the operating room as well as the methods of sterilising equipment and materials in the theatre sterile supply unit.

2. Sterile Technique in the Operating Room

Sterility is the "absence" of microorganisms including spores (Groah, 1990). Sterility is attained by the process of sterilisation. Aseptic technique is the procedure of ensuring that an item remains sterile after sterilisation and at the time of use for the patient. It is the responsibility of the surgical team to ensure that only sterile items are used during surgery (Atkinson and Fortunato, 1996).

The skin is a barrier to microbial infection. A surgical incision is a potential port of entry for microorganisms (Groah, 1990). Therefore, items used during surgery must be sterile as non-sterile item carries with it pathogenic microorganisms which may cause wound infections.

Aseptic technique is the method by which contamination of microorganisms is prevented. The activities of the sterile team that ensures sterility include scrubbing, preparation of trolley, antiseptic cleaning of patient, draping procedure, aseptic technique during surgery, cleaning and dressing of wound after surgery, and post-surgical procedures.

For illustration, the procurement of the head of femur will be used as the example. Aseptic technique is not an easy concept to grasp. To aid in the visualisation of this technique, concepts from Kolb's

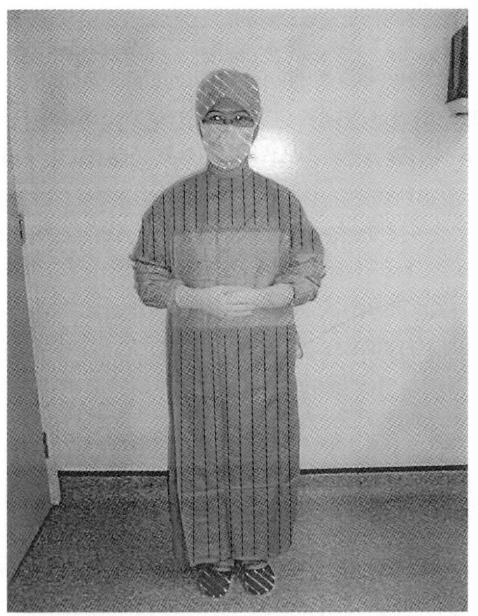

Fig. 1. Sterile person.

(1984) experiential learning theory and neurolinguistic programming (1980) theory will be used. For visualising the concept of sterility, colours will be used. Yellow is denoted as non-sterile areas of a scrubbed person, blue as sterile and red as the safety margin (Fig. 1). The safety margin is an area that is sterile but considered non-sterile. The safety margin is always present wherever there is a non-sterile area and a sterile area. Basically, in aseptic technique, "blue" (sterile) can only touch another "blue", "yellow" (non-sterile) can only touch "yellow" and "red" (safety margin) can only touch "red".

2.1. Scrubbing

Prior to scrubbing, the nurse will gather the requisites necessary for the surgery. The scrub nurse places the draping pack onto the instrument trolley, instrument set and cleansing set onto a stand. The scrub nurse then perfors the scrubbing, gowning and gloving procedure.

The Association of Operating Room Nurse (AORN, 1996) which recommended practice for maintaining a sterile field, recommends that a sterile gown be considered sterile in front from the chest to the level of the sterile field, and the sleeves from two inches above the elbow to the cuff. In a scrubbed sterile person, the safety margin would include areas at the neckline, shoulders, under the arms, back and the sleeve cuff, and below the waist level (trolley level). The hands and arms, which are denoted by the blue colour, must remain within the sterile zone (blue zone) of the operating gown (Fig. 1). Unguarded sterile areas must be considered as non-sterile. The back of the gown, which cannot be monitored, becomes the "red" zone even though a wrap-around gown is used. Other safety margins include areas 5 cm below the neckline of the gown and areas of the gown below the waistline.

2.2. Preparation of sterile trolley

The sterile trolley should be prepared as close as possible to the time of surgery. All linen or paper-wrapped items used for surgery should be double wrapped (Atkinson and Fortunato, 1996).

It is the responsibility of the operating room nurse to ensure that items used fulfils the criteria for sterility. Prior to opening any item, the non-sterile person checks for expiry date, change in colour of chemical indicator, that the packaging remains intact with no visible punctures and that the items remain dry. In some institutions, event-related sterility is practised, making expiry date not applicable.

The circulating nurse (non-sterile person) unwraps the outer wrapper of the draping pack, instrument and cleansing set. The scrub nurse (sterile-scrubbed person) unwraps the inner wrapper of the draping pack, making sure that her gloved hands does not go beyond the level of the trolley as she unfolds the wrapper. The scrub nurse proceeds to unfold the inner layers of other items, places the items on the sterile trolley and arranges receptacles, drapes and instruments onto the sterile trolley. The circulating nurse provides the necessary items for the scrub nurse. The scrub nurse counts the instruments, blades and needles prior to the surgery (Fig. 2). The circulating nurse documents all counts made.

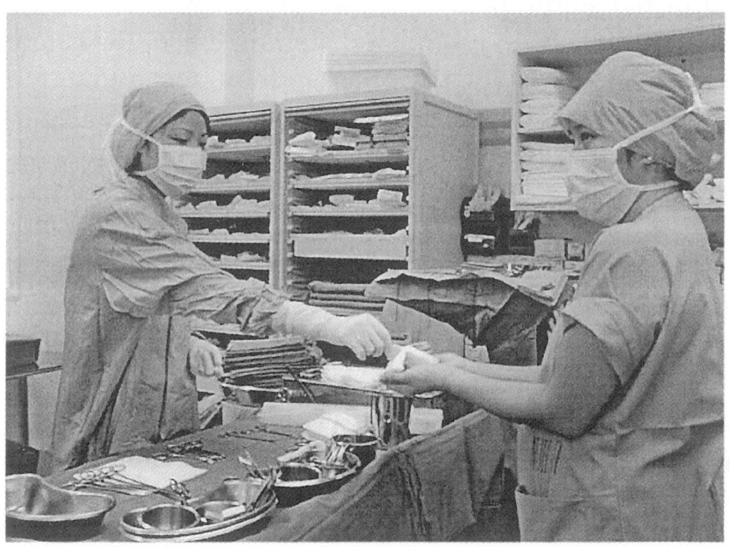

Fig. 2. Trolley preparation.

2.3. Antiseptic cleansing of patient

The presence of hair may interfere with exposure, closure and dressing of the wound. If hair gets into the surgical would, this may be a foreign body and may exacerbate infection. Hair removal may be required within the perimeter of the incision. Hair removal is best performed using either a depilatory cream (if there is no allergy) or clippers. If shaving is used as a method for hair removal, it should be performed as close as possible to the time of surgery. Presence of nicks and abrasions becomes a source of infection.

2.3.1. Procedure

- Appropriate germicidal solution is used to decrease the microbial counts. A choice of chlorhexidene with 70% alcohol or povidone-iodine may be used. A sufficient volume of cleansing solution is poured into a galipot. The gauze is folded and mounted onto the sponge-holding forceps. Additional gauze is placed into the galipot or into the kidney dish.
- The area is exposed only when the surgical team is ready to cleanse the patient. Modesty should be maintained and only a minimal area is exposed.
- Standing at the foot of the operation table, the technician will assist to lift the lower limb by holding the heel.
- Place towels on the table beneath the limb to collect run off solutions.
- Dip the gauze in the antiseptic solution, squeeze excess solution and commence scrubbing from the surgical site outward towards the periphery in a circular motion. Sufficient pressure and friction should be applied to remove dirt and microorganisms from the skin and pores. The gauze is discarded. Repeat the procedure with a new piece of gauze in the same manner.
- The receptacles for the skin preparation are discarded.
- If run-off solution is expected, place towels along the incision site to prevent wetting of the sheet. The non-sterile person, upon completion of the skin preparation, removes the side towels as

the cleansing solution can cause irritation to the skin. Pooling of alcoholic based solutions can cause chemical or diathermy burns.

2.4. Draping

"Sterile drapes should be used to establish a sterile field" (AORN, 1996). Sterility must be maintained during the draping procedure. The requisites include five protective drapes (Mackintosh or cellulose paper sandwiched between folded dressing towel), two abdominal towels, two trolley towels, one cotton bandage, one stockinette, one adhesive U-drape (3M), and one Ioban adhesive drape (iodine-impregnated drape).

The operating theatre technician will continue to lift up the limb during this procedure.

- Arrange drapes in sequence of use.
- Place sterile protective drape beneath the limb, at the side at the hip region, covering the abdomen and the pubis area.
- Take the abdominal towel and stand on the other side of the OT table facing the surgeon. Carefully pass one end of the folded abdominal towel to the surgeon beneath the limb. Grab other end of the folded abdominal towel. Simultaneously pull the towel taut while supporting the mid-portion of the towel to prevent the towel from touching the non-sterile table. Unfold the towel by gathering the folds in the hand. Spread the towel and cover the lower portion of the table.
- Perform the same motion but this time cover the upper part of the patient. Two towel clips, one on each side, will be clipped to secure the two towels together.
- Take the trolley towel and again stand on the opposite side of the OT table. Unfold the towel. The technician will lower the limb onto the towel. Wrap the limb with the towel. Secure with cotton bandage, bandaging from the foot to slightly beyond the proximal end of the towel. Tie the bandage to secure the towel in place.
- A sterile member lifts the limb. Scrub nurse places an unfolded trolley towel beneath the limb to reinforce the drapes.

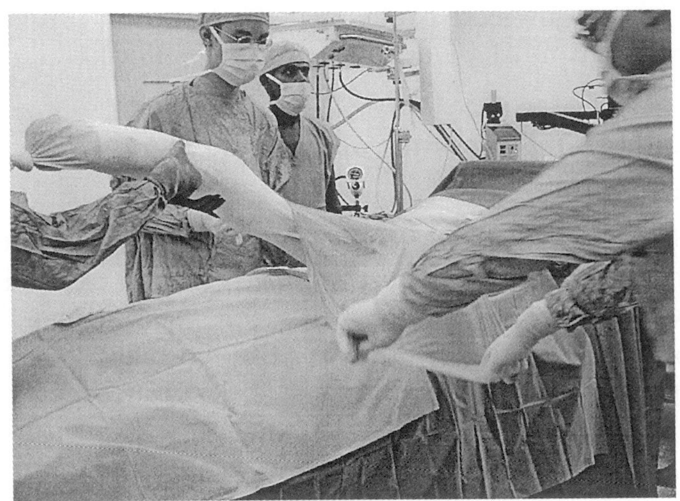

Fig. 3. Draping procedure.

- A U-drape adhesive drape may be used. This drape should be placed beneath the limb. The two slits are to go around the proximal limb and cross at the anterior (NUH, 1995) (Fig. 3).

2.5. Aseptic technique during surgery

Sterility must be maintained throughout the whole surgical procedure. The surgical team must remain vigilant for any breaks in sterility. Items used during surgery must remain sterile (Atkinson and Fortunato, 1996).

- Drapes must remain dry. Reinforce as soon as it is wet.
- Non-sterile items or persons must be one foot away from a sterile field.
- Drapes below the table level are considered non-sterile.
- Sterile person always faces the sterile drapes. Never turn the back towards the sterile table. Principle of "blue touching or facing blue" (sterile), "yellow touching or facing yellow" (non-sterile) and "red touching or facing red" (safety margin) applies.

- Changing of gowns if contaminated.
- Surgical team must be on the lookout for breaks in sterility.

2.6. Cleaning and dressing of wound after surgery

- The wound is cleansed with saline after closure of the skin. The gauze is soaked in saline. Start cleaning from one end of the suture line and end at the other. Use another gauze to clean around the wound.
- Drying of the wound is done in a similar manner beginning at the wound, followed by drying of the surrounding area.

2.7. Post-surgical procedures

- Remove all instruments from the field.
- Discard soiled swabs into the biohazard carrier.
- The drapes are removed from the patient and discarded into the appropriate linen carrier.
- Check that the underlying towel is clean and dry.
- Patient is covered and modesty maintained (NUH, 1995).

3. Sterile Scrub (Surgical Hand Scrub)

A surgical hand scrub is performed prior to a surgical procedure. Scrubbing is the act of application of antiseptic solution on the fingers, nails and forearms using a specific technique (AORN, 1999). This technique may be a brush-stroke or time-based hand-rubbing technique.

The skin harbours transient and resident microorganisms. These microorganisms are pathogenic when skin integrity is compromised. Thus, surgical hand scrubs effectively

- Remove debris and transient microorganisms from the nails, hands and forearms.
- Reduce the resident microbial count to a minimum.
- Inhibits the rapid rebound growth of microorganisms (Atkinson and Fortunato, 1996, AORN, 1999).

3.1. Choice of antiseptics

Common antiseptics used for scrubbing at this centre include 4% chlorhexidene gluconate and 7.5% povidone-iodine. Choice of antiseptic is dependent on the user and whether there is any user allergy. Antiseptics should never be used in combination. Chlorhexidene has been shown to be more effective in decreasing the bioburden and is effective against gram-positive and some gram-negative microorganisms. Upon application, chlorhexidene is effective for approximately eight hours. Chlorhexidene also has substantive effect. A study by Paulson (1994) found chlorhexidene gluconate to be the most effective antimicrobial agent with regard to its immediate, persistent and residual effect. Povidone-iodine is effective against gram-negative and some gram-positive microorganisms. Once applied, povidone-iodine is effective for approximately five hours (Atkinson and Fortunato, 1996).

3.2. Preparation prior to scrubbing

- Fingernails should be kept short and clean.
- Nail polish should not be used (Wynd *et al.*, 1994).
- Hands are inspected for cuts and abrasions
- Jewelry should be removed from hands and arms.
- Hair must be well covered.
- Mask adjusted snugly and comfortably over nose and mouth.
- Fluidshield mask or goggles to be worn where blood splashing is expected.
- Disposable plastic aprons are worn where blood, fluid or water splashing is expected (NUH, 1995).

There are two methods in current practice in Singapore — the brushing method and the hand-rubbing method. This centre's operating theatre department has recommended the 3-minute surgical hand-rubbing technique to be the effective method although orthopaedic surgeons and other surgeons prefer the brushing method. A study by Loeb *et al.*, (1997) found the surgical hand-rubbing method to be similar or slightly more effective than the surgical brushing method.

3.3. Surgical brushing method

The brushing method uses a brush-stroke technique (Gruendemann, 1992). The brushing procedure can be divided into two phases.

3.3.1. Phase I

  (i) Adjust the tap to provide water with a suitable temperature and moderate flow.

  (ii) Wet hands and forearms up to 5 cm above the elbow (Fig. 4(a)).

 (iii) Dispense approximately 5 ml of hospital approved antiseptic agent onto the palm (Fig. 4(b)).

 (iv) Perform hand-washing procedure to remove superficial soil.

Using friction, rub the hands backwards and forwards in the following manner:

  (a) Palm to palm.

  (b) Right palm over left dorsum and vice versa.

  (c) Palm to palm with fingers interlaced.

  (d) Rub the backs of fingers to opposing palms with fingers interlocked.

  (e) Rotational rubbing of right thumb clasped in left hand and vice versa (Fig. 4(c)).

  (f) Rotational rubbing of left palm backwards and forwards with clasped fingers of right hand and vice versa.

  (v) Clasp right hand around left arm. Rub in an upward and downward motion. Ensure that every area of the arm is rubbed till 5 cm above the elbow (Fig. 4(d)). Do the same with the other arm.

 (vi) Rinse thoroughly starting from the fingers, to the hands and forearms. Keep hands and forearms elevated at all times.

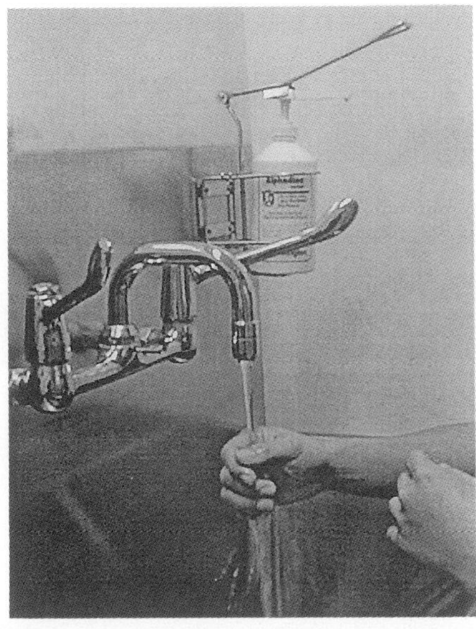

Fig. 4(a). Rinse hand and arm thoroughly.

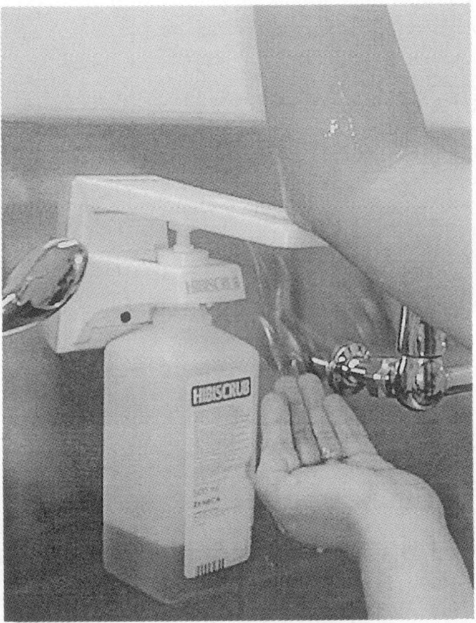

Fig. 4(b). Apply generous amounts of antiseptic.

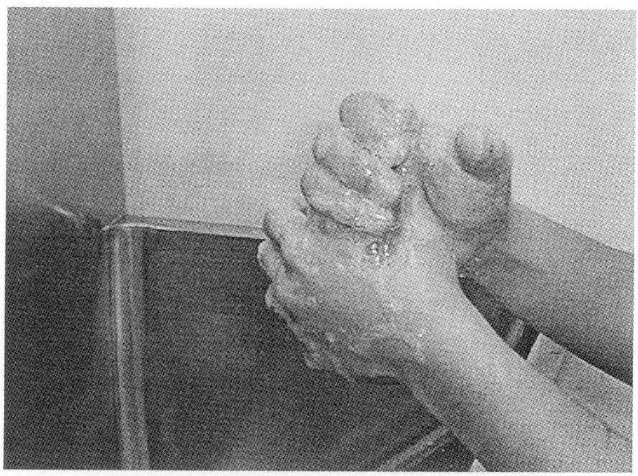

Fig. 4(c). Rotational rubbing of thumb.

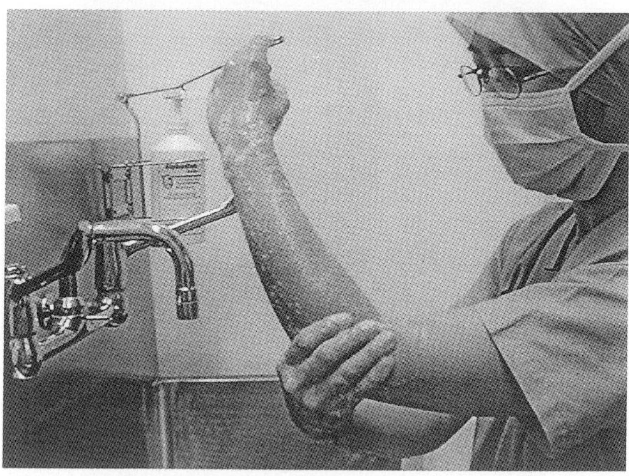

Fig. 4(d). Application of antiseptic to 5 cm above the elbow.

3.3.2. Phase II

(i) Wet brush and apply sufficient amount of antiseptic solution onto the brush.

(ii) Visually divide each finger into four planes. Brush each plane with 30 strokes of the brush. For the anterior and posterior aspects of the fingers, extend the stroke to include the palm and dorsum of the hand, respectively (Fig. 5(a)).

(iii) Visually divide the arm into two sections. Each section is further divided into four planes.

(iv) Brush section 1 first from the wrist to mid forearm. Brush each plane with an upward and downward stroke of the brush for 30 times.

(v) Proceed to brush section 2 from mid-forearm to 5 cm above the elbow in the same manner.

(vi) Rinse thoroughly, starting from the finger tips and ending at the elbows with arms elevated at all times. Proceed to the gowning trolley.

(vii) Pick up the hand towel without contaminating any other sterile items on the trolley.

(viii) Begin by drying the fingers, palms and dorsum of the hands.

(ix) Continue to dab dry the arm from the wrist to the elbow (Fig. 5(b)). Discard the hand towel. Do the same for the other arm.

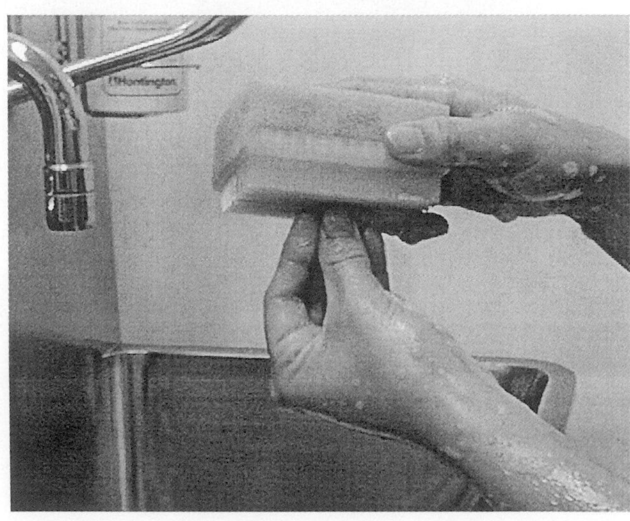

Fig. 5(a). Brushing of finger tips.

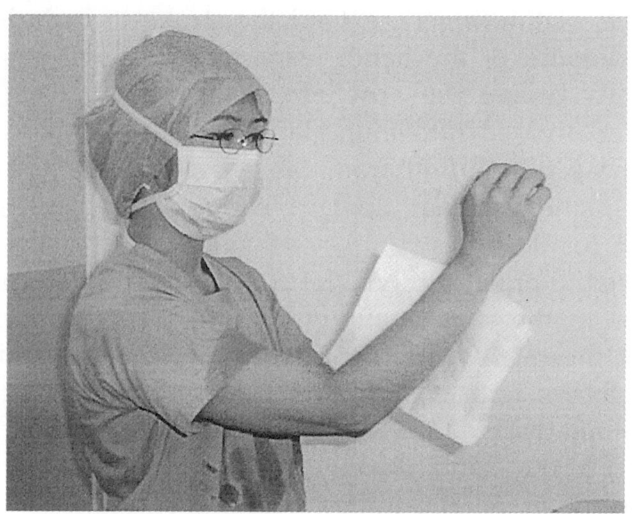

Fig. 5(b). Dab dry the arm.

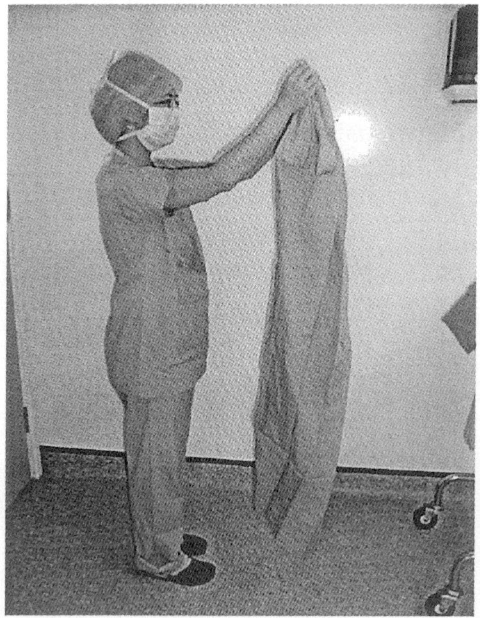

Fig. 5(c). Unfolding of sterile operating gown.

3.4. Gowning

(i) Pick up the gown and stand slightly away from the trolley.

(ii) Lift the gown up and away from the body. Holding the corners of the collar, allow the gown to unfold (Fig. 5(c)).

(iii) Slip both arms simultaneously into the armholes and stretch the arms outward momentarily. Do not spread arms higher than shoulder level.

3.5. Gloving

The close-donning method is recommended by AORN (1999) when gloving prior to surgery.

(i) Open and orientate the gloves (fingers must remain within the cuff of the gown during this procedure). Pick up the glove by the cuff and place glove onto the palm of the opposite hand. Orientate the glove with the thumb facing the palm and the opening of the glove cuff in line with the opening of the gown cuff.

(ii) Pinch the centre of the cuff of the glove. Flip the glove over the fingers. Simultaneously tug the glove and push fingers through the cuff and into the glove (Fig. 5(d)).

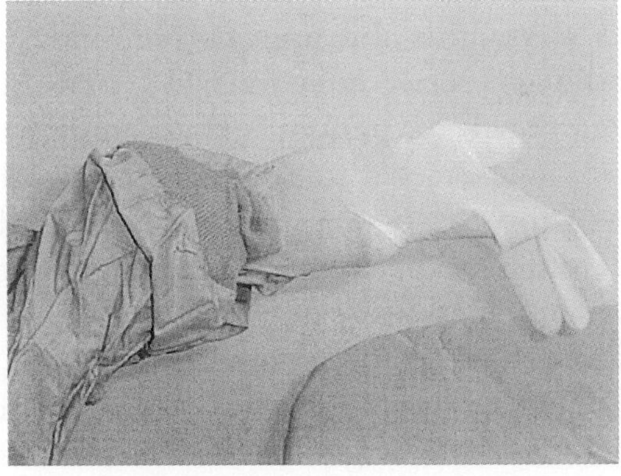

Fig. 5(d). Close-donning method.

4. Monitoring of Sterility in the Operating Room

The skin serves to protect against the invasion of pathogenic micro-organisms. When an operation is performed, the skin is first incised. Skin integrity is therefore compromised. In addition, patients who require surgery may be immunologically weakened because of the disease process. Monitoring of sterility in the operating room is therefore crucial in controlling the propagation of infection in the operating room.

The sources of contamination in the operating room include human factors, air circulation, environmental controls and supplies used during surgical intervention.

4.1. Human factors

The main source of contamination comes from humans because they harbour the most pathogenic microorganisms and are the means by which microorganisms are introduced into the wound.

4.2. Health and hygiene

Groah (1990) advocates that personnel working in the operating room must be free from transmissible bacterial infection such as URTI, carbuncles, dermatitis and unhealed wounds, and infection of mouth, eyes and ears. Most infections are transmitted via direct contact from personnel to patient or via indirect contact from personnel to inanimate objects to patient. Handwashing procedure eliminates most of the pathogenic microorganisms that are present on the hands. It must be performed consistently before and after each patient contact. Handwashing is one of the most effective methods to halt further propagation of infection. AORN (1996) advocates that patients should have a shower and/or shampoo prior to surgery to remove organic debris from the skin, thereby reducing the risk of contamination.

4.3. Attire

The operating room suite is a clean environment. The use of clean attire reduces contamination of the operating room from extraneous infection. The operating room suite is sectioned into three zones (Earl, 1996).

The unrestricted zone is the "grey-area" where personnel or public may mingle with personnel in operating room garb. The grey area refers to the reception and recovery area, and the top-up store, where consumable and pharmaceuticals are replenished from external source.

The semi-restricted zone refers to the corridors, administrative office, storage rooms and the theatre sterile supply unit (TSSU) in the operating room suite. All personnel entering the operating room suite must change into freshly laundered operating theatre outfit. Changing into fresh attire reduces particle count of shedding from the body (Atkinson and Fortunato, 1996). Hair covers are worn to prevent dandruff and hair from being shed onto the scrub clothing and wound. Clean footwear is worn.

The restricted zone is the operating room suite where surgery is performed. It includes the operating room, preparation room, scrub room and induction room. In addition to the operating room attire, a mask must be worn prior to entering this zone.

4.4. Air circulation

Opening of doors results in mixing of clean operating room air with that of the outside corridor air, which has a higher microbial count. Traffic in and out of the operating room must be kept to a minimum during surgery. In the construction, it is preferable that doors should open from a clean room (double-door concept). Only authorised personnel and surgical team are allowed within the operating rooms. The number of people within the operating room must be limited. Movement within the operating room creates air turbulence, which can circulate lint, dust and microbes onto the wounds.

4.5. Environment

Methods employed in controlling the environment in the operating room complex are aimed at reducing the microorganism count in the operating rooms.

The design of the operating theatre suite includes considerations for:

- The flow of personnel and equipment within the operating room complex. Movement of "clean" and "dirty" items prevent contaminated items from mixing with clean and sterile items.
- Siting of the TSSU, storage rooms, pantry, decontamination area and disposal rooms.
- The size of the operating room must be adequate to allow the surgical team to move freely within the operating room and for surgical procedures to be performed without untoward contamination.
- Toilet facilities must not be located within the vicinity of the operating room complex.
- Flooring and walls should not inhibit cleaning.

Considerations for mechanical and engineering control of the environment include air-conditioning and ventilation system, air exchanges, temperature control, and humidity.

- Dust and lint from fresh air that is sucked into the ventilation system is removed. Recirculation with fresh air takes place. Just before the air enters the operating room, it passes through a high-efficiency particulate air (HEPA) filter. Atkinson and Fortunato (1996) stated that the use of HEPA filters can remove as much as 90% of particles larger than 0.5 μm. Air sampling is said to improve the bacteriological quality of air during surgery. It assists in limiting the colony-forming units and the bacteria-carrying particle counts (Edminston *et al.*, 1999). However, it has not been shown to directly affect the infection rate. Holton *et al.* (1990) and Humphreys (1992) recommended its use only during commissioning and following major refurbishment of the operating theatre. The purpose of doing air sampling is to identify engineering faults.

* Air conditioning in each operating room is supplied from the ceiling and is exhausted via vents, which is located near the floor. This system creates positive pressure within the operating rooms and air is forced out of the operating room. Air exchanges in the operating room are maintained at 20 to 30 air exchanges per hour. Relative humidity should be maintained at 50 to 60% (Atkinson and Fortunato, 1996).

Housekeeping is essential in maintaining cleanliness of the operating room environment.

At the beginning of the day's list, a general inspection of the overall cleanliness and dryness of the operating rooms and suite are conducted by the operating room personnel. It is essential to perform a housekeeping audit of the operating room to ensure that standards of cleanliness are maintained (NUH, 1991).

Daily routine cleaning is performed with detergent and warm water. Tabletops, equipment, fixtures and stools are damp dusted to control airborne microorganisms that are on dust and lint. Corridors and operating room floors are mopped.

Standard operating procedures for housekeeping must also be followed (NUH, 1991) to ensure that the operating room environment is maintained clean in between cases and at the end of the day's operating list.

Thorough cleaning of the operating theatre environment and equipment is also performed on a weekly basis, including damp dusting walls and ceiling with soap and water and cleaning of trolleys and drip stands.

Monthly cleaning schedule includes chemical restripping and polishing of the floor, cleaning air-conditioned vents and changing of filters at regular intervals.

5. Methods of Sterilisation of Equipment and Materials

The term "sterile" means items are free from any microorganism including spores (Groah, 1990). Atkinson and Fortunato (1996) defines sterility as the "probability that an item is not contaminated". Sterilisation is the process by which an item is rendered sterile. In a hospital setting, the sterilisation process occurs in the Theatre Sterile Supply Unit (TSSU). The TSSU is an important part of an operating room setting where invasive procedures are performed. The processes of sterilisation include decontamination, preparation, packaging, loading, sterilisation and sterile storage. Certain criteria must be fulfilled at every stage in order to attain complete sterilisation.

5.1. Decontamination

Prior to any method of sterilisation, items must be cleaned to reduce the bioburden. The sterilisation process is time based. Therefore, the more microorganisms there are on an item, the longer it takes to destroy them completely or near completely. Furthermore, presence of blood or soil on an item will prevent the surface of the item from direct exposure to the sterilising agent. Figure 6(a) shows personnel arranging utensils into an open basket to allow water and detergent

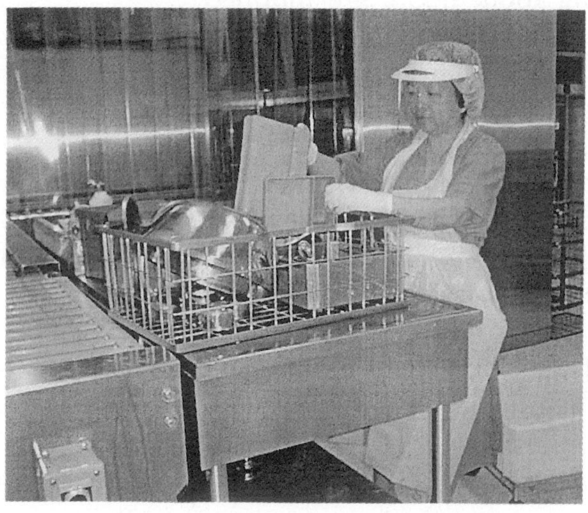

Fig. 6(a). Decontamination — Arranging of utensils and instruments into the basket to ensure that water and detergent can get to all surfaces.

to get to the surfaces of the items in the washer steriliser. All instruments are unclamped and removable parts are disassembled.

5.2. Preparation

In the preparation area (Fig. 6(a)), instruments are inspected for integrity and functioning. All instruments are counted and arranged in sequence in the basket.

5.3. Packaging

Appropriate packaging materials are used. Proper technique of wrapping also affects the effectiveness of the sterilisation. Tapes if used must be sufficient to secure wrappers. Container is the most efficient method of packaging instruments set. It eliminates linen wrappers, which require careful inspection for minute holes. In addition, there would be fewer problems with linting when using containers (Fig. 6(b)).

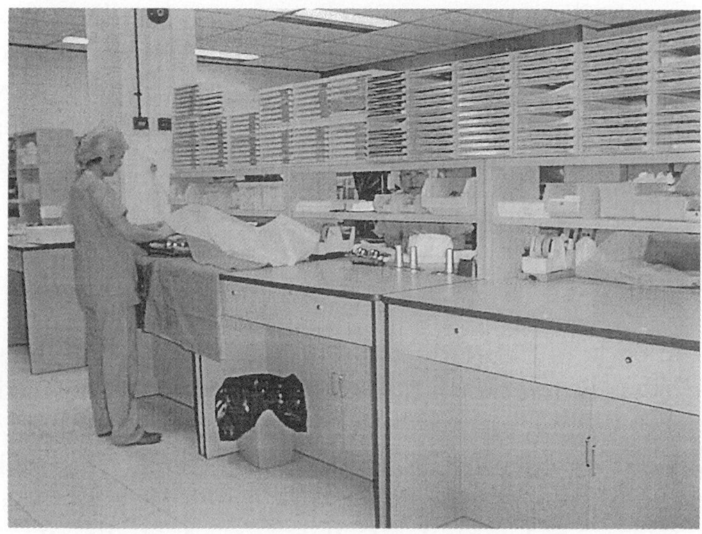

Fig. 6(b). Preparation and packaging area.

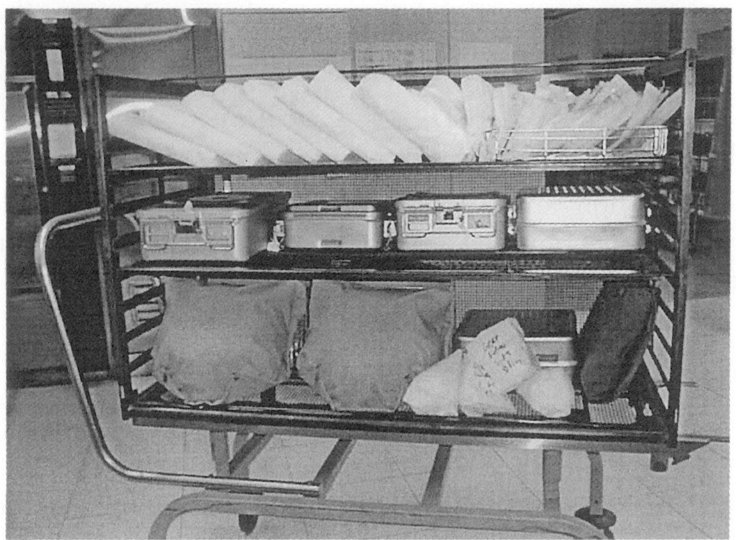

Fig. 6(c). Arrangement of items for sterilisation (loading procedure).

5.4. Loading

For effective sterilisation to occur, all surfaces of an item must come in direct contact with the sterilising agent. Arrangement of items in the steriliser chamber determines adequate contact with the sterilising agent. Placement of an item in a chamber is dependent on the material, the type of equipment employed, and the sterilisation method (Fig. 6(c)).

5.5. Unloading

Upon completion of the sterilisation process, the door of the steriliser is opened slightly (cracked). Opening of the door widely will allow cool air to enter the chamber, resulting in condensation. An item that is wet allows microorganisms to travel freely, thus making the item non-sterile. When the temperature in the chamber has cooled, the load is removed and the trolley is pushed directly into the storage area.

5.6. Storage

The load is allowed to cool further. The chemical indicators are checked to ensure that the items have undergone sterilisation. The sterile items are distributed and placed in a cool, clean, dry, low-humidity area (Fig. 6(d)).

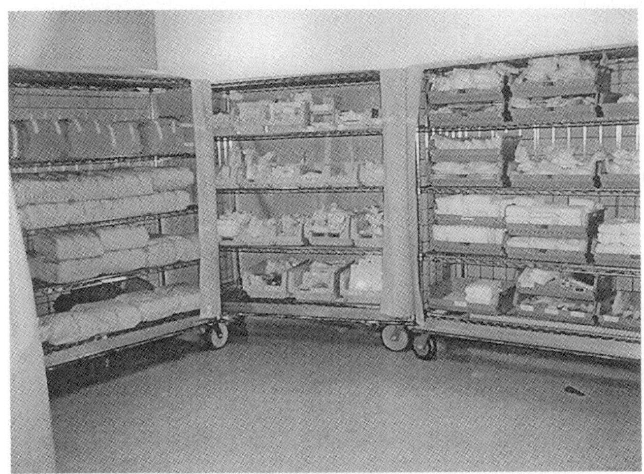

Fig. 6(d). Sterile storage area.

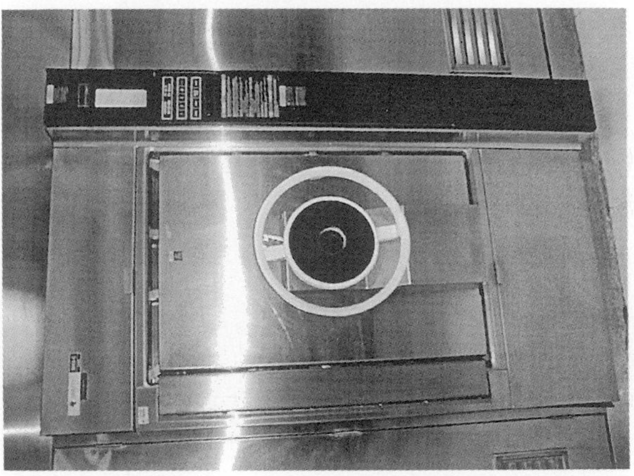

Fig. 7(a). Steam steriliser.

5.7. Sterilisation

Sterilisation can be classified into two groups — physical and chemical methods. Physical sterilisation includes steam and hot air (Figs. 7(a) and 7(b)). Chemical sterilisation methods include hydrogen peroxide, ethylene oxide, paracetic acid and glutaraldehyde

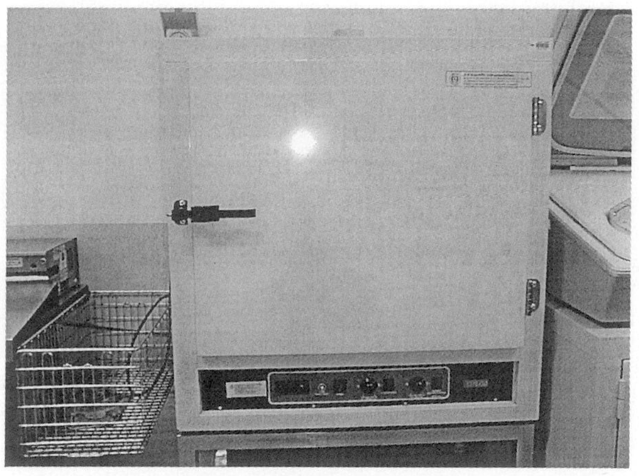

Fig. 7(b). Hot air steriliser.

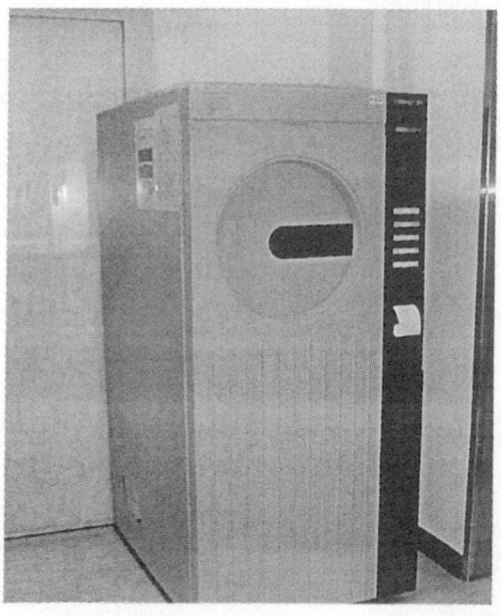

Fig. 8(a). Hydrogen peroxide steriliser (Sterrad).

(Figs. 8(a), 8(b), 8(c) and 8(d)). The description for each type of sterilisation method is displayed in Table 1.

It is the responsibility of TSSU to ensure that items sent out for use are sterile. Mechanical, physical and chemical monitoring of the

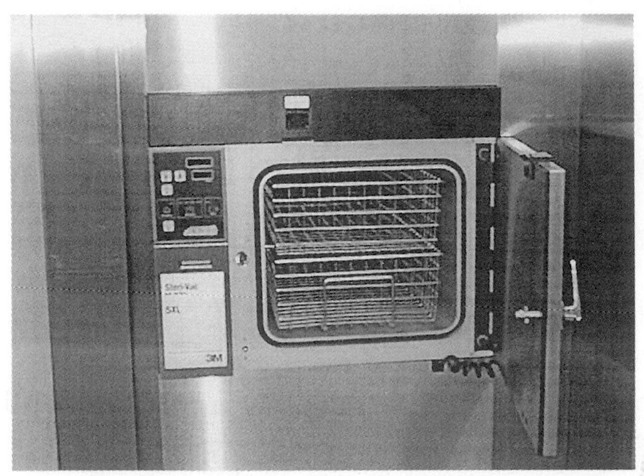

Fig. 8(b). Ethylene oxide steriliser.

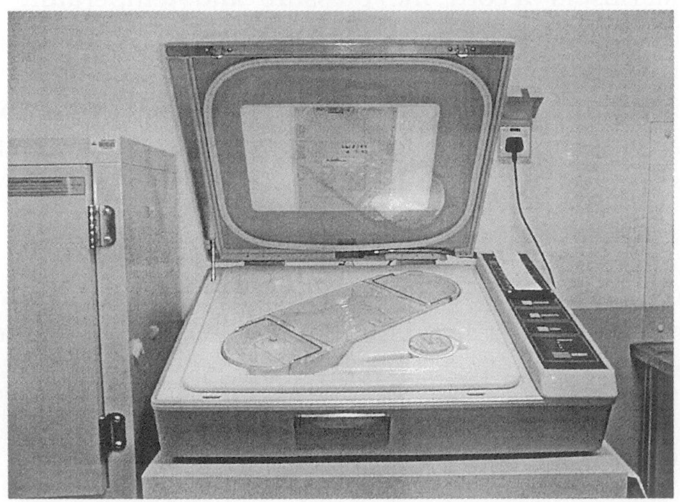

Fig. 8(c). Paracetic acid steriliser (Steris).

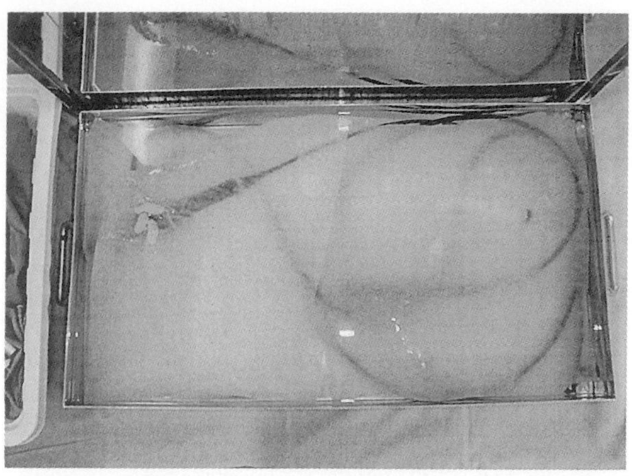

Fig. 8(d). Glutaraldehyde.

sterilisation process must fulfil the criteria fully before the items are considered sterile.

5.8. Mechanical monitoring

Modern sterilisers record the pressure and temperature at every stage of the sterilisation process. At the end of the sterilisation process, TSSU personnel will check the printout for correct pressure, temperature and exposure time. The printouts are filed for quality assurance. Mechanical monitoring is performed at every load.

5.9. Physical monitoring

TSSU and operating theatre personnel check the items for absence of wet load for steam-sterilised items. Items are discarded when discovered to be wet.

5.10. Chemical monitoring

Bowie Dick's test is performed daily to test the efficacy of steam sterilisers. Chemical indicator is placed on every item. TSSU personnel check for change in the colour of chemical indicators to confirm that the item has undergone the process of sterilisation.

5.11. Biological monitoring

Biological indicator is the ultimate test and gold standard to test the sterility of an item. For steam sterilisers, the vial is placed on the bottom shelf. For other types of sterilisers, it can be placed anywhere within the chamber. After the sterilisation, the vial is cracked, dated and placed in the incubator at a temperature of 37°C (ASP, 1998). A non-sterilised vial is cracked and marked "control". The results are read 24 to 48 hours later. The control will change colour, indicating growth of microbes whereas the sterilised vial is not affected, indicating conditions for sterilisation has been met.

6. Acknowledgements

- Ms. Lee Yee Kew, Director of Nursing, Nursing Department, National University Hospital.
- Ms. Tan Soh Chin, Senior Manager, Nursing Administration, Nursing Department, National University Hospital.
- Mr. Mohd. Osman bin Hussain, Registered Nurse, Physician Assistant.
- Ms. Ong Hong Yar, Senior Nursing Officer, Theatre Sterile Supply Unit, Operating Theatre Suite, Nursing Department, National University Hospital.
- Ms. Leow Chai Choo, Senior Nursing Officer, Operating Theatre Suite, Nursing Department, National University Hospital.
- Ms. Helen Goh, Nursing Officer, Infection Control Nurse, National University Hospital.
- Ms. Ho Swee Fook, Wendy, Nursing Officer, Central Sterile Supply Department, National University Hospital.
- Ms. Ong Ah Hua, Senior Lecturer, Nursing Division, Nanyang Polytechnic.

7. References

ADVANCED STERILIZATION PRODUCTS (ASP) (1998) *Sterrad Biological Indicator II: Instructions for Use*. Johnson & Johnson, USA.

ANSELL MEDICAL (1995) Reducing infection by disinfection and sterilisation. *Infection Control*, Issue 2, May, MediMedia Asia.

AORN (1996) Recommended practices for maintaining a sterile field. *AORN J.* **64**(5), 817–821.

AORN (1991) Recommended practices: Aseptic technique, *AORN J.* **54**(4), 819–824.

AORN (1994) Proposed recommended practices for chemical disinfection. *AORN J.* **60**(3).

AORN (1994) Proposed recommended practices for surgical attire. *AORN J.* **60**(2), 282–292.

AORN (1996) Recommended practices for traffic patterns in the perioperative practice setting. *AORN J.* **63**(3), 655–658.

AORN (1998) Recommended practices for environmental cleaning in the surgical practice setting. *AORN J.* **67**(2), 448–452.

AORN (1999) Recommended practices for standard and transmission-based precautions in the perioperative practice setting. *AORN J.* **69**(2), 404–411.

AORN (1999) Recommended practices for surgical hand scrubs. *AORN J.* **69**(4), 842–876.

ATKINSON, L.J. and FORTUNATO, N.H. (1996) *Berry & Kohn's Operating Room Technique*, 8th edn., Mosby, USA.

EARL, A. (1996) *APIC Infection Control and Applied Epidemiology: Operating Room*. Mosby, USA.

EDMISTON, C., SINSKI, S., SEABROOK, G., SIMONS, D. and GOHEEN, M. (1999) Airborne particulates in the OR environment. *AORN J.* **69**(6), 1169–1183.

GROAH, L. K. (1990) *Operating Room Nursing: Perioperative Practice*, 2nd edn., Appleton & Lange, USA.

GRUENDEMANN, B.J. (1992) *Hand Hygiene: A Manual for Health Care Professionals Professional Education & Services*. January, Johnson & Johnson Medical Inc., Arlington, Texas.

HARRISON, S.K., EVANS, W.J., LEBLANC, D.A. and BUSH, L.W. (1990) Cleaning and decontaminating medical instruments. *J. Healthcare Mat. Mget.* **8**(1).

HOLTON, J., RIDGWAY, G.L. and REYNOLDSON, A.J. (1990) A microbiologist's view of commissioning operating theatres, *J. Hosp. Infec.* **16**, 29–34.

HUMPHREYS, H. (1992). Microbes in the air — When to count!: The role of air sampling in hospitals. *J. Med. Microbiol.* **37**, 81–82.

J & J (1992) *FACTS: Glutaraldehyde and Ventilation Recommendations*. Johnson & Johnson Medical Inc., Arlington, Texas.

J & J (1992) *FACTS: Healthcare Workers Safety and Glutaraldehyde*. Johnson & Johnson Medical Inc., Arlington, Texas.

J & J (1992) *FACTS: Instrument Safety with Glutaraldehyde*. Johnson & Johnson Medical Inc., Arlington, Texas.

J & J (1994) *FACTS : Glutaraldehyde and Endoscopes*. Johnson & Johnson Medical Inc., Arlington, Texas.

J & J (1995) *FACTS: The Importance of Monitoring Glutaraldehyde Solutions During Reuse*. Johnson & Johnson Medical Inc., Arlington, Texas.

KOLB, D.A. (1984) *Experiential Learning: Experience as the Source of Learning and Development*. Prentice-Hall, New Jersey.

LANKTON, S. (1980) *Practical Magic: A Translation of Basic Neuro-Linguistic Programming into Clinical Psychotherapy*. Meta Publication, California.

LOEB, M.B., WILCOX, L., SMAIL, F., WALTER, S., and DUFF, Z. (1997) A randomized trial of surgical scrubbing with a brush compared to antiseptic soap alone. *AJIC* **Feb**, 11–15.

NUH (1991a) *Infection Control Manual: Sharps Injury and Body Fluid Exposure.* National University Hospital, Singapore.

NUH (1991b) Operating theatre policy. Environmental cleaning in the Operating Theatre Department (8.1). *Policy and Procedure Manual,* National University Hospital, Singapore.

NUH (1991c) Operating theatre policy. Perioperative safety measures in handling blood & body fluids (8.3). *Policy and Procedure Manual,* National University Hospital, Singapore.

NUH (1995a) Scrubbing, gowning and gloving. *Clinical Nursing Procedures* 7(2.2), National University Hospital, Singapore.

NUH (1995b) Operating theatre nursing standards: Draping technique. *Clinical Nursing Procedures* 7(2.3). National University Hospital, Singapore.

PAULSON, D.S. (1994) Comparative evaluation of five surgical hand scrub preparations. *AORN J.* **60**(2), 246–256.

RUTALA, W.A. (1996) APIC guidelines for infection control: APIC guideline for selection and use of disinfectants. *Am. J. Infect. Control* **24**(4), 313–341.

STERIS (1996) Sterile processing just in time. *Steris System1 Steris 20D Sterilant Operator Manual,* Steris Corporation, USA.

WYND, C.A., SAMSTAG, D.E. and LAPP, A.M. (1994) Bacterial carriage on the fingernails of OR nurses. *AORN J.* **60**(50), 796–804.

16 STERILE PROCUREMENT OF BONES AND LIGAMENTS

A. NATHER

NUH Tissue Bank, National University Hospital
5 Lower Kent Ridge Road
Singapore 119074

Abstract

Bones can be procured from:

- Living donors
- Deceased donors

In Singapore, as in most Asia Pacific countries, legally, consent is needed from the donor or next-of-kin. This follows the Medical Therapy, Education and Research Act of 1972.

In addition to obtaining consent for donating the tissue, the living donor must also give consent to allow blood to be taken for screening of HIV1, HIV2, hepatitis B, hepatitis C and syphilis. The patient is required to fill a separate consent form from the tissue bank incorporating agreement to donate tissues as well as consent for performing the laboratory serological testing.

With living donors, bones are procured sterile in the operating theatre.

With deceased donors, some tissue banks perform non-sterile, clean procurement in the mortuary. In this situation, one must note that the tissues must be procured within 12 hours of death if the body is not kept in a refrigerated room. However, if it is kept refrigerated at 4°C, procurement must be done within 24 hours.

In Singapore, sterile procurement from deceased donors is performed in the operating theatre. No procurement is performed from deceased donors in the mortuary.

1. Living Donor Procurement

1.1. Potential donors

Potential living donors include:

- Elderly patients with fracture neck of femur undergoing hemiarthroplasty
- Elderly patients with osteoarthritis of the hip undergoing total hip replacement
- Elderly patients with osteoarthritis of the knee undergoing total knee replacement
- Less commonly, patients with vascular ischaemia of the lower limb without infection undergoing above-knee amputation

One of the commonest bones procured is the femoral head from hemiarthroplasty for patients with fracture neck of femur. In Singapore, total hip replacement is not so commonly performed. In contrast, total knee replacement is commonly carried out for osteoarthritis of the knees. However, the bone slices obtained from TKR are not as good as the femoral head.

In NUH Tissue Bank, many TKR bone slices collected are not used. Surgeons prefer and ask for femoral heads instead. In order to save running costs of the bank, a policy was adopted to stop collecting TKR bone slices from August 1999. Only femoral heads are now collected from living donors.

1.2. Surgical instruments and other materials required

A separate sterile trolley must be prepared in the operating room where the living donor is being operated for collection of the procured bone. The trolley must have the following instruments and consumables:

- Kidney dish (2)
- Jug (1)
- Squirt (1)
- Bone nibbler small
- Blade holder and sterile surgical blade
- Dissecting forceps teeth
- Curved scissors Metezenbaun
- Normal saline
- Ampicillin
- Cloxacillin
- Sterile inner jar
- Sterile outer jar
- Sterile culture bottle (yellow cap)

1.3. Femoral head procurement

The technologist must change into hospital attire with cap, mask, theatre sandals and enter the operating theatre with sterile double jars, culture bottle and the Living Donor Form, Consent Form and Laboratory Investigation Form. The inner and outer sterile jars and a culture bottle are passed in sterile fashion to the scrub nurse to be placed on the procurement trolley. The surgeon performing the operation passes the femoral head removed after measuring its diameter for prosthesis sizing to the scrub nurse (Fig. 1). The latter flushes the bone with normal saline until all blood and fat globules have been washed away (Fig. 2). Next, a small piece of bone is nibbled from the neck of the femoral head to be sent for culture and sensitivity tests. The tissue is then soaked in a kidney dish containing 500 ml of normal saline with 500 mg each of ampicillin and cloxacillin.

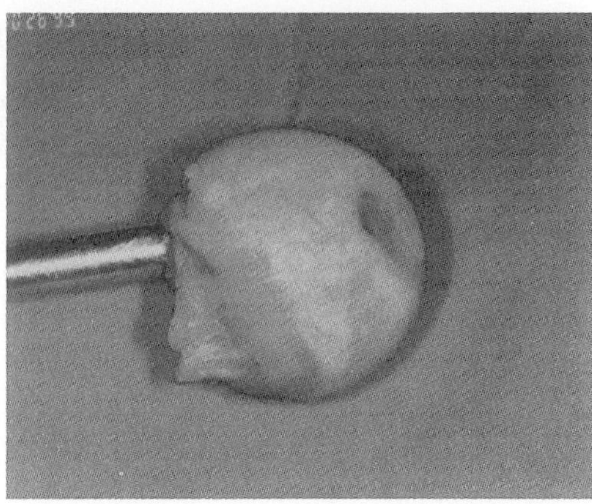

Fig. 1. Femoral head procured from patient removed with corkscrew instrument.

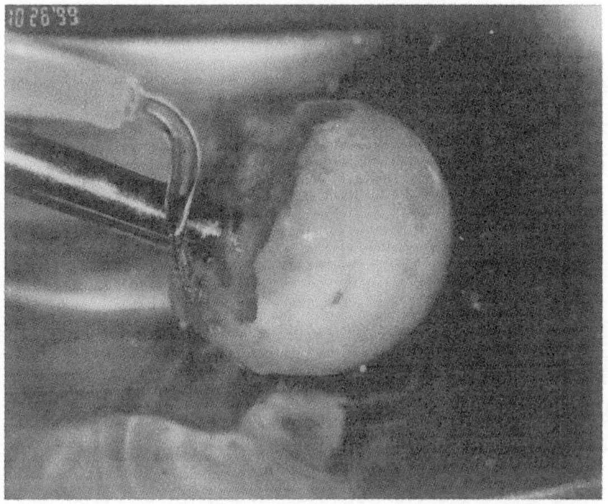

Fig. 2. Femoral head flushed with normal saline.

The femoral head is then placed inside the sterile inner jar and the jar closed with its lid. The inner jar is in turn placed into the sterile outer jar, closed and passed on together with the culture bottle to the tissue-bank technologist waiting to receive the specimen procured.

The technologist labels the sterile double jar (Fig. 3) and the culture bottle with the particulars of the patient using adhesive labels. The technician leaves the operating theatre with the double jar and the culture bottle. Upon returning to the tissue bank, the double jar is immediately stored in the "Quarantine Freezer" or in the "Quarantine Section" of the deep freezer at a temperature of −80°C (Fig. 4). The culture bottle is sent as soon as possible to the Department of

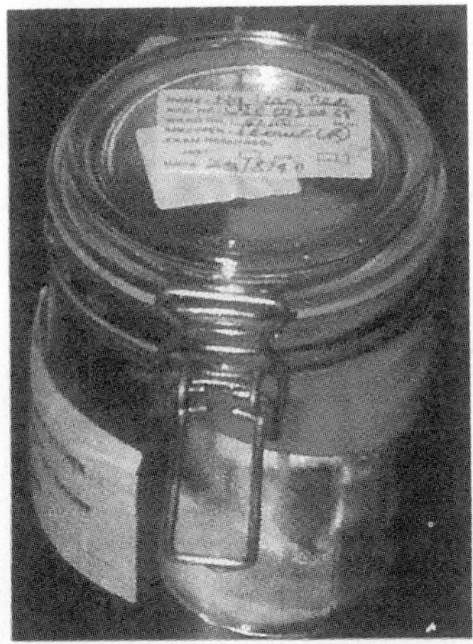

Fig. 3. Femoral head in sterile double jar.

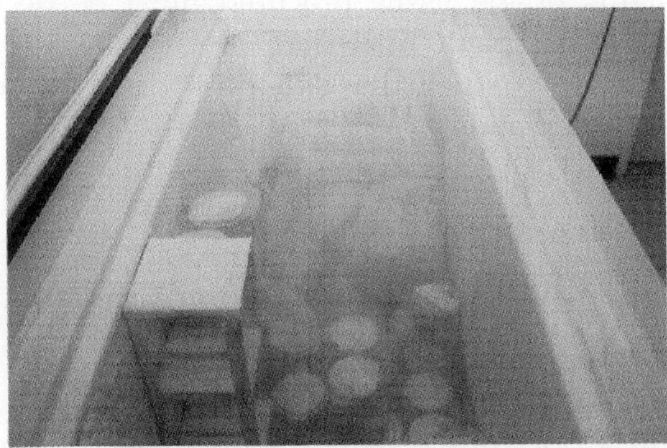

Fig. 4. Double jar placed in "Quarantine Section" of deep freezer (−80°C).

Laboratory Medicine for culture and sensitivity tests for both aerobic and anaerobic organisms.

1.4. Documentation

The technologist must document each tissue procurement with meticulous detail and accuracy using the Living Donor Form which must include the following details:

- Date of operation
- Donor number
- Donor particulars (name, identification number sex, age, etc.)
- Type of tissue procured
- Name of surgeon
- Name of hospital/ward number
- Medical history
- Test results
- Status of tissue procured
  - Awaiting results
  - Ready for use
  - To be discarded

The results of all laboratory serological tests, including culture and sensitivity results, must be accurately recorded in the Living Donor Form. The status of the tissue procured must be decided by the director of the tissue bank.

The Consent Form of the living donor must also be properly filled for proper documentation.

2. Deceased Donor Procurement

2.1. Multi-organ and tissue procurement system

In Singapore, bone procurement from deceased donors is part of a multi-organ and tissue procurement system coordinated by the Ministry of Health. Under this system, the organs and tissues procured include kidneys, liver, heart, cornea and bones. The programme is coordinated by a National Transplant Coordinator who is responsible for approaching the donor or his relatives for the necessary consent for procurement and for performing all the laboratory screening tests — blood grouping, HLA typing, anti-HIV1 and anti-HIV2, HbsAg, anti-HCV, RPR (TPHA) and anti-CMV.

All potential donors with sudden but known causes of death are approached. All consenting donors usually agree to donate both kidneys. Only 10 to 20% of consenting donors also agree to donating bones. In these cases, the consent form indicates the limb or limbs from which the bones and ligaments could be procured.

Upon receiving consent, the National Transplant Coordinator activates the various teams concerned to perform the procurement. With bone procurement, the National Transplant Coordinator informs the NUH Transplant Coordinator, who in turn activates the NUH Tissue Bank to assemble the bone procurement team immediately.

2.2. Bone procurement team

The bone procurement team consists of at least two orthopaedic surgeons, two residents and three technicians. Wherever possible, the director himself is the leader of the team (orthopaedic surgeon). When the director is not available, the deputy director (another orthopaedic surgeon) will lead the team.

Upon activation by the NUH Transplant Coordinator for donor procurement, the manager of the bank alerts the director and all members of the procurement team. The orthopaedic surgeons and residents are provided by the Department of Orthopaedic Surgery in the National University Hospital.

2.3. Surgical instruments and other materials required

2.3.1. Surgical instruments

- Major orthopaedic surgical instrument set containing:

Artery forceps	Dissecting forceps teeth
Straight kockers	Dissecting forceps lane

Curved scissors Metezenbaun
Nurses scissors
Needle holders
Sponge holders
Towel clips
Blade handles No. 4
Bone rongeur small
Bone hook kocker
Gigli saw holders

Lengenback retractors
Mollision self-retaining
Weitlaner self-retaining
Bone levers
Periosteal elevators
Hibbs osteotome
Bone rongeur Olivercrona
Mallet
Gigli saw blades

- Major cleansing set containing:

  Basin (1)
  Kidney dish (4)
  Gallipots (5)
  Jug (1)
  Squirt (1)

- Powered Portable Osteotome (electric-driven)

2.3.2. Consumable items

- Disposable sterile surgical gowns
- Disposable sterile surgical drapes
- Sterile penny towels
- Sterile raytex gauze
- Sterile surgical blades (size 21)
- Sutures 1-0 coated vicryl, 1-0 Dexon or 1-0 Mersilk
- Primapore dressings
- Povidone-iodine solution
- Hibiscrub solution
- Sterile normal Saline
- Ampicillin
- Cloxacillin
- Sterile cotton bandage
- Sterile double jars (inner jar and outer jar)
- Sterile triple wraps

    — sterile polyethylene bags
    — sterile cotton tapes
    — sterile linen wrappers

- Sterile culture bottles (yellow cap)
- Sterile surgical gloves
- Surgical aprons
- Disposable sterile scrub brushes
- Head caps
- Surgical masks
- Masking tape
- Permanent fine point marker
- Adhesive labels for labelling specimens

Where the donor is not in NUH and is in another hospital, the NUH ambulance is booked immediately for transportation of staff and instruments and equipment.

2.4. Bone procurement system

The tissue bank is fully equipped with operating instruments, trolleys, sterile disposable gowns, sterile disposable drapes and all consumables for performing sterile procurement of bones and ligaments from the deceased donor.

Following all procedures spelt out in detail in the Procedure Manual, the NUH Tissue Bank at any one time has all the necessary equipments and consumable items ready to be transported immediately to any hospital for procurement from one deceased donor.

One major orthopaedic surgical instrument set including a powered portable osteotome, a major cleansing set and two trolleys are ready for mobilisation — already autoclaved and ready for use.

All consumable items are also ready for use — pre-packed in polylite containers — sterile disposable drapes, sterile disposable gowns, sterile gloves, sterile penny towels and Raytec gauze, sterile disposable blades, povidone-iodine solution, normal saline solution and vials of ampicillin and cloxacillin.

Following the Procedure Manual, all sterile double jars, sterile linen, autoclaved cotton tapes and sterilised polyethylene bags as well as sterile culture and sensitivity bottles have also been pre-packed in polylite containers ready to be used. The normal protocol is to have ready at any one time all containers, bags and culture bottles to receive specimens from two lower limbs. This is because the majority of donors give consent for procurement from both lower limbs. Occasionally, consent is given for procurement from one lower limb and one upper limb. On two occasions, consent is given to donate "all bones" from the donor. Operating within the confines of a multi-organ and tissue procurement system, time is the limiting factor. The kidney team procures the vital organs first, followed sometimes by the liver team. The cornea team goes next and the bone procurement team is the last to operate on the donor. It is given a maximum of two hours to complete all its procurement procedures. Even if the donor consents to give all bones, it is usually wise to restrict procurement from two lower limbs only. In addition, when a donor pledges two lower limb,s to save time and to perform the procurement efficiently, two surgical teams will scrub up and operate on the patient simultaneously, each team consisting of a surgeon, a resident and a technician.

The tissue bank also has ready all items required for proper reconstruction of the limbs to be operated upon. These include plastic bones (femur, tibia), sutures and primapore dressings.

Adhesive labels are prepared beforehand to help more efficient labelling of the large number of specimens which will be retrieved during the procurement. This preparation is started upon activation of the tissue bank team as soon as all laboratory test results of the donor have been received and the procurement confirmed. Donor number, date of procurement and type of tissue procured are typed on each adhesive label.

3. Plan For Procurement of Tissues

This is also clearly spelt out in the Procedure Manual. Deceased donors are very scarce. It is very important to procure tissues in the best planned manner to maximise the possible utilisation of tissues obtained from one deceased donor. It is wasteful to procure the whole femur as one bone. The femur is procured as three specimens — the femoral head, a proximal half and a distal half. The tibia is likewise to be procured in two portions — a proximal half and a distal half. The patella tendon is procured in two longitudinal halves for two recipients. Likewise, the calcaneum tendon is also procured in two longitudinal halves. Other soft tissues procured include the tibialis anterior and tibialis posterior tendons. A large piece of the iliac crest is also procured from each iliac wing.

4. Bone Procurement Itself

All procurement staff must change their attire into theatre attire, including theatre caps, masks and surgical boots or surgical sandals.

The two trolleys, one containing the major orthopaedic surgical instrument set and the other containing the major cleansing set are prepared by the tissue-bank technicians (who have been trained in sterile technique and in nursing procedures).

The surgeons and the residents scrub up for the operation, wear sterile gowns and double pairs of sterile gloves.

Each technician lifts the lower limb by the toes for cleansing. Each surgeon cleanses one lower limb with povidone-iodine solution from the hind foot all the way to the groin and including the iliac crest region. Each limb is then carefully draped using disposable sterile drapes. The foot is then wrapped with sterile linen and then placed on the draped operating table. The technicians then scrub up to join the two surgical teams.

5. Operative Procedure for Lower Limbs

A midline vertical incision is made over the front of the lower limb (A) from the middle of the groin above to the middle of the ankle joint below (Fig. 5).

The incision is deepened using sharp blades to reach the deep fascia which is then incised. Every member of each team is clearly

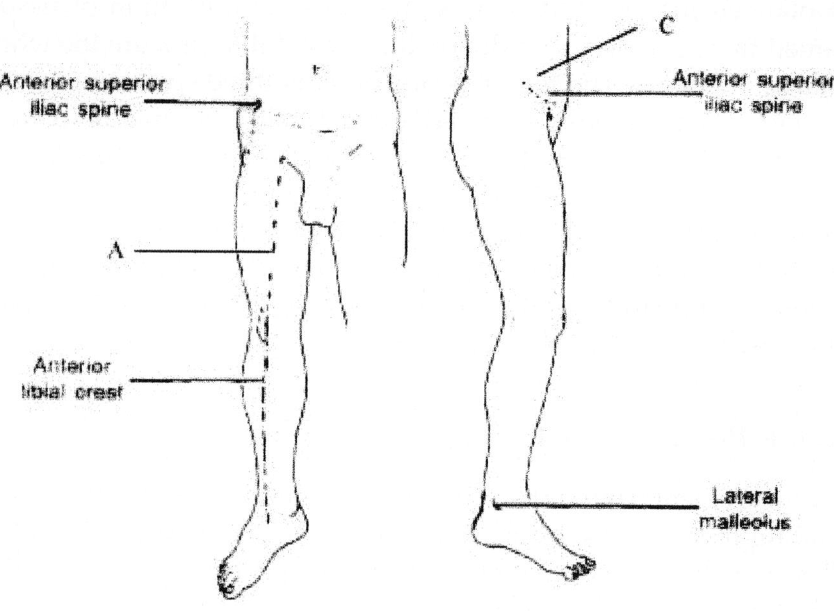

Fig. 5. Incision made over front of thigh and leg (A). Incision made over curved iliac crest (C).

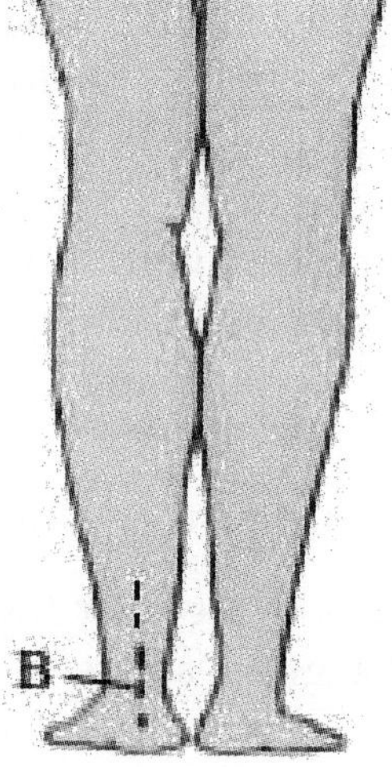

Fig. 6. Incision made over back of heel (B).

reminded before starting as to the importance of using "no touch technique" to avoid accidental injuries occurring to any member of the surgical team. This means that during the operation, no one is allowed to touch or hold any tissue with fingers — to avoid being accidentally cut by the surgeon. An instrument must be used instead when there is a requirement to hold any tissue.

The key to easy procurement of bones in the lower limb is to operate on the knee joint first. The patella-tendon–tibial-tuberosity complex is procured first (Fig. 7). The portable electric-powered osteotome is used to split the patella and the tibial tuberosity into two equal halves.

This is best done *"in situ"* instead of dissecting the patella tendon completely first and then splitting the free patella tendon into two halves (medial and lateral halves). After the longitudinal splits in the bones using the powered osteotome, the split in the tendon is completed using a large surgical blade. The patella tendon is then dissected completely free to be removed for collection.

The menisci are not procured. The medial and lateral collateral ligaments are divided at the joint line. Only after this dissection could

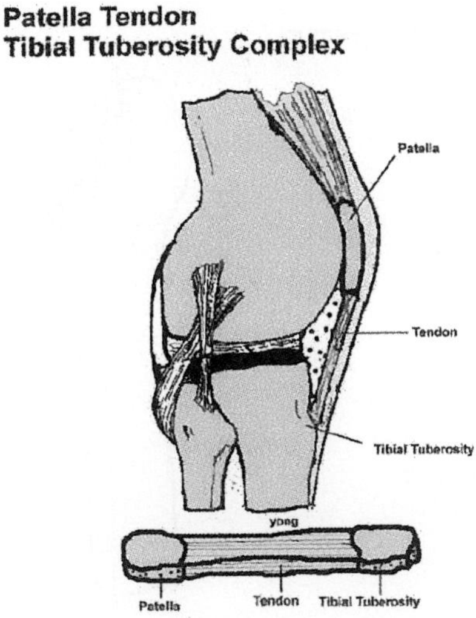

Fig. 7. Patella-tendon–tuberosity complex.

the articular lower end of the femur be delivered out easily. Using a periosteal elevator and sharp knife dissection, all muscles are stripped off the surface of the femur. Sharp knife dissection is especially required to free the soft tissues from their attachment to the thick linea aspera posteriorly.

At the upper end, the ligamentum teres is divided and the femoral head dislocated from the acetabular socket.

Using the portable electric-driven osteotome, the femoral head is cut at the base of the neck and the femoral shaft osteotomised in the middle to give an upper and a lower half (Figs. 8 and 9). The three specimens of the femur are then removed for collection.

Below the knee, the dissection in the leg is likewise deepened to the deep fascia. The muscles are likewise stripped off the tibia and fibula bones using the periosteal elevator and sharp knife dissection.

The key to dissection in the leg is first to remove the fibula intact as one bone by disarticulation at the proximal tibio-fibular joint above and cutting the interosseous ligament between the tibia and the fibula below as well as the calcaneo-fibular ligament inferiorly. The fibula is then removed and retrieved as one bone (Fig. 10).

Proximal Femur

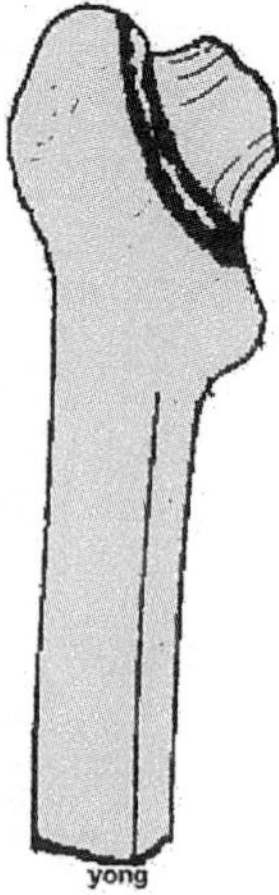

Fig. 8. Proximal femur.

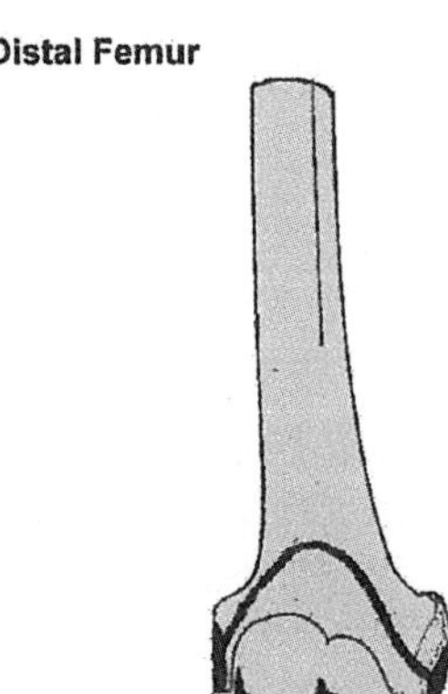

Fig. 9. Distal femur.

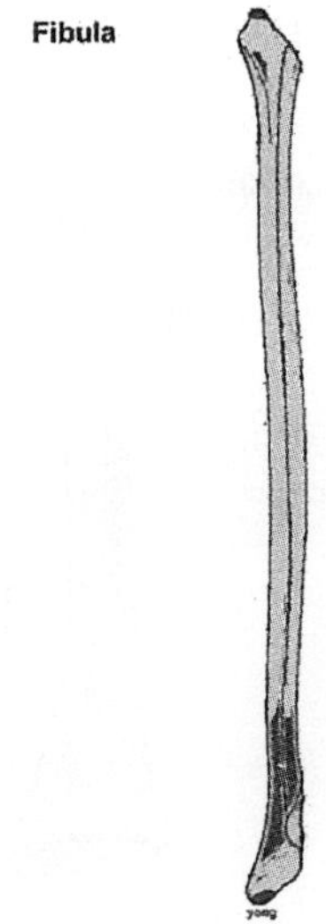

Fig. 10. Fibula.

Once the fibula has been excised, it is then easy to remove the tibia. The tibia is osteotomised into two halves for collection (Figs. 11 and 12).

A small incision is then made posteriorly to expose the calcaneum (B) (Fig. 6). The tendinous part of the tendo-achilles is excised in

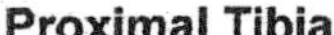

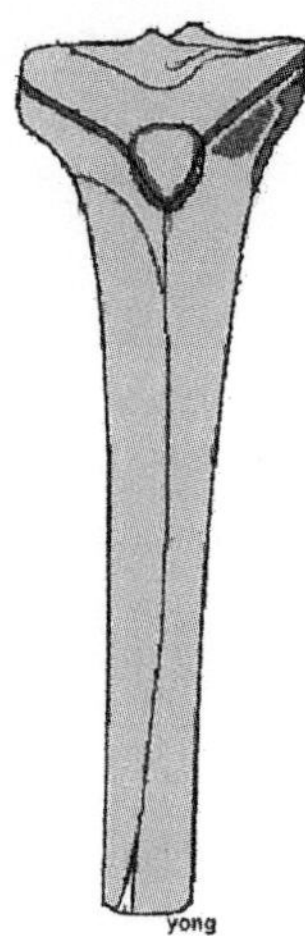

Fig. 11. Proximal tibia.

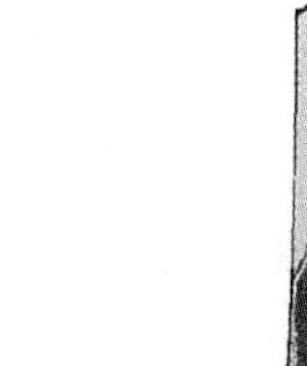

Fig. 12. Distal tibia.

continuity with a large piece of the calcaneum tendon (Fig. 13). This is first split into two longitudinal halves, as for the patella tendon, for collection as two specimens.

Other soft tissues are procured at this stage. In the thigh, a large rectangular piece of fascia lata about 24 cm × 6 cm is procured. In

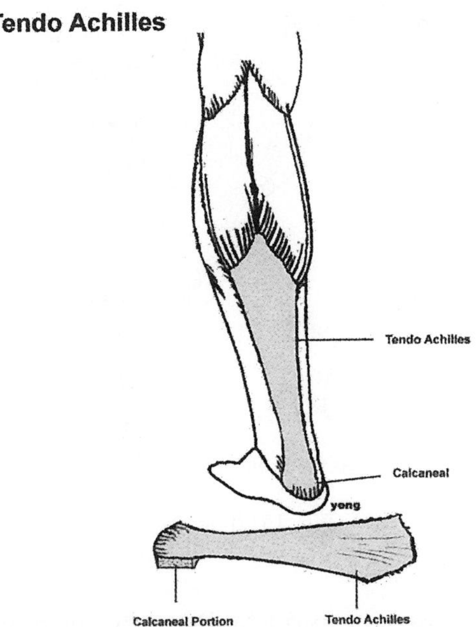

Fig. 13. Calcaneum tendon.

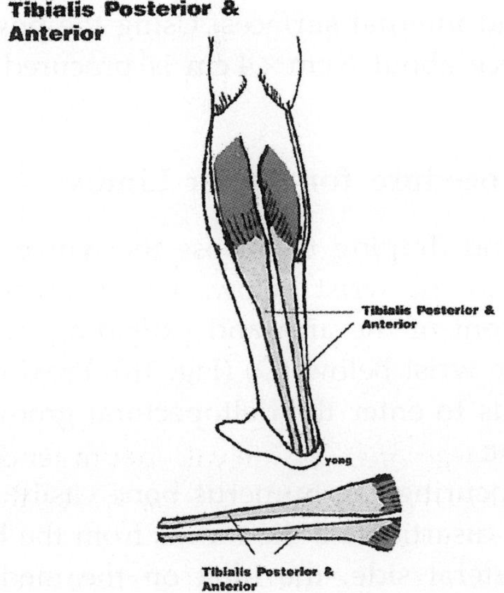

Fig. 14. Anterior and posterior tibialis tendons.

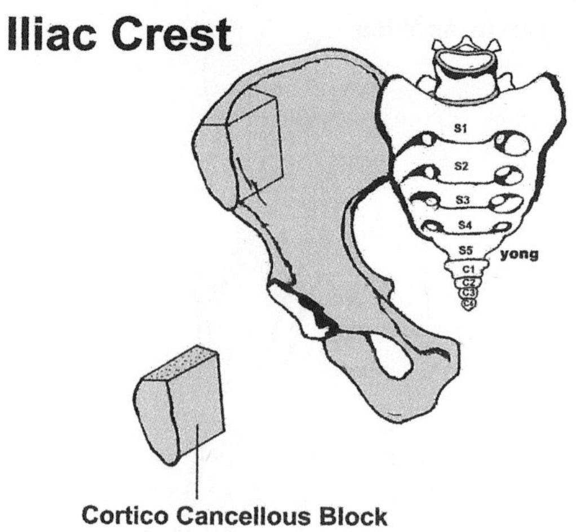

Fig. 15. Iliac crest.

the leg, the tibialis anterior and tibialis posterior tendons are procured (as long a tendon as possible) (Fig. 14).

A separate curved incision is made over the crest of the iliac wing (C) (Fig. 5). The iliac bone is exposed, stripping the muscles on its external and internal surfaces. Using the powered osteotome, a rectangular piece about 6 cm × 4 cm is procured (Fig. 15).

6. Operative Procedure for Upper Limbs

After cleansing and draping to expose the whole upper limb from the axilla above to the wrist below, a vertical midline incision is made over the front of the arm and extending over the middle of the forearm to the wrist below (D) (Fig. 16). Proximally, the incision is curved upwards to enter the deltopectoral groove to the front of the shoulder joint.

The key to procuring the humerus bone easily is to first dissect the ellow joint to disarticulate the radius from the humeral articular surface on the lateral side, the ulna on the medial side and the olecranon from the humeral articular surface posteriorly.

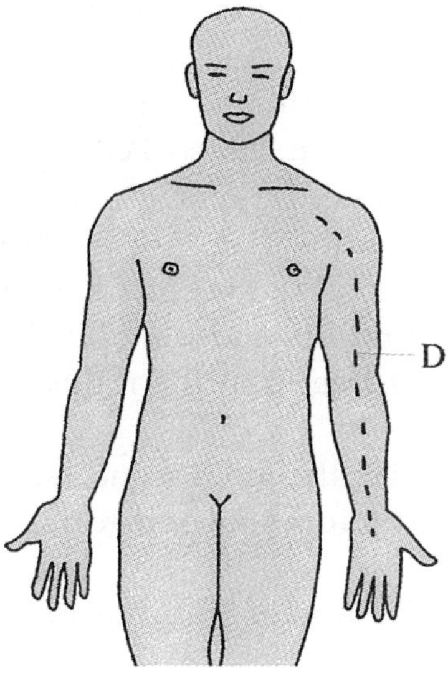

Fig. 16. Incision made over the front of the arm and forearm (D).

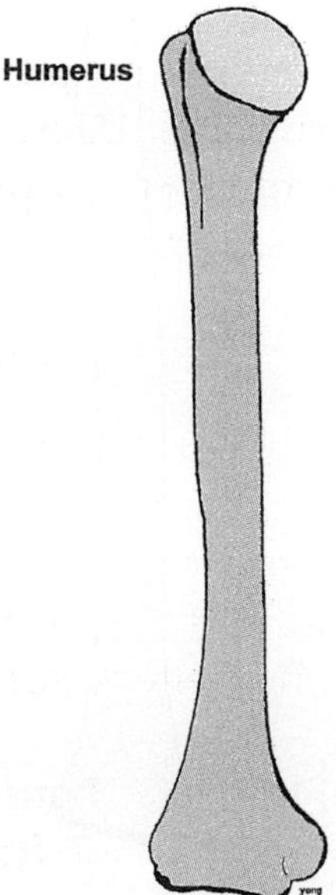

Fig. 17. Humerus.

The humeral bone (Fig. 17) is then delivered readily. All muscles and soft tissues are Proximally, the capsule of the shoulder joint is cut to leave a cuff attached to the neck of the humerus and the humeral head dislocated from the socket (glenoid articular surface of the scapula) of the shoulder joint.

In the forearm, the radius (Fig. 18) is dissected free from the ulna (Fig. 19) at the proximal radio-ulnar joint and the interrosseous membrane between the radius and ulna bone incised. Likewise, all soft tissues are dissected free from the radius and ulnar surfaces in similar fashion.

At the level of the wrist, the inferior radio-ulnar joint is dissected. The capsule of the wrist joint is incised to free the radius and ulna bones.

All three bones in the upper limb are procured as whole bone specimens.

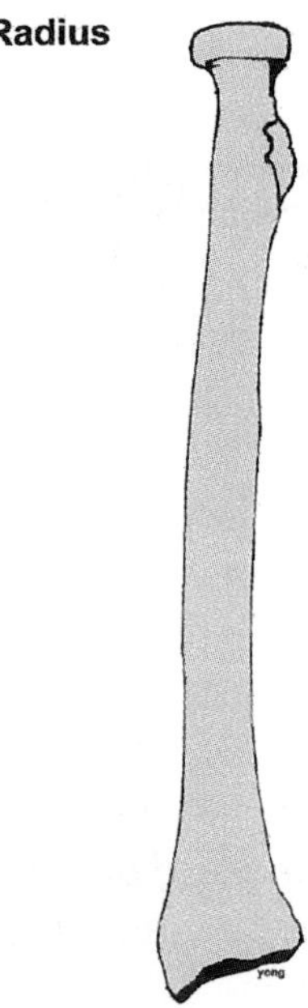

Fig. 18. Radius.

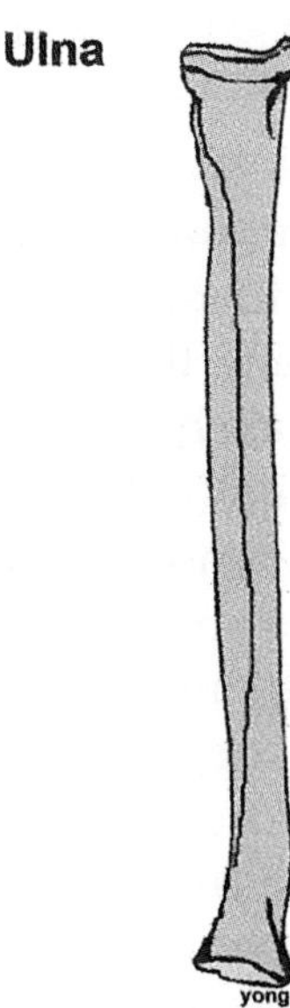

Fig. 19. Ulna.

Usually consent is not obtained to extend the incision into the palm and therefore, usually flexor tendons could not be procured.

7. Specimen Collection

The director or the manager of the tissue bank is responsible for this very important role to ensure that specimens are collected in the most sterile and organised fashion and that they are also labelled correctly.

This is done on a separate sterile trolley containing the major cleaning set. Specimens are received in kidney dishes on the trolley. Each specimen, including the long bones and the smaller specimens, are flushed with copious amounts of sterile normal saline. After thorough cleaning, a small piece of tissue is obtained from each specimen and placed in a small bottle for culture and sensitivity tests. The specimen is then soaked in a wash basin containing a solution of two litres of sterile normal saline with four vials each of ampicillin and cloxacillin (2 grams each).

After soaking in the antibiotic solution for about 10 to 20 minutes, the smaller specimens — femoral heads, patella-tendons, calcaneum tendons, tibialis anterior and tibialis posterior, tendons and fascia lata are collected in sterile jars using the "sterile double jar-technique" as is used for collection of small bones from living donors.

A sterile metal ruler is first used to measure the length of the tendinous part of the patella-tendon and the calcaneum tendon, and also the lengths of the tibialis anterior and tibialis posterior tendons. The length and breadth of all long bone specimens are also measured and documented. This is meticulously and accurately documented by the third technician who does not scrub for the operation. The role of this technician is to receive the collected specimens in their proper containers and to label them properly and correctly using the adhesive labels already prepared beforehand.

The large specimens, femur, tibia, iliac crest are collected using the "sterile triple-wrap technique" — inner polyethylene bag, a middle linen-wrap tied with two sterile cotton tapes and an outer polyethylene bag (Figs. 20–22).

All specimens are labelled immediately to avoid mistakes, including the culture bottles accompanying each specimen and stored in the polylite container. Care is taken to make sure that each

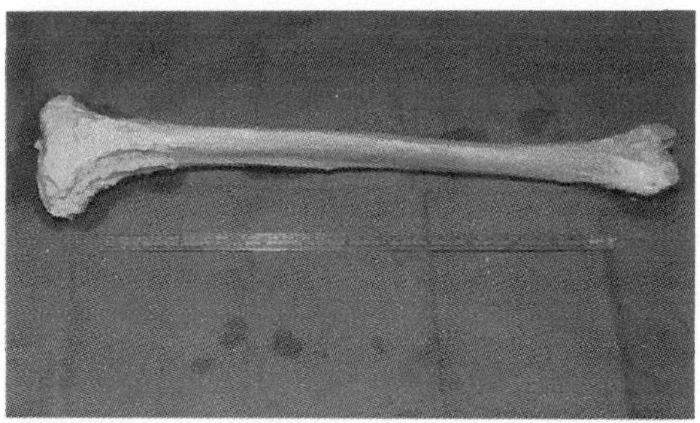

Fig. 20. Tibia specimen being measured with a ruler.

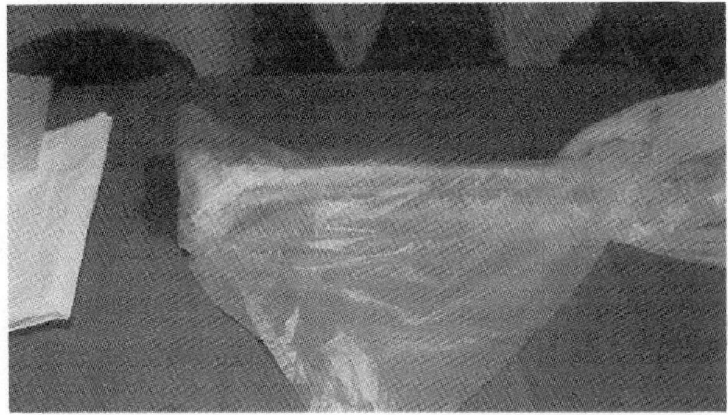

Fig. 21. Tibia placed in first layer of triple wrap — a sterile polyethylene bag.

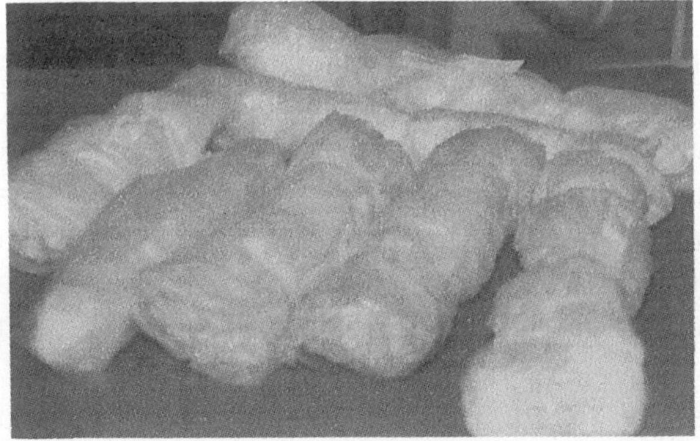

Fig. 22. Long bones procured from a single, deceased donor using sterile triple wrap technique.

specimen is accompanied by a corresponding culture bottle containing tissue from that specimen.

8. Reconstruction

8.1. Lower limb

Upon completion of retrieving the last specimen from each lower limb — usually the iliac crest, reconstruction of both lower limbs is

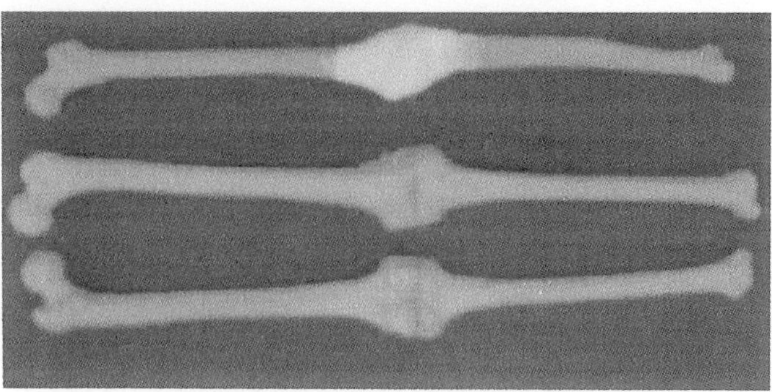

Fig. 23. Reconstruction is done using a plastic femur and plastic tibia arthrodesed at the knee with plaster of Paris.

begun. A plastic femur and a plastic tibia arthrodesed at the knee by two rolls of four inches of plaster of Paris is used (Fig. 23). The length of this construct may have to be trimmed using the powered osteotome to ensure a snug fit. The tissues in the incision are then closed in two layers, the muscles and fascia lata with 1-0 prolene or 1-0 vicryl and the skin stitched with 1-0 prolene using a well-knitted running stitch. The wounds are then dressed with primapore dressings.

Care must be taken that all bleeding has stopped and that a clean dressing remains.

8.2. Upper limb

For reconstruction, plastic humerus, and radius and ulna bones are used. The soft tissues are again closed in two layers, the muscles and fascia lata with 1-0 coated vicryl or 1-0 prolene and the skin with similar suture using a well-knitted running stitch. Primapore dressing is then applied over the whole incision wound.

It is important to procure tissues in a manner which shows the utmost respect for the deceased donor. Every cadaveric body must be treated with respect. In the case of a deceased donor, we must take further into account the good deed he has done by donating tissues.

It is therefore very important to reconstruct the limb as best as can be done to give a cosmetically acceptable reconstructed lower limb to allow for open casket funerals.

At the end of the procurement, the leader of the team should thank the relatives who are usually waiting outside the operating room chanting prayers with the Buddhist monk whilst waiting to start funeral procedures. (All donors in Singapore are Buddhists.)

9. Transportation of Procured Tissues

Upon completion of procurement, all specimen bottles and culture bottles are immediately transported back to the tissue bank. The specimen bottles are stored in the "Quarantine Freezer" or in the "Quarantine Section" of the freezer immediately, whilst the culture bottles are immediately dispatched to the Department of Laboratory Medicine where the culture and sensitivity for aerobic and anaerobic organisms will be performed.

10. Documentation

Each specimen is documented using a separate Donor Form (Deceased Donor Form). All results including the culture and sensitivity tests must be meticulously and accurately recorded in each form. A copy of the consent form must be properly filed for proper documentation.

Detailed documentation must be carried out using the Deceased Donor Form which must include the following information:

- Donor number
- Donor particulars (name, identification number, sex, age)
- Date of death
- Cause of death
- Name of hospital/ward number
- Medical history
- Serological test results
- Details of tissue procurement (date, time, surgeons, residents, technicians)

- Description and size measurements of allograft
- Status of tissues
  — Awaiting quarantine
  — Ready for use
  — To be discarded

The status of the tissue must be decided by the director of the tissue bank.

11. Procedure in the Event of Personnel Accident

- Upon an accident in which the technologist suffers from fresh cuts or abrasion during processing, the technologist should immediately rinse the wound thoroughly under running water, wash the wound with povidone and then dress the wound with a bandage.
- If the wound is large, the technologist is brought to the Accident & Emergency section of the hospital where a debridement, and toilet and suture are done. The technologist will be given a course of antibiotics in addition to injection of the tetanus toxoid.
- The technologist must be tested for the following:
  — Anti-HIV$_1$ and Anti-HIV$_2$
  — HbsAg
  — Anti-HCV
  — RPR (TPHA)

The tests are repeated at six-monthly intervals up to 18 months.

12. Acknowledgements

The author would like to record his gratitude to Mr. S.C. Yong for drawing all the illustrations, and also Dr. Wang Lihui and Mrs. D.P. Vathani for the secretarial assistance provided.

17 STERILE PREPARATION OF TISSUE GRAFTS DURING TRANSPLANTATION

A. NATHER

NUH Tissue Bank, National University Hospital
5 Lower Kent Ridge Road, Singapore 119074

1. Introduction

As allograft transplantation is increasingly used by more orthopaedic surgeons, it is important to ensure that surgeons know how to
use the bone and soft tissue allografts. Professional education is
required regarding the proper indications for allograft transplantation, the biological and biomechanical behaviour of different types
of processed allografts and the preparation procedures required for
different types of processed tissues before they can be transplanted.
Surgeons must be made to understand that it is only by paying
meticulous attention to such detail that good clinical outcomes could
be obtained with tissue transplantation and the complications that
would otherwise result from such transplantation could be minimised or avoided.

2. Reception of Tissue Allografts For Transplantation

All allografts received from the tissue bank must be carefully checked
before use. The donor number, graft number, description of type of
graft and expiry date must be closely scrutinised. The condition of

the jars for "double-jar" deep-frozen specimens must be checked to ensure that the jars are not broken and sterility not already breached. With "triple-wrap" deep-frozen specimens, the integrity of the outer plastic layer must be carefully inspected. In the case of freeze-dried specimens, the polyethylene packing must be closely scrutinised for loss of vacuum (with vacuum-sealed specimens) or for minute cracks or tears in the outermost plastic layer. The latter indicates a breach of sterility. Furthermore, the cerric-cerrous dosimeter must be verified to be red in colour indicating that gamma irradiation sterilisation has indeed been performed. Instructions accompanying all specimens sent by the tissue bank must also be carefully read and complied with.

3. Donor and Recipient Teams During Tissue Transplantation

To maintain proper discipline in using the allografts, there must be a donor team which receives and prepares the graft on a donor trolley specially draped and reserved for this purpose. The donor team should be headed by a surgeon, at least a registrar and assisted by a resident. This team is responsible for carrying out all preparations for the tissue graft in a sterile manner before the allograft is ready to be passed to the recipient team for transplantation. The recipient team is headed by the consultant in charge of the recipient.

4. Preparation For Tissue Allografts

Different preparation techniques are required for different types of tissue allografts which has been processed differently — small deep-frozen bone allografts, large cortical deep-frozen allografts, cryopreserved osteoarticular allografts, freeze-dried bone allografts and deep-frozen soft tissue allografts.

4.1. Small deep-frozen bone allografts

The femoral head in the "sterile double jar" is taken out of the freezer and allowed to thaw for at least one hour before the start

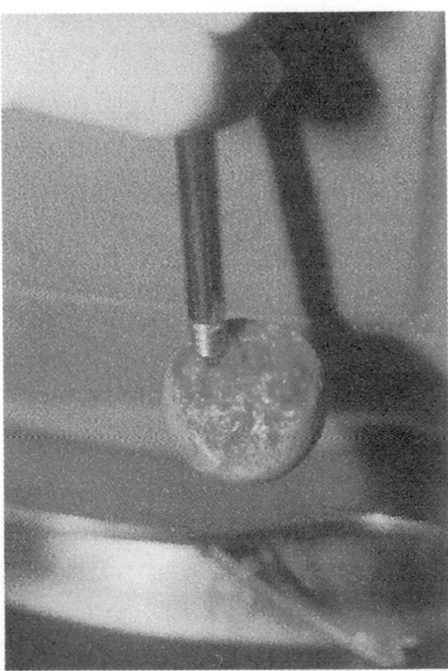

Fig. 1. Femoral head held with a corkscrew transferred to a kidney dish containing normal saline for thawing.

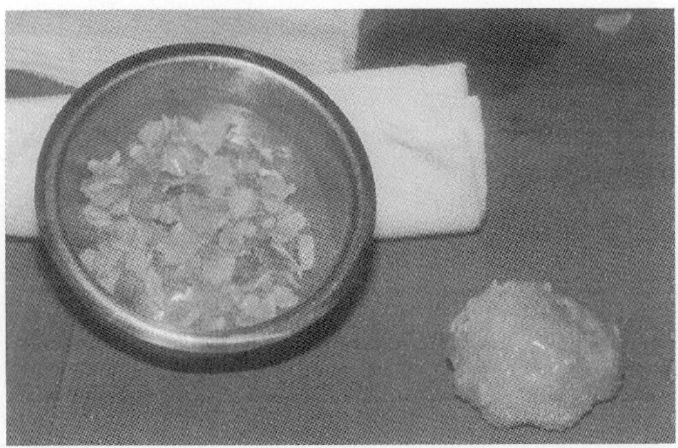

Fig. 2. All cartilage nibbled off from the femoral head. The cartilage pieces to be discarded are contained in the gallipot and the denuded femoral head is on the right side of the picture.

of the operation. The circulating nurse opens the lid of the outer jar without contaminating the inner jar and passes the sterile inner jar to the scrub nurse. The scrub nurse then opens the lid of the inner jar and removes the allograft. This is transferred into a kidney dish containing normal saline with 500 mg of ampicillin and 500 mg of cloxacillin placed on a separate sterile trolley specially draped for preparation of the allograft (Fig. 1) by the donor team. Using a bone nibbler, the surgeon or his assistant meticulously removes all cartilage from the femoral head (Figs. 2 and 3). It is extremely important to remove all cartilage since cartilage left behind will impair proper bone fusion and incorporation. All soft tissues must also be removed from the bone. Using a manual osteotome, the femoral head is then cut into small pieces (Fig. 4). As oscillating saw could also be used for this purpose. The bone pieces are then flushed with normal saline using jet lavage to remove all blood and fat globules (Fig. 5). A swab is taken and sent for culture and sensitivity testing (Fig. 6). The bone pieces are then soaked in another kidney dish containing 500 ml of normal saline and 500 mg of ampicillin and 500 mg cloxacillin for about 30 minutes. (For patients allergic to penicillin, 500 mg of erythromycin is used instead.)

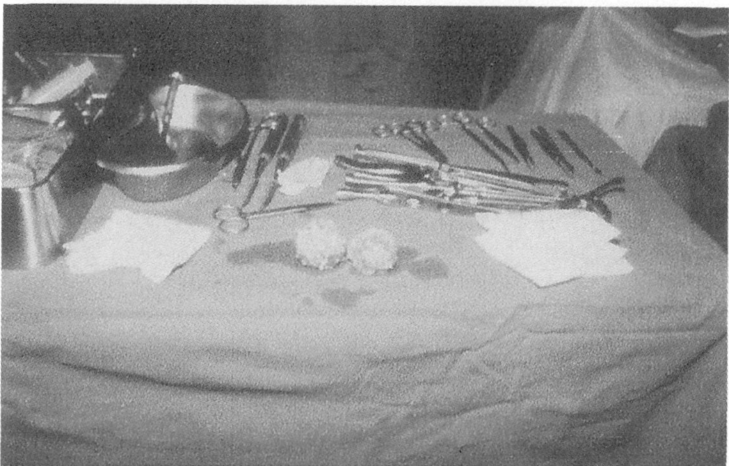

Fig. 3. Two femoral heads denuded of cartilage on the donor trolley.

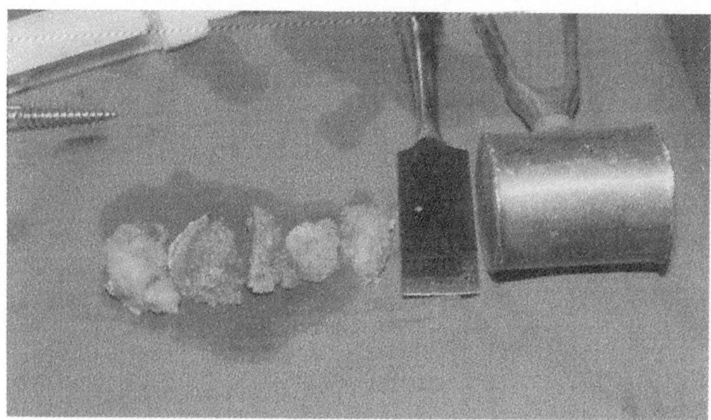

Fig. 4. The femoral head osteomised into small pieces using a manual osteotome.

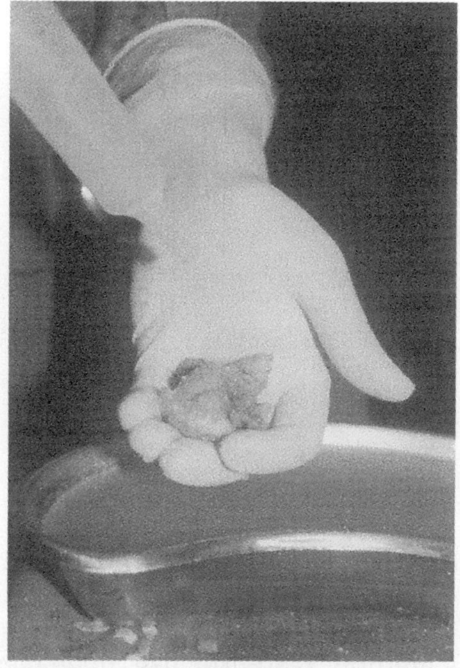

Fig. 5. The small pieces are flushed with sterile normal saline. The blood and fat globules removed in this lavage could be seen in the kidney dish holding the effluent wash.

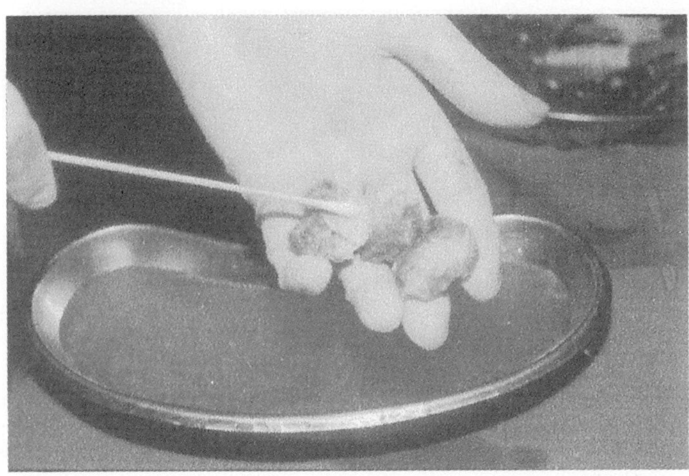

Fig. 6. A swab is taken from the washed grafts for culture and sensitivity testing.

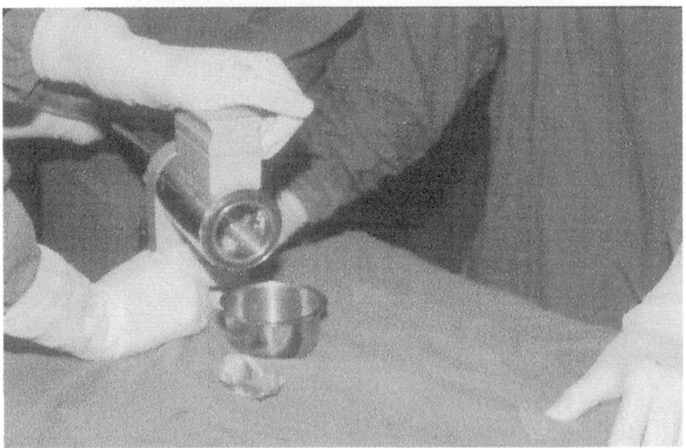

Fig. 7. Grinding the bone pieces into smaller pieces using a sterile bone mill.

The bone grafts are now ready for use. If smaller bone pieces are required, the bone pieces are then ground into smaller pieces using a sterile bone mill (Fig. 7). On the recipient side of the operation, at the start of operation, the recipient is given a prophylactic dose of

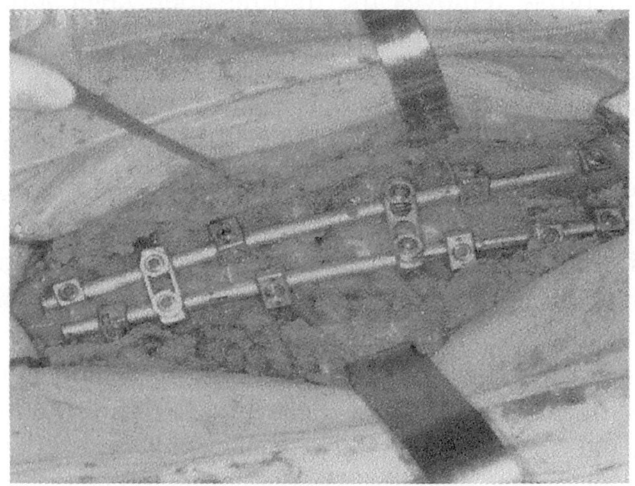

Fig. 8. Bone grafts from two femoral heads inserted in the fusion bed on either side of implant used for correction of scoliosis in a 12-year-old girl.

1 g of cefazoline intravenously. A redivac drain is usually inserted into the operation site before closure of the wound. For scoliosis cases (Fig. 8), no drain is inserted. Post-operatively, the patient is continued on intravenous cefazoline (1 g) six-hourly for 48 hours. This is then followed by oral antibiotics — ceporex (500 mg) six-hourly for two weeks until the wound has healed completely. (Cyclosporin C is not used.)

4.2. Long bone, deep-frozen allografts

The long bone in the "sterile triple wrap" stored at −80°C must be taken out of the freezer and allowed to thaw for at least one hour before the start of the operation. The circulating nurse opens the outermost plastic layer without contaminating the sterile middle linen layer and passes the bone wrapped with middle linen layer and inner plastic layer to the scrub nurse. The latter places the graft on a separate trolley draped separately for preparation of the graft by the donor team.

The scrub nurse removes the middle linen layer and the inner plastic layer and soaks the long bone in a basin containing two litres of normal saline. Amounts of 1 g of ampicillin and 1 g of cloxacillin powder are added to this solution. After further thawing for half an hour, the surgeon preparing the transplant places the bone on a sterile towel and dissects all soft tissues and periosteum from the bone. This is done meticulously using sharp cuts with a scalpel and further stripping using a periosteal elevator. At the ends of the bone, tough small parts of the periosteum are removed using a bone nibbler. Upon completion of this procedure, the bone is washed with sterile normal saline. It is extremely important to remove all periosteum and soft tissues since these are the tissues that render the allograft immunogenic.

The cleaned bone is then placed on a sterile towel and the required portion of the bone (intercalary) is marked with sterile methylene blue dye to mark the two sites for the osteotomy (Fig. 9). The osteotomies are then made using an oscillating saw (Fig. 10). The large intercalary segment cut is then manually reamed using a manual reamer to remove all marrow contents from its medullary canal (Fig. 11). This must also be done meticulously as the marrow

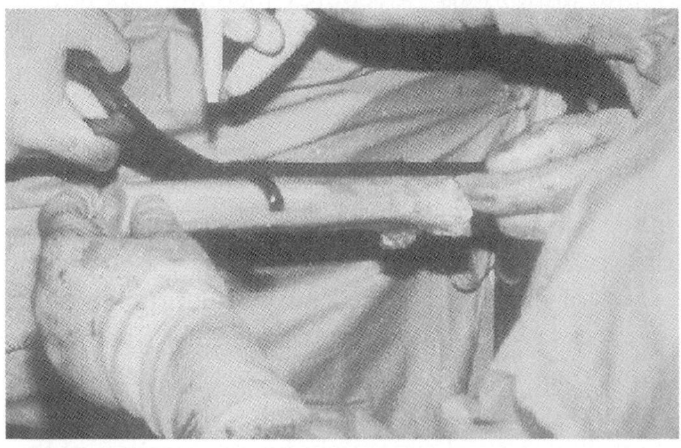

Fig. 9. Marking one osteotomy site with sterile methylene blue.

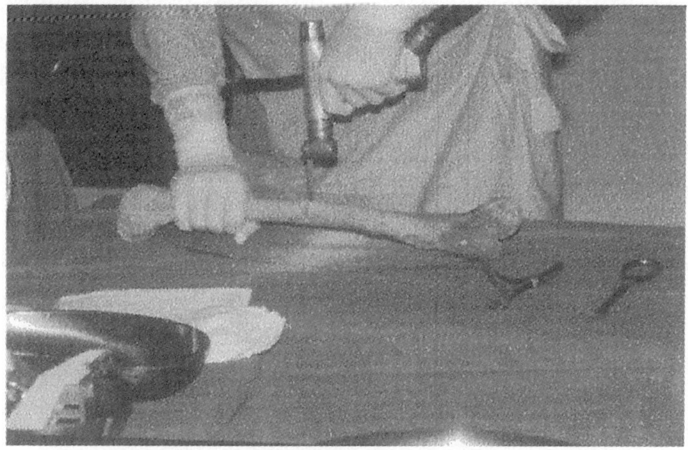

Fig. 10. Osteotomising the long bone using an oscillating saw.

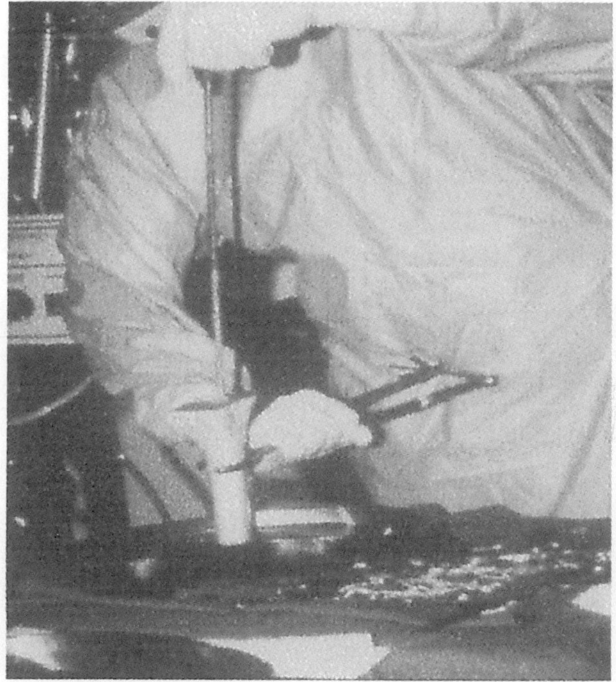

Fig. 11. Reaming the medullary canal of the long bone segment with a manual reamer.

is the most immunogenic part of the deep-frozen allograft. Upon completion of the reaming, jet lavage is done using normal saline to ensure that all marrow contents have been totally flushed out.

The cut bone allograft specimen is then finally soaked in a kidney dish containing one litre of normal saline (Fig. 12) with 500 mg of ampicillin and 500 mg of cloxacillin (Fig. 13) for at least 30 minutes.

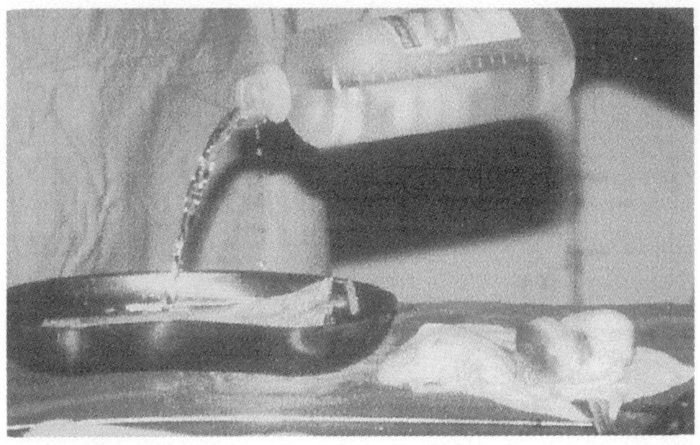

Fig. 12. Prepared allograft placed into new kidney dish and one litre of normal saline is poured.

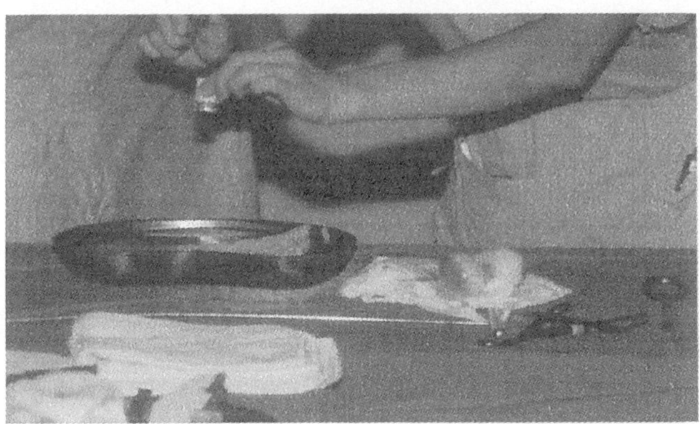

Fig. 13. Antibiotics powder being added to this solution.

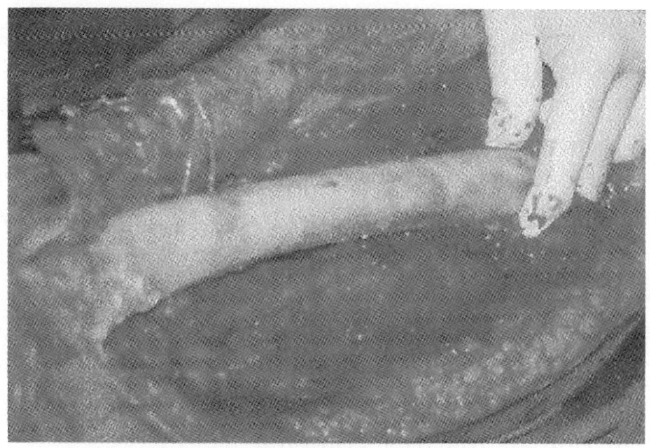

Fig. 14. Prepared intercalary allograft being placed into defect in a patient after resection of osteogenic sarcoma of the patient's femur.

The intercalary bone allograft is now ready for use by the recipient team (Fig. 14). The same antibiotic regime described for the use of small deep-frozen bone allografts is used. A drain must be inserted before closure of the wound. The same post-operative antibiotic regime is used. (Cyclosporin C is not used.)

4.3. Cryopreserved, osteo-articular allografts

The long bone in the "triple wrap" cryopreserved at −160°C with 10% glycerol used as cryoprotectant for the articular surface of the long bone must likewise be taken out of the freezer and be allowed to thaw for at least one hour before the start of the operation. In a similar fashion, the circulating nurse removes the outer plastic layer and hands the graft to the scrub nurse who places it on a special trolley reserved for preparation of the graft by the donor team.

The scrub nurse removes the remaining two layers and washes the articular end of the bone with running sterile normal saline until the gauze wrapping the end with 10% glycerol could be removed. The bone is then also soaked in a basin containing two litres of normal saline with antibiotics as described in the preparation of long bone deep-frozen allograft. After soaking for another 30 minutes, the bone allograft is placed on a sterile towel and a similar dissection of all soft tissues and periosteum from the bone is meticulously performed. The bone is again washed with sterile normal saline.

The cleaned bone is again placed on a new sterile towel and the site for osteotomy in the diaphysis of the bone is marked with sterile methylene blue. The osteotomy is then made using an oscillating saw.

Taking care not to damage the articular cartilage at the end of the bone, a manual reamer is used gently to ream out marrow contents of the diaphysis. The reaming must not enter the distal one inch of the end of the bone where the articular surface is. Jet lavage is again used to flush out all marrow contents.

The bone is then soaked in a kidney dish containing 500 ml of normal saline with antibiotics for at least 30 minutes before it is ready for use by the recipient team for transplantation.

4.4. Freeze-dried bone allografts

With cortical freeze-dried allograft (Fig. 15), the outer layer is removed by the circulating nurse and the graft contained in the sterile inner polyethylene layer is passed to the scrub nurse who places it

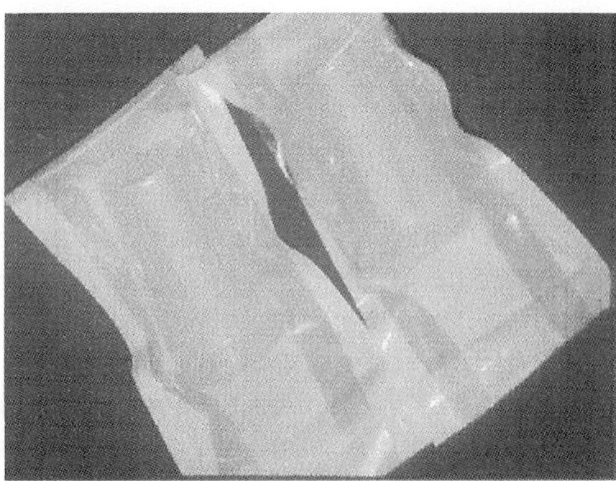

Fig. 15. Cortical femoral ring lyophilised allografts used for anterior spinal reconstruction.

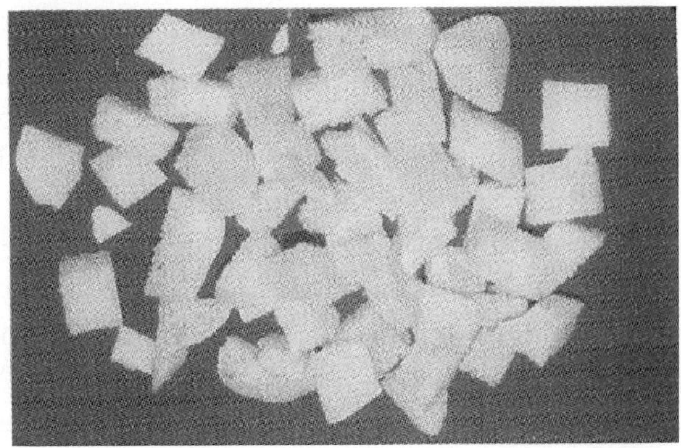

Fig. 16. Cancellous femoral head lyophilised chip allografts used for packing small bone cavities.

on the donor preparation trolley. The graft is soaked in a kidney dish containing 500 ml of sterile normal saline and 500 mg of ampicillin and cloxacillin for about one hour before use. The exact length of the graft is cut using an oscillating saw by the donor team.

With small cancellous freeze-dried chip allografts (Fig. 16) it is best not to rehydrate the grafts for more than ten minutes before they are used. Rehydration is done using the sterile normal saline containing antibiotics. Our experience showed that prolonged rehydration in such cases weakens the grafts substantially. It is not uncommon to find that the grafts have turned into powder if they were left to be re-hydrated for more than one hour. Some surgeons prefer to use such grafts without rehydration. The serum from the recipient bed is sufficient to rehydrate such grafts.

4.5. Deep-frozen, soft tissue allografts

Tibialis posterior and anterior tendons, patella tendons, calcaneal tendons and fascia lata are processed deep-frozen at −80°C without gamma irradiation and stored in "sterile double jars".

The same procedure is used in their preparation as for small deep-frozen bones. The graft is allowed to thaw for at least one hour before the start of the operation. The circulating nurse passes the inner sterile bottle to the scrub nurse who then soaks the graft in a kidney dish containing 500 ml of sterile normal saline, and 500 mg of ampicillin and 500 mg of cloxallin on the donor preparation trolley. Using tooth forceps and dissecting scissors, all the fats and other soft tissues are meticulously dissected to leave only the tendon for use by the surgeon. The graft is then flushed with normal saline and finally soaked into a clean kidney dish containing sterile normal saline with 500 mg of cloxacillin and 500 mg of ampicillin for at least 30 minutes. It is now ready for use by the recipient team.

In the case of fascia lata, several tissue forceps are clipped to the edges of the sheet to spread the fascia over an inverted kidney dish (Fig. 17) to allow dissection of all fats from the fascia. After completion of the dissection, the graft is rolled tightly using two artery forceps held at each end (Fig. 18). Upon completion of rolling this tissue, the solid tubular graft is maintained in this configuration by stitching the free end using a running stitch of 3-0 Dexon (Fig. 19).

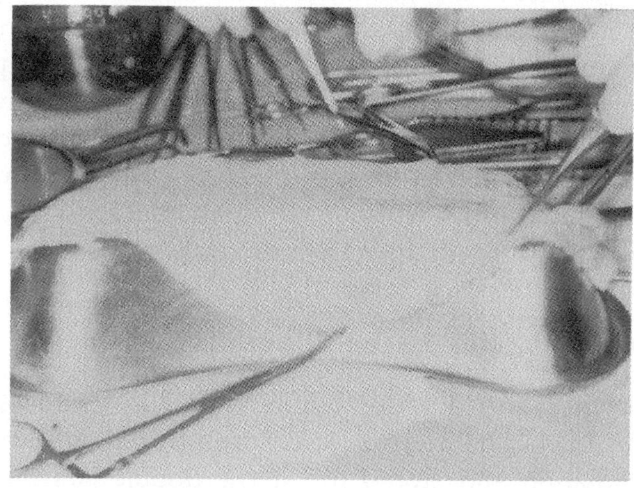

Fig. 17. Fascia lata held by tissue forceps at various edges and spread over an inverted kidney dish for dissection of all fats from its surface.

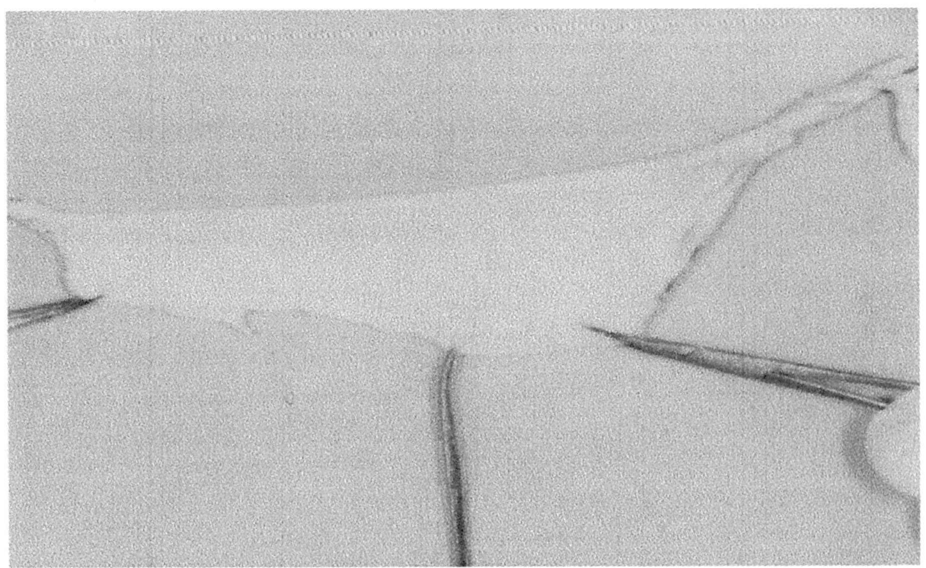

Fig. 18. Fascia lata gripped by an artery forceps at each end rolled to form a solid tube.

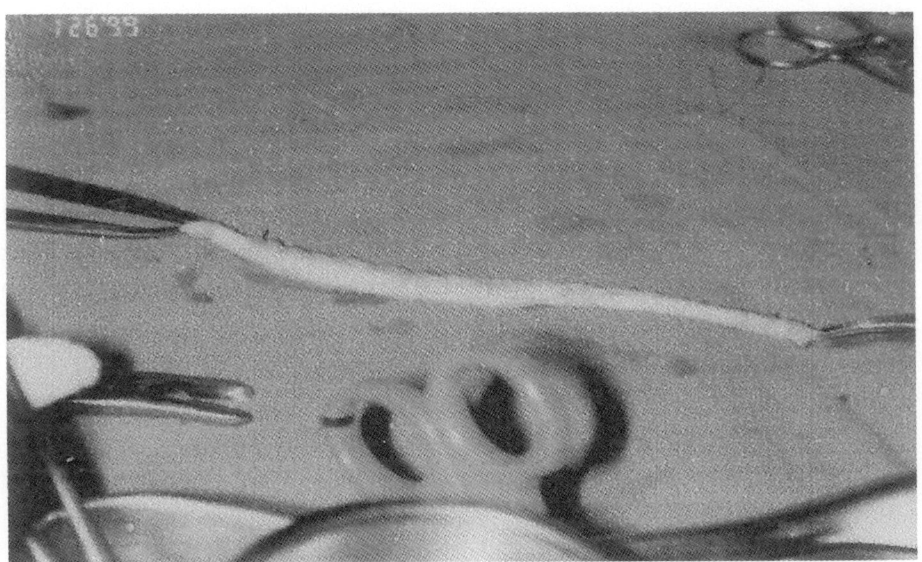

Fig. 19. Fascia lata roll or "tendon" stitched with running 3-0 Dexon.

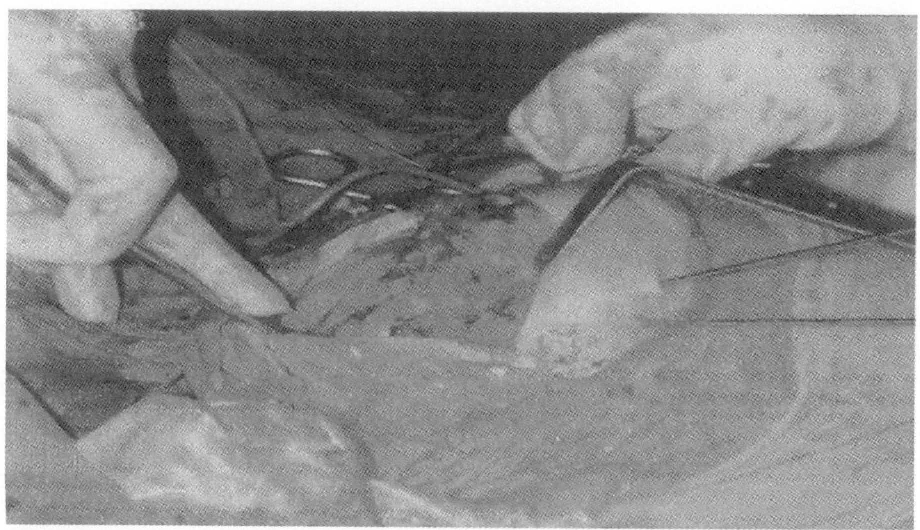

Fig. 20. Fascia lata used as a "figure of eight" sling for reconstruction of acromic-clavicular dislocation of the shoulder

The fascia lata "tendon" is then ued for reconstruction (Fig. 20). This gives increased strength to an otherwise weak sheet of fascia.

5. Acknowledgements

The author would like to thank Mr. S.C. Yong for all the technical assistance provided, Mr. B.K. Tan and Mr. S.S. Moorthy for excellent photography, and Mrs. D.P. Vathani and Dr. Wang LiHui for the secretarial assistance provided.

SECTION V:

RADIATION SCIENCES

Advances in Tissue Banking Vol. 5
© 2001 by World Scientific Publishing Co. Pte. Ltd.

18 RADIATION SCIENCES

KHAIRUL ZAMAN HAJI MOHD DAHLAN

Radiation Processing Technology Division
Malaysian Institute for Nuclear
Technology Research (MINT)
Bangi, 43000 Kajang, Selangor, Malaysia

1. Introduction to Ionising Radiation

Ionising radiation is defined as radiation that has sufficient energy to dislodge electrons from atoms and molecules and to convert them to electrically-charged particles called ions. Further reactions of these species, ions and electrons, give rise to the formation of free radicals that are usually highly reactive, which eventually lead to chemical reactions. The study of chemical changes in the system that is produced by absorption of ionising radiation is known as radiation chemistry.

1.1. Types of ionising radiation

1.1.1. Electromagnetic radiation

There are two types of ionising radiations, i.e. electromagnetic radiation and high-energy charged particles. Figure 1 shows the series of electromagnetic radiation that comprises radiowaves, microwaves, visible light, ultraviolet, X-rays and gamma-rays. However, only

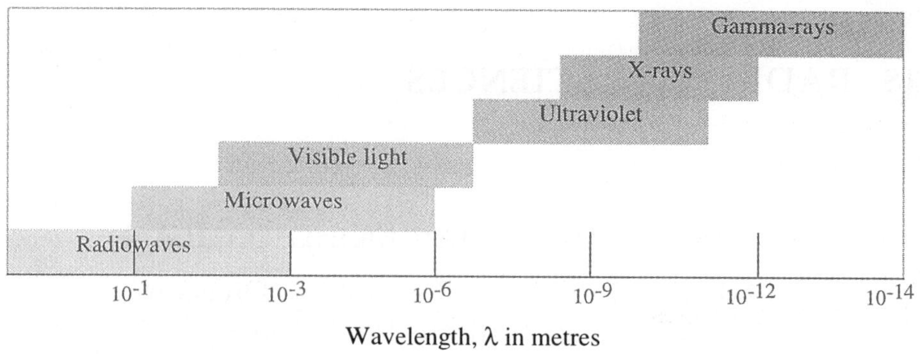

Fig. 1. Series of electromagnetic radiation.

X-rays and gamma-rays which have short wavelengths and energy ($E = hc/\lambda$) of higher than 50 eV are capable of ionising atoms and molecules. Therefore, X-rays and gamma-rays have the same properties and effects on materials. However, the origins of X-rays and gamma-rays are different. X-rays are generated from machines and gamma-rays are emitted from radioisotopes.

Electromagnetic radiation of longer wavelength, e.g. ultraviolet, may initiate chemical changes in the system not via ionisation but via electronically excited species. This is called photochemistry.

In photochemistry, each photon (light) excites only one molecule. By using monochromatic light, it is possible to produce a single, well-defined excited state in a particular component in the system.

In radiation chemistry, each photon or particle can ionise or excite a large number of molecules, which are distributed along its track.

1.1.2. High-energy charged particles

High-energy charged particles can be negatively charged or positively charged. They can be generated by machines, such as electrons from electron accelerator and H, He, Ar, C and positron from ion beam accelerator. However, high-energy charged particles can also be obtained from radioisotopes such as beta particles — β (electron), and alpha particles — α (helium). Unlike X-rays and gamma rays, charged particles have limited penetration power. They can be stopped by a substrate such as paper. However, increasing the energy of the particles from a few keV to MeV can increase the penetration power of charged particles. Beam current of charged particles can vary from a few µA to several mA. High current will increase the number of charged particles and hence increase dose rate. Since charged particles have sufficient energy to ionise atoms and molecules, their chemical effects are the same as X-rays or gamma-rays.

1.2. Source of ionising radiation

Ionising radiation can be obtained from two different sources, such as radioisotopes and electrical discharge machines. The most common radioisotopes used commercially are cobalt-60 and caesium-137. Both of these radioisotopes are gamma (γ) emitters. Other sources of ionising radiation are electron accelerator, X-ray machine and positively-charged particle accelerator or ion beam accelerators.

1.2.1. Radioisotopes

Radioisotopes, which are also known as radioactive isotopes or radionuclides, occur naturally. They can also be produced artificially in a nuclear reactor. Radioisotopes are unstable elements which have excess of neutrons or protons in their nuclei and emit radiation — alpha, beta, gamma (α, β, γ) as they spontaneously disintegrate or decay to a stable state. The time taken by radioisotopes to decay to half the level of radioactivity originally present is known as its half-life, and is specific for each radioisotope of a particular element. The decay scheme of radioisotope such as cobalt-60 is shown in Fig. 2.

Cobalt-60 and caesium-137 are the industrial sources of gamma radiation which have different half-lives as shown in Table 1. They

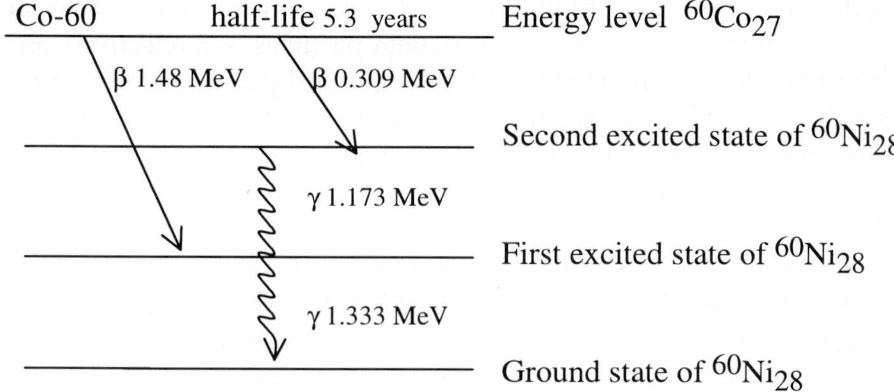

Fig. 2. Decay scheme of radioisotopes, cobalt-60.

Table 1. Radioisotopes — Radiation sources.

Source	Half Life (Year)	Type of Radiation	Energy of Radiation (MeV)
^{60}Co	5.27	β	0.341
		γ	1.332
		γ	1.173
^{137}Cs	30	β	0.520
		γ	0.662

are generally housed in lead cells (also known as gamma cells) or in concrete cell with walls of a few metres thick. Cobalt-60 is the most popular industrial source of gamma radiation due to its higher energy of radiation compare to caesium-137. It is used for sterilisation of medical products, herbs, cosmetic items and pharmaceutical raw materials, for food irradiation, decontamination of sewage sludge and waste water, vulcanisation of rubber latex and other applications where the greater penetration of gamma radiation is an advantage.

1.2.2. Electron accelerator

Electron accelerators are generally the preferred radiation source for curing or crosslinking of polymeric-based materials, such as plastic films, heat-shrink film, heat-shrink tubing, hot water pipe, wire and cable and many other applications whereby the materials are not too thick and require high-speed processing.

Electron accelerators are manufactured in a variety of forms and can be designed to produce electron beams with electron energies ranging from 80 keV to 10 MeV for commercial applications. Beam powers, the product of beam current versus electron energy, range from a few kW to 300 kW, although more powerful accelerators up to 500 kW are expected to be produced in the future. Electrons have less penetration than gamma radiation, but the advantage that electron accelerators have is that electron penetration can be tailored to the application by controlling the energy of the electrons. For example, electron energies of about 80–350 keV are used for curing of printing inks, coatings and adhesives on various type of substrates, while energies of between 500 keV to 5 MeV are used to crosslink polyolefins, such as insulation of wire, tubes and plastic films. Energies of electron accelerators from 5 to 10 MeV are used to sterilise medical products. The low-energy electron accelerators up to 800 keV can be self-shielded (i.e. the necessary lead shield is built into the accelerator itself).

1.3. Radiation unit

Radioactivity means the property of a material to emit radiation. It also indicates the strength of the radiation source. The standard international unit of radioactivity is "Bq" (Becquerel), although the old unit "Ci" (Curie) is still being used.

Energy of ionising radiation is as follows:

The energy unit is electron volt (eV, keV, MeV)
$1\,eV = 1.6021 \times 10^{-19}$ joule or $1\,J = 6.2418 \times 10^{18}\,eV$

Gamma radiation from cobalt-60 source has two energies, 1.17 and 1.33 MeV, whereas energies of X-rays and electron beam vary from a few keV to 10 MeV.

Radiation dose is defined as follows:

The absorbed dose (Grays, Gy) is the amount of energy absorbed per unit mass of the irradiated product. The old unit is the "rad". The standard unit is the "Gray".

$$1.0\,\text{Gy} = 1.0\,\text{J/kg}\ (= 100\,\text{rad})$$
$$= 6.2418 \times 10^{18}\,\text{eV/kg}$$
$$= 6.2418 \times 10^{18}\,\text{eV/dm}^3 \text{ for water (dm}^3.\text{litre)}$$

The absorbed dose rate is the absorbed dose per unit time e.g. Gy/sec or kGy/min or kGy/hr.

Relation of radiation dose to calorie:

$$1.0\,\text{cal} = 4.185\,\text{J} \quad 1\,\text{J} = 0.2389\,\text{cal}$$
$$1.0\,\text{kGy} = 1 \times 10^3\,\text{J/kg} = 238.9\,\text{cal/kg (about 0.24°C increased)}$$

G value is the number of molecules/radicals produced per 100 eV absorbed energy.

One curie of Co-60 source means 37 thousand million (3.7×10^{10}) of its radioactive atoms are disintegrating in one second. The new unit of Becquerel equals to one disintegration per second (1 Bq = 1 disintegration per second).

2. Interaction of Radiation with Matter

2.1. Electromagnetic radiation (gamma-rays)

The interaction of radiation with matter is essential for the understanding of radiation-induced chemical changes which are the direct consequences of the absorption of energy from the radiation by matter. When electromagnetic radiations, such as gamma-rays, pass through matter, the absorption of gamma-rays by matter obeys the fundamental Lambert–Beer law; $I = I_0 e^{-\mu x}$, where I and I_0 are the intensities of the transmitted and incident radiations, respectively, x is the thickness of the absorber and μ is the linear absorption coefficient. If the thickness of the absorber is expressed in cm, μ will have the units cm^{-1}.

The linear absorption coefficient depends on the density of the absorber and it is defined as the mass absorption coefficient by $\mu_{mass} = \mu_{linear}/\rho$, where ρ is the density of the absorber.

The total absorption coefficient is the sum of three separate coefficients representing the three main processes of energy absorption by gamma-rays. These processes are the photoelectric effect, the Compton effect and pair production.

2.1.1. Photoelectric effect

In this process, the photon or electromagnetic radiation (gamma-rays) is completely absorbed by atom. The energy of photon is transferred to an inner orbital of electron (usually from the K-shell) that is then ejected from the atom. An electron from the outer atomic orbit subsequently fills the inner orbital vacancy with consequent liberation of energy. This energy may appear as X-rays. The ejected electron will travel with energy equivalent to the energy of photon less the binding energy of electron to the atom to undergo further interaction with other atoms. The photoelectric effect is greatest for low photon energies, < 0.1 MeV, or for matters of high atomic number.

2.1.2. Compton effect (Compton scattering)

Interaction between a high-energy photon or electromagnetic radiation and a free or loosely bound electron will cause the diversion of direction of the photon and a loss in energy. The energy loss is transferred to the electron which will travel with an energy equivalent to the energy loss by the photon. The scattered photon may then undergo subsequent absorption either by the photoelectric effect or Compton effect. Compton absorption is more important for photons of higher energies, 0.1 to 10 MeV. Compton effect is the only process for the interaction of Co-60 gamma-rays with water.

2.1.3. Pair production

Pair production is the simultaneous formation of a positive electron (positron) and an electron as a result of the interaction of electromagnetic radiation of sufficient energy (≥ 1.02 MeV) with the field of an atomic nucleus of the atom. The electron and positron, after being slowed down, recombine with each other, resulting in the production of two 0.51 MeV gamma-rays (annihilation radiation).

The relative importance of the three absorption processes on the energy of the incident gamma radiation may be seen in Fig. 3. Whatever the mechanism of energy loss of the gamma radiation, secondary electrons with considerable kinetic energy are produced. Subsequent energy absorption processes, which will account for most of the energy of the incident radiation, will be those characteristic

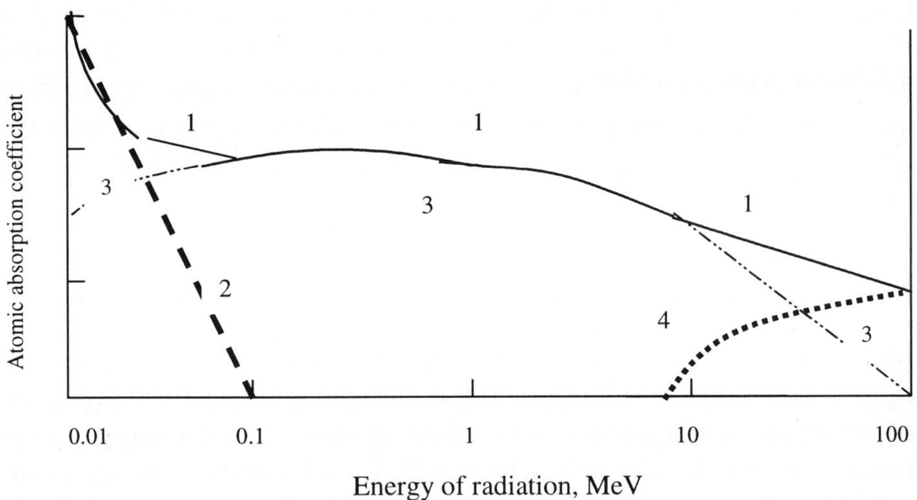

Fig. 3. Atomic absorption coefficients for water: total absorption (1), photoelectric effect (2), Compton effect (3), pair production (4).

of electrons. These electrons are similar to those electrons generated from electron accelerator.

2.2. Electrons

Electrons interact with matter in several ways which mainly are:

- Emission of electromagnetic radiation,
- Inelastic collisions, and
- Elastic collisions.

2.2.1. Emission of electromagnetic radiation

Electron passing close to the nucleus of an atom is decelerated with the subsequent emission of energy as X-ray. This radiation is known as *bremsstrahlung* radiation. *Bremsstrahlung* radiation can be absorbed by matter similar to that of electromagnetic radiation which can lead to chemical changes. *Bremsstrahlung* emission is the predominant mode of energy loss for electron energies in the range 10–100 MeV but it is negligible below 0.1 MeV.

2.2.2. Inelastic collisions

At lower energy, electrons lose their energies by inelastic collisions with electrons of the target materials resulting in ionisation and

Table 2. The range and LET values for electrons.

Energy (MeV)	Range in air (cm, 15°C, 760 mmHg)	Range in Aluminium (mm)	Range in Water (mm)	Average LET in Water (keV $\mu - 1$)
1	405	1.5	4.1	0.24
3	1400	5.5	15	0.20
10	4200	19.5	52	0.19

excitation. The rate of loss of energy with distance is known as the linear energy transfer (LET). The LET of all particles increases as the energy decreases, i.e. as the electrons are slowed down in the medium (Table 2).

2.2.3. Elastic collisions

Electrons, because of their small mass, are readily deflected by the coulomb field of nucleus. There is no energy loss in elastic collision. However, such a collision will result in a non-linear passage of electron through the medium. Elastic collisions are important for low-energy electrons in materials of high atomic number.

2.3. Ionization and excitation along radiation tracks

Excitation and ionisation occur when gamma radiation from Co-60 source (1.33 and 1.17 MeV) interact with matter mainly via Compton effect. As a result, the electrons ejected from the atoms will travel at high energy and cause further excitation and ionisation along their path, mainly via inelastic collisions. The scattered gamma-rays continue to interact with other atoms resulting in excitation and ionisation via Compton effects, photoelectric effect or pair production, depending on the energy of the scattered radiation.

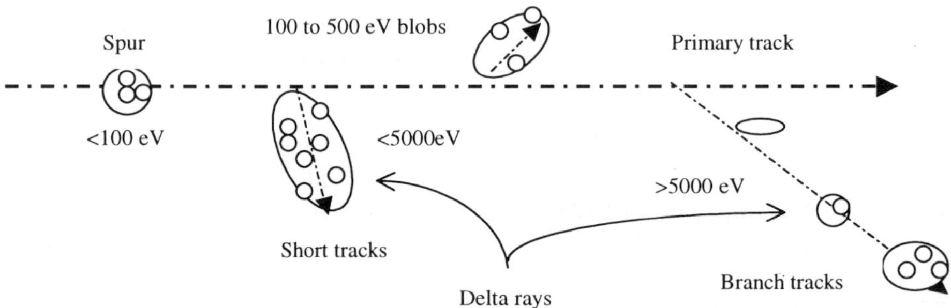

Fig. 4. Distribution of ions and excited molecules in the track of a fast electron.

The effects (excitation and ionisation) of secondary electrons produced from gamma interaction on matter are similar to those of the electron accelerator. If the energy of the secondary electrons is relatively small, ≤ 100 eV, their range in liquid or solid materials is short (2 cm in water) and the secondary ionisation occurs close to the primary ionisation track, giving a small cluster called a "spur".

The energy required to produce an ion pair is about 30 eV and about three ion pairs are produced within a spur. Some of the secondary electrons have enough energy to travel further and form tracks of their own, branching from the primary track, which are known as delta rays. Towards the end of the track, when the energy of the electron falls below 500 eV, the LET becomes higher and the region of ionisation and excitation become bigger and denser and this is called "blob".

All ionising radiations give rise to qualitatively similar effects. However, radiations of different types and energies will lose energy in matter at different rates. Consequently, they form tracks that may be densely or sparsely populated with the active species (ions, electrons and excited molecules). The different densities of active species in the particle tracks lead to differences in the quantities and proportions of the chemical products. Track effects of this sort are more important in the case of liquid, where active species are hindered from moving apart by the proximity of other molecules, than in gases, where they can move apart relatively easy. Therefore, the active species may recombine to give the initial molecules or they may diffuse out into the bulk of the solution where they may react with other solutes. The yields of species recombining and diffusing out are known as the molecular and radical yields, respectively.

2.4. Time scale of chemical reactions in radiation chemistry

The ionisation and excitation processes which lead to the chemical reactions occur within a short time scale.

Table 3. Time scale of chemical reaction in radiation chemistry.

Time (sec)	Event
10^{-18}	Ionising radiation traverses one molecule
10^{-15}	Time interval between successive ionisation
10^{-14}	Dissociation of electronically excited species Transfer of energy to vibration modes Ion–molecule reactions begin
10^{-13}	Electron reduced to thermal energies
10^{-12}	Radicals diffuse into the medium
10^{-11}	Electron is solvated in polar media
10^{-10}	Faster diffusion-controlled reactions are complete

3. Interaction of Radiation with Aqueous System

In elastic collision of high-energy electrons or secondary electrons, $E \geq 100\,\text{eV}$, with water molecules, excitation and ionisation of the water molecules occur predominantly. Depending on how close the high-energy electrons pass the water molecules and the velocity of their motion, the electron in the shell of the water molecule takes up a large or small amount of energy and momentum. Consequently, the shell electron changes its position and motion. If the energy absorbed by the electron is larger than the ionisation potential, it may part with the molecule leaving the positive ion.

In a stable molecule in the ground state, electrons are normally coupled into pairs with opposite spins. However, excitation into an excited singlet state leads to the quantum transition of an electron to a higher energy level, but in such a way that the spin orientation does not change. If the spin changes direction, it is in an excited triplet state which is formed by the interaction of ionising radiation with matter. Triplet-excited molecules are important in radiation chemistry, both because of their relatively long lifetimes and diradical character, which favour chemical reaction with the substrate and because they are formed in the tracks of charged particles in rather greater number than might be anticipated by photochemistry. Ionising radiation can produce excited molecules in water directly and also indirectly by neutralisation of the ions formed.

Therefore, the interaction of radiation with the aqueous system is as follows:

$$H_2O \rightsquigarrow \longrightarrow H_2O^*, H_2O^+ + e^- \quad \text{excitation \& ionisation} \quad (1)$$

Electron ejected from a water molecule may be thermalised before it could escape the coulomb attraction of the parent positive ion and recaptured to give an excited state molecule which subsequently decomposes to give hydrogen and hydroxyl radicals

$$H_2O^+ + e^- \longrightarrow H_2O^* \quad \text{recombination} \quad (2)$$

$$H_2O^* \longrightarrow H\cdot + \cdot OH \quad \text{decomposition} \quad (3)$$

A considerable number of hydrogen and hydroxyl radicals recombine to give water molecules

$$H\cdot + \cdot OH \longrightarrow H_2O \quad \text{recombination} \quad (4)$$

A hydrogen radical may react with a water molecule to produce hydrogen gas.

$$H\cdot + \cdot H_2O \longrightarrow H_2 + \cdot OH \quad (5)$$

However, the presence of molecular hydrogen is also explained by the following reaction:

$$H_2O^* \longrightarrow H_2 + O \quad (6)$$

An electron ejected from the water molecule may also possess sufficient energy to produce further ionisation and excitation. The energy is dissipated until it becomes lower than the threshold of electronic excitation and it ultimately ends as thermalised electron. The thermalised electron which is surrounded by water molecules is also known as a hydrated electron.

$$e^- \longrightarrow e_{aq}^- \quad \text{hydrated electron} \quad (7)$$

The water molecule ions may undergo proton transfer reaction with neighbouring water molecules,

$$H_2O^+ + H_2O \longrightarrow H_3O^+ + {\cdot}OH \qquad (8)$$

$$H_3O^+ \longrightarrow H_3O^+_{aq} \qquad (9)$$

The time scale of the above reactions is very fast, i.e. in the range of 10^{-16}–10^{-11} sec.

$$H_2O \leadsto\longrightarrow H_2O^*, H_2O^+ + e^- \qquad \sim 10^{-16}\text{–}10^{-15} \text{ sec}$$

$$H_2O^+ + H_2O \longrightarrow H_3O^+ + {\cdot}OH \qquad \sim 1.6 \times 10^{-14} \text{ sec}$$

$$H_2O^+ + e^- \longrightarrow H_2O^* \qquad \sim 10^{-13} \text{ sec}$$

$$H_2O^* \longrightarrow H{\cdot} + {\cdot}OH \qquad \sim 10^{-14}\text{–}10^{-13} \text{ sec}$$

$$e^- \longrightarrow e^-_{aq} \qquad \sim 10^{-12}\text{–}10^{-11} \text{ sec}$$

The diffusion control reaction will take place around 10^{-10} sec, whereby the active species started to diffuse out from the spur or blob, or its track, and to react with each other such as follows:

reaction	rate constant
$e^-_{aq} + e^-_{aq} \longrightarrow H_2 + 2OH^-$	$5.5 \times 10^9 \text{ M}^{-1} \text{ sec}^{-1}$
$H + H \longrightarrow H_2$	$1.5 \times 10^{10} \text{ M}^{-1} \text{ sec}^{-1}$
$OH + OH \longrightarrow H_2O_2$	$6.0 \times 10^9 \text{ M}^{-1} \text{ sec}^{-1}$
$e^-_{aq} + H_3O^+ \longrightarrow H + H_2O$	$2.06 \times 10^{10} \text{ M}^{-1} \text{ sec}^{-1}$

The primary products of radiolysis of water are:

$$H_2O \leadsto\longrightarrow H_3O^+_{aq}, OH, e^-_{aq}, H, H_2O_2, H_2.$$

These products are found in the irradiated water about 10^{-9} sec after the passage of high-energy radiation, when reactions in the spurs, blobs and short tracks are terminated. The number of radicals or molecules produced per 100 eV energy of radiation absorbed (G-value), the so-called primary product yields, can be determined and they are influenced by many factors.

Table 4. G-value or yield of primary radicals and molecular products of water radiolysis.

$G\,e^-_{aq} + G_H$	$G\,e^-_{aq}$	G_H	G_{OH}	G_{H_2}	$G_{H_2O_2}$	G_{-H_2O}	pH
3.65	0	3.65	2.90	0.4	0.78	4.45	0.46
3.67	2.63	0.55	2.72	0.45	0.78	4.08	3–13

To maintain a material balance, the radical and molecular yields must be related by:

$$G_{-H_2O} = 2G_{H_2} + G_H + G\,e^-_{aq} = 2G_{H_2O_2} + G_{OH}$$

3.1. The reducing species (e^-_{aq}, H, H$_2$)

Earlier, there were two views on the fate of electron ejected from a molecule.

- The electron would be thermalised before it could escape the coulomb attraction of the parent positive ion and thus recaptured to give an excited molecule which subsequently decomposes to produce hydrogen atom and hydroxyl radical.
- Alternatively, the electron would escape the parent ion but would react rapidly with a neutral water molecule to produce a hydrogen radical (atom).

However, it was later found that the electron after being thermalised is surrounded by the water molecules which aligned themselves in the electric field of the electron — polarisation. The electron can only occupy certain prescribed orbits in this field, i.e. it has quantum energy levels. Transitions between these energy levels give rise to the optical absorption spectrum. Hart and Boarg were the first to identify the absorption spectrum of the hydrated (solvated) electron with the absorption peak at 700–720 nm, which has blue colour (at 720 nm, the extinction coefficient, $\varepsilon = 1.58 \times 10^4$ dm^3 mol^{-1} s^{-1}).

The principal features of the reactions of hydrated electron (transfer of charge):

- Positive inorganic ions are more reactive than negative ones, and the higher the charge, the higher the rate constant ($Cu^{2+} + e_{aq}^- \longrightarrow Cu^+$)
- Organic acids react most rapidly when they are not dissociated. The higher the degree of dissociation, the lower the rate constant for reaction with the hydrated electron ($CH_3COOH + e_{aq}^- \longrightarrow CH_3COO^- + H$)
- Reaction with reactive groups in aliphatic compounds such as C–Cl, C = O, C = S and S–S ($CHCl_3 + e_{aq}^- \longrightarrow .CHCl_2 + Cl^-$)
- Aromatic compounds (benzene and phenol) react slowly, but some of their derivatives (such as nitrobenzene, benzonitrile and benzoate ion) may react rapidly
- Some biological compounds are very reactive (purine, cystamine, etc.) but some react slowly (amino acid)
- Derivative of aromatic compounds display higher reactivity as the character of the ring becomes more positive.

The role of the H atom (radical) as reducing species in the radiolysis of aqueous solution is considerably less than that of hydrated electron. This is due to the fact that the number of H atoms is substantially less than that of e_{aq}^- and that their reactivity is in general considerably weaker.

However, in certain cases such as in acidic condition, e_{aq}^- is converted into H atom ($e_{aq}^- + CH_3COOH \longrightarrow .H + CH_3COO^-$). The value of the rate constant for the reaction is rather high ($k = 1.8 \times 10^8$ dm^3 mol^{-1} s^{-1}). In this connection, the H atom plays a considerable role as a reducing species. However, since the rate of reaction of H atom is generally much lower than e_{aq}^-, it may give chemically different products from e_{aq}^-.

H atoms reacts via additional reaction and abstraction:

$$H + CH_3C \equiv N \longrightarrow CH_3CH = N. \quad \text{additional reaction}$$

$$H + CH_3OH \longrightarrow H_2 + .CH_2OH \quad \text{abstraction reaction}$$

In a strongly basic solution, pH > 10, the H atom may react with OH^- to form e_{aq}^-.

$$H + OH^- \longrightarrow e_{aq}^- + H_2O, \quad k = 2.3 \times 10^7 \text{ dm}^3 \text{ mol}^{-1} \text{ s}^{-1}$$

3.2. The oxidising species (OH, HO_2, H_2O_2)

The hydroxyl radical, OH, is the main oxidising species when aqueous solution is irradiated.

$$H_2O^+ + H_2O \longrightarrow H_3O^+ + OH$$

$$H_2O^* \longrightarrow H + OH$$

$$G(OH) = 2.7$$

Saturating the aqueous solution with N_2O converts e_{aq}^- into OH radical ($k = 9.8 \times 10^9 \text{ dm}^3 \text{ mol}^{-1} \text{ s}^{-1}$), resulting in a rather clean OH radical source (90% OH, 10% H).

$$N_2O + e_{aq}^- + H_2O \longrightarrow OH + N_2 + OH^-.$$

Both the hydroxyl and perhydroxyl radicals behave as weak acids, and in solution are in equilibrium with their anions, O^- and O_2^- superoxide ions, respectively. The relative proportion of acid and anion depends on the pH of the solution.

In a strong basic solution (pH 14), the OH radical is converted into O^-,

$$OH + OH^- \longrightarrow O^- + H_2O, \quad k = 1.2 \times 10^{10} \text{ dm}^3 \text{ mol}^{-1} \text{ s}^{-1}$$

With high LET radiation, considerable inter-radical reaction occurs in the particle track, producing H_2O, H_2 and H_2O_2. Reaction of OH with the latter creates a small yield of perhydroxyl radicals, HO_2, before the track disperses.

$$OH + H_2O_2 \longrightarrow H_2O + HO_2, \quad k = 2.7 \times 10^7 \text{ dm}^3 \text{ mol}^{-1} \text{ s}^{-1}$$

Large yields of HO_2 are formed in aerated solution by reactions of e_{aq}^- and H atom with oxygen.

$$e_{aq}^{-} + O_2 \longrightarrow O_2^{-}, \quad k = 1.9 \times 10^{10}\,dm^3\,mol^{-1}\,s^{-1}$$

$$H + O_2 \longrightarrow HO_2, \quad k = 1.9 \times 10^{10}\,dm^3\,mol^{-1}\,s^{-1}$$

3.2.1. Properties of hydroxyl, perhydroxyl and their anions

<u>Hydroxyl radical</u>

Absorption maximum

OH	230 nm, $\varepsilon = 530\,M^{-1}\,cm^{-1}$
O^{-}	240 nm, $\varepsilon = 240\,M^{-1}\,cm^{-1}$
pK (OH $\rightleftharpoons$ O^{-} + OH)	11.9 ± 0.2

<u>Perhydroxyl radical and anions</u>

Absorption maximum

HO_2	240 nm, $\varepsilon = 1150\,M^{-1}\,cm^{-1}$
O_2^{-}	245 nm, $\varepsilon = 1970\,M^{-1}\,cm^{-1}$
pK (HO_2 $\rightleftharpoons$ O_2^{-} + H^{+})	4.88 ± 0.10
pK (H_2O_2 $\rightleftharpoons$ HO_2 + H^{+})	1.0 to 1.2

Types of reactions of OH with stable species or free radicals are:

- Electron transfer is the most frequent mechanism of OH-induced oxidation of both inorganic anions and cations

$$Fe^{+2} + OH \longrightarrow Fe^{+3} + OH^{-}$$

$$S^{-} + OH \longrightarrow S + OH^{-}\ (S\ is\ Cl,\ Br,\ I)$$

- Hydrogen abstraction and OH addition are the most common types of reactions with organic molecules.

$$(R)_3CH + OH \longrightarrow H_2O + (R)_3C\bullet\ abstraction$$

$$C_6H_6 + OH \longrightarrow (OH)C_6H_6\ addition$$

- Addition reactions also occur with free radicals

$$OH + OH_2 \longrightarrow H_2O_3\ (in\ acid\ medium,\ 0.02\ M\ H_3O^{+})$$

$$H_2O_3 \longrightarrow H_2O + O_2$$

4. Effects of Radiation on Packaging Materials

Most of the packaging materials are polymer-based and contain mainly light elements, such as C, H, O, N and Cl, with which the energetic gamma photon of Co-60 undergo predominantly Compton scattering. The resulting energetic electrons ionise and excite the polymer molecules which then undergo specific reactions, such as crosslinking and degradation. The extent of the reaction depends on molecular structure and elemental composition of the plastic.

Crosslinking is the process in which two polymer chains link up in a chemical bond. Polymers with units $CH_2 - CHR - $ (R is either CH_3 or bigger group), with at least one H on the alternate carbon atom, crosslink predominantly. Crosslinking increases molecular weight, decreases solubility and raises the softening point to a higher temperature.

Degradation is the process leading to scission of a polymer chain and reduction of molecular weight. In halogenated polymers, dehydrohalogenation may occur. In polymers of units, $- CH_2 - CR_1R_2 -$, where alternate carbon atoms are fully substituted, degradation predominates.

4.1. Types of packaging materials

- Glass — has no effect except changes in colour to dark brown or violet at the sterilisation dose of 25 kGy and higher doses.
- Plastic materials can undergo crosslinking and/or chain scission (degradation) at the decontamination (5–15 kGy) and sterilisation (25 kGy) doses. It depends very much on the type of plastic material used.
- Cellulosic-based materials, such as paperboard or cardboard, usually experience some scissioning of bonds in the cellulose chain. At the decontamination and sterilisation doses, the physical properties of the paperboard or cardboard are only slightly affected, hence not impairing the performance of the packaging.
- Metals, such as steel cans, aluminium foils and metallised papers, are unaffected by radiation at the levels used for decontamination

and sterilisation. However, the sealing compounds and coating materials used may have some effects upon irradiation.

4.2. Product qualification

For sterilisation of medical products, the process validation in accordance to ISO 11137 requires *product qualification* which include *product and packaging material evaluation* and *sterilisation dose determination*. Amongst the items to be considered for product and packaging material evaluation are the following:

- the effect of radiation on the materials that make up the products and packaging
- the quality, safety and performance of the product throughout its shelf life exposed to radiation
- a maximum acceptable dose for each product and packaging.

Prior to selecting the radiation sterilisation process for medical products, it is important to consider the effect of radiation on the stability of the materials that make up the product components or packaging materials. There are several rules that apply for the selecting or designing of radiation-stable materials. A general rule is that all plastics that predominantly crosslink with radiation tend to have higher radiation stability and vice versa.

4.2.1. General guidelines for selection of radiation stable materials

(i) Aromatic materials are more stable than aliphatic materials.
(ii) Phenolic antioxidants contained in most plastics are a cause of discolouration.
(iii) Most polypropylene and polytetrafluoroethylene are unstable with irradiation. Polyvinylchloride and polypropylene should be stabilised to improve radiation compatibility.
(iv) Polymer processing conditions and materials that lead to brittleness of medical products or packaging materials should be carefully evaluated for radiation sterilisation (e.g. the use

of plastic regrind or nucleated polymers; the use of high temperatures during moulding; the creation of high-level crystallinity in semi-crystalline polymers in slow cooling and autoclaves).

(v) High level of antioxidants improve radiation stability. In general, the level of antioxidant should be doubled if the packaging is going to be radiation sterilised.

(vi) For semi-crystalline polymers, processing conditions that lead to low degrees of crystallinity will improve stability.

(vii) The elastic modulus of plastic is not significantly affected with a sterilising dose of irradiation.

(viii) Within a given polymer class, the lower the density the greater is the radiation stability, e.g. irradiation causes less brittleness in low-density polyethylene (0.92 g/cm^2) than in high-density polyethylene (0.95 g/cm^2).

The quality, safety and performance of the products, product components and packaging throughout the shelf-life should be assured. It can be determined by carrying out a series of tests on the materials or products/packaging. Testing should include any specific property essential to the intended function of the products, such as tensile property, tear strength, burst strength, flexural property, clarity, colour, biocompatibility and package integrity. The test should also include all variations of manufacturing processes, tolerance, radiation doses, radiation source, raw materials and storage conditions. With these tests, the maximum acceptable dose for that particular product shall be established.

The effects of radiation dose on the materials/products might not be immediately apparent. Therefore, the test should also include accelerated aging at extreme conditions for initial indication of material suitability, as well as at ambient real-time aging (e.g. 60°C for 7 days equivalent to 180 days of ageing at ambient conditions). The time interval for accelerated aging test is one to four weeks and at ambient conditions for 0, 3, 5, 9, 12 months.

The radiation dose between 10–100 kGy can be used throughout the tests. The dose of ~100 kGy determines the maximum tolerable dose for the materials after they are subjected to various tests.

Table 5. General guide to radiation stability materials.

Material	Radiation Stability	Comments
Thermoplastics		
Polystyrene	Excellent	
Polyethylene	Excellent	
Polyamides	Excellent	
Polyimides	Excellent	
Polysulfone	Excellent	
Polyphenylene sulphide	Excellent	
Aromatic polyester	Excellent	
Polyvinyl chloride (PVC)	Good	Yellow—antioxidants and stabilisers prevent yellowing. High molecular weight organotin stabilisers improve radiation stability
Styrene/acrylonitrile	Good	
Polycarbonate	Good	Yellow—mechanical properties not greatly affected
Paper, card, corrugated, fibres (cellulose)	Good	
Polypropylene	Poor	Must be stabilised—physical properties greatly reduced when irradiated
Fluropolymers (PTFE, PCTFE)	Poor	Significantly damaged.
Thermoset		
Phenolics	Good	Very good with the addition of mineral fillers
Polyesters	Good	Very good with the addition of mineral or glass fibres
Polyurethane—aliphatic	Excellent	
Elastomer		
Urethane	Excellent	
EPDM	Excellent	
Natural rubber	Good	
Nitrile rubber	Good	Discolours

In addition to the physical and mechanical testing, some materials might need to undergo biocompatibility testing. Biocompatibility testing of the radiation-sterilised products is dependent on the end use of the products. This test is required to ensure that any chemical changes in the chemical structure of the polymer and/or additives, as well as gaseous products liberated during irradiation, will not alter the material's biocompatibility for medical product applications (ISO 10993 gives the basic biological screening testing).

Products and packaging material evaluation is the responsibility of the primary manufacturer. The manufacturer is responsible for ensuring the suitability of the materials, design and packaging for irradiation. The irradiator operator can only, if requested, provide advice in general terms and perform test irradiation. Primary manufacturers of the medical products are also responsible for ensuring that they inform the suppliers of the materials and components of any changes in the formulation and/or manufacturing process of the materials that could affect radiation stability.

5. Overview of Radiation Sterilisation, Facilities and Methods

5.1. Radiation facilities

Radiation sterilisation was first introduced commercially in USA in 1957 using electron-beam accelerator. However, until now, the number of radiation sterilisation plants using Co-60 gamma radiation is much higher than those using electron-beam accelerators, due to the high penetration of gamma radiation and hence sterilisation of bulk products can easily be carried out. Nevertheless, electron-beam sterilisation using high-energy accelerator, 5 to 10 MeV, is again beginning to receive wide application in the industry. Figures 5 and 6 show the gamma-sterilisation and electron-beam plants for sterilisa-tion, respectively. For comparison, Table 6 provides the characteristics of gamma radiation and electron beam.

In the Asia Pacific region, radiation sterilisation technology is well established and currently, there are about 90 units of Co-60

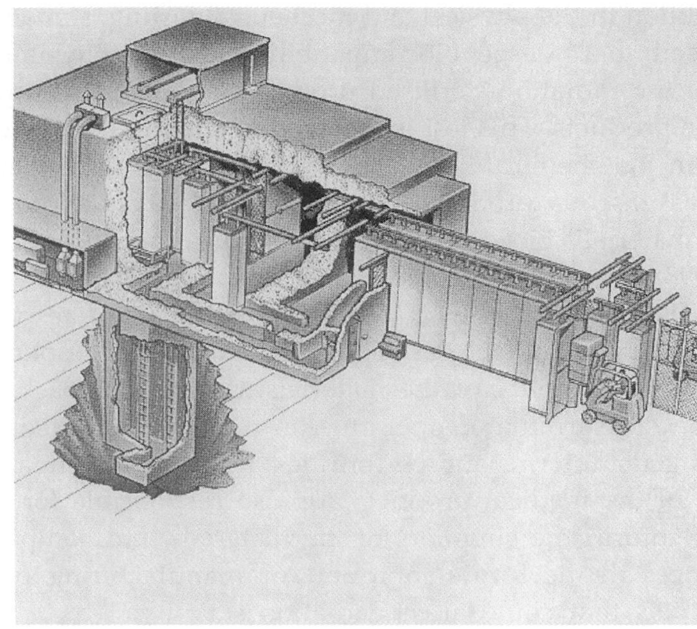

Fig. 5. Diagram of Co-60 gamma sterilisation plant using carrier system.

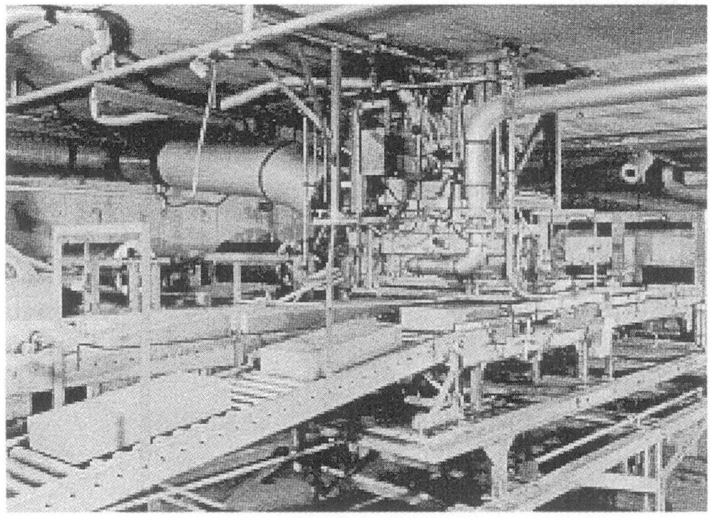

Fig. 6. Electron-beam facility for sterilisation of medical products.

Table 6. Comparison of gamma-rays from Co-60 and electron-beam.

Characteristic	Gamma-Rays	Electron-Beams
Energy	1.17–1.33 MeV	Variable 0.2–10 MeV
Power	1.48 kW/100 kCi	Variable 4–400 kW/unit
Dose rate	Low (kGy/hr)	High (kGy/sec)
Penetration	High (43 cm in water)	Low (~0.35 cm/MeV)
Energy utilisation efficiency	Low (~40%)	High (~90%)
Production rate	Low	High
Maintenance	Replenishment of Co-60 source	Replenishment of electronic parts
Others	Source decay 1% per month	Shut-off power source

sterilisation plants. X-rays generated from the bombardment of electrons on metals with high atomic number, such as tungsten, are another source of radiation which has the potential to be used for sterilisation. However, the conversion factor of electron energy to X-ray is in the range of 5–8% for a 3–5 MeV accelerator and 20–23% for a 10 MeV accelerator. Table 7 shows the various sources of industrial gamma, electron-beam and X-ray radiations.

5.2. Sterilisation process

Radiation sterilisation is an integral part of the overall manufacturing process of any medical product that is required to be sterile. It is very important to have in place, at every step of the development of the product, good practices that meet International Standards such as the Standard ISO 9000 series and Standard ISO 11137: Sterilisation of Health Care Products — Requirement for Validation and Routine Control — Radiation Sterilisation. What is more important is that these good manufacturing practices are not only in place, but are strictly adhered to during normal everyday operations.

Table 7. Radiation sources of industrial gamma, electron-beam and X-ray radiations.

Gamma source

Several hundred kCi to several Mci of Co-60 source (e.g. 100 kCi–5.0 MCi)

Useful energy range: 1.17–1.33 MeV
Power range: 1.48–72.4 kW

Electron-beam sources

- Insulating core transformer (ICT)
- Multistage rectifier circuits. Series-coupled cascade system (Cockroft Walton type)
- Multistage rectifier circuits. Paralell-coupled cascade system (Dynamitrons)

Useful energy range: 1–5 MeV
Power range up to 200 kW

- Microwave linear accelerator (linac)
- Resonant-cavity accelerator

Useful energy range: 5–10 MeV
Power up to 200 kW

X-ray (brehmsstrahlung) source

Brehmsstrahlung is a highly penetrating form of ionising radiation when energetic electrons are slowed down or stopped in a suitable target (tungsten, uranium)

Conversion factor:
$\varepsilon \equiv 5$–8% for 3–5 MeV electrons
$\varepsilon \equiv 20$–23% for 10 MeV electrons

The same rules apply to the irradiation sterilisation portion of the manufacturing process. Radiation sterilisation is usually the last process that the product goes through. Consequently, the next step is for the product to be used on a patient who will have complete faith in the safety and integrity of the product.

Radiation sterilisation must have good radiation practices (GRP) and these must be contained in a precise written form called a Standard Operating Procedure (SOP).

Good radiation practice (GRP) involves the following:

- *Irradiator commissioning* — To characterise the magnitude, distribution and reproducibility of absorbed dose in homogenous material for a typical range of density and to relate these parameters with operating conditions.

- *Irradiator* — To ensure the irradiator's electro-mechanical systems are functioning correctly and reproducibly prior to performing the commissioning dosimetry study.
- *Dose mapping* — Initial commissioning must include extensive dose mapping, using actual or simulated product at the upper and lower limits of the density range for which the irradiator is to be used. The dose absorbed by the product is influenced by several factors:

  ☆ Product density — The gamma-ray is a high-frequency electro-magnetic wave that has high penetration power that can penetrate through the products. However, the absorbed dose is affected by the density of the product (bulkiness) and therefore, it must be taken into account in the validation process. The product density is calculated by dividing the weight over the volume;

$$
\begin{aligned}
\text{Box weight} &= 5000 \text{ g} \\
\text{Box volume } (25 \times 25 \times 25 \text{ cm}^3) &= 15\,625 \text{ cm}^3 \\
\text{Product density} &= 5000/15\,625 \text{ g/cm}^3 \\
&= 0.32 \text{ g/cm}^3
\end{aligned}
$$

  This method is also used to consequently determine the product density of each carrier or tote and then the product density of all carriers/totes in the irradiation room at a given time during the sterilisation process.

  ☆ Product loading pattern — The manner in which a group of boxes is loaded into the carrier/tote will also have an influence on the absorbed dose (Fig. 7). If products of high density are positioned on either side of products of lower density, then radiation shielding will occur and this will result in a lower absorbed dose. Consequently, the weight and size of each box to be processed must be known and a suitable product loading must be determined to ensure homogenous carrier/tote, with maximum space utilisation for economic and productivity purposes.

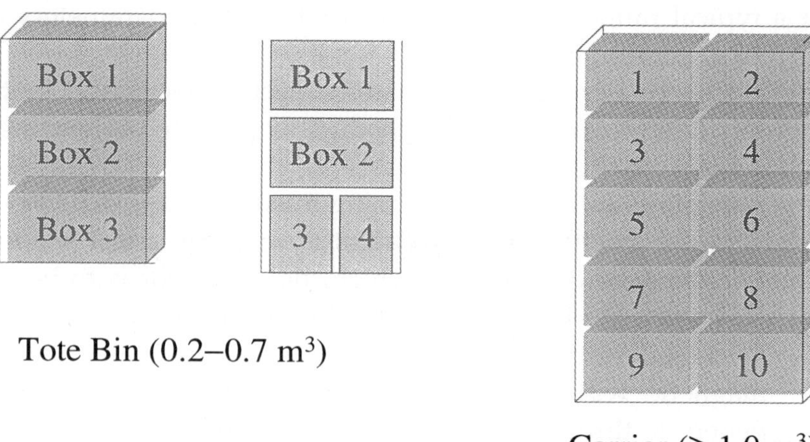

Tote Bin (0.2–0.7 m^3)

Carrier ($\geq$ 1.0 m^3)

Fig. 7. Product loading pattern in tote bin or carrier for gamma sterilisation.

- *Dose uniformity (DU)* — This is the ratio of minimum dose to maximum dose received in any carrier/tote, and this ratio should be as close to one as possible.
- *Dosimetry* — Routine dosimeter, such as ceric-cerrous sulphate solution is acceptable for use in commissioning of the irradiator. However, reference dosimeter, such as ferrous sulphate solution (Fricke dosimeter) should be placed in parallel with routine dosimeters at selected positions in order to compare the response of the routine dosimeter in the production environment.

     For electron-beam accelerator, cellulose triacetate (CTA) film or radiochromic film can be used as routine dosimeter, and water or graphic calorimeter as the reference dosimeter. The CTA film is used to determine the minimum and maximum doses within the product geometry, as shown in Fig. 8.
- *Dosimeter placement* — Dose mapping requires the placement of dosimeters throughout a representative product load. For consistency in positioning and ease of locating the dosimeters, it is helpful to define a three-dimensional grid throughout the product load. The points of planar intersection provide reference locations.

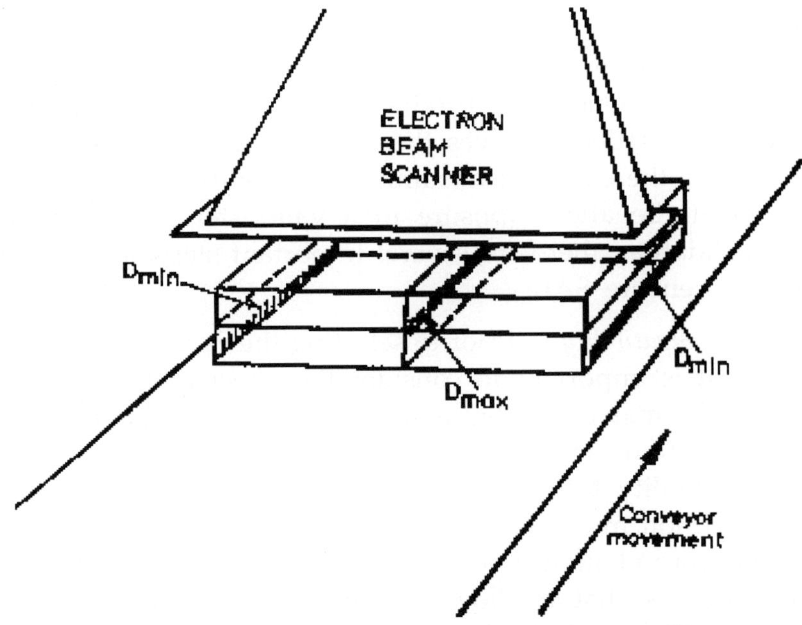

Fig. 8. Measurement of dose uniformity in a box irradiated by electron beam.

The use of multiple dosimeters at a given location will increase the confidence in the dose reading at that location.

- *Irradiation and dose measurement* — After irradiation, the dosimeters are removed and read (UV spectrophotometer or potentiometer). The maximum and minimum doses are identified, and dose uniformity and processing parameters are determined.
- *Recommissioning* — In theory, the minimum and maximum dose locations do not change significantly when the source is reloading or upgrading. However, a dose-mapping study can be done in these locations and the surrounding regions to demonstrate the data continued validity. If the result of this study is in disagreement with the prior result, or if the source configuration has been changed, an extensive dose-mapping study, such as the performed during the initial commissioning, is required.

5.3. Process validation

Process validation is the process that provides reliable and reproducible evidence that product items which are subjected to radiation sterilisation achieves the desired sterility assurance level (SAL). SAL is the expected maximum probability of a product item being non-sterile after exposure to a valid sterilising process. In process validation, there are several important steps which need to be taken to ensure SAL:

- *Material compatibility* — Prior to selecting the radiation sterilisation process, it is important to consider the effect that radiation will have on the materials. The material should be evaluated in terms of its radiation stability. Some materials may need to undergo biocompatibility testing.

  Attention must also be given to the suitability of packaging materials for radiation exposure. One of the advantages of radiation sterilisation is that it allows the use of non-porous packaging materials, such as polyethylene.
- *Selection of SAL* — An SAL of 10^{-6} is widely accepted for sterile medical products. However, other levels are also being used. The selection of this level is a function of the end use of the product.
- *Selection of sterilising dose* — It is a basic assumption that the product to be sterilised is manufactured under conditions that comply fully with the requirements of GMP. A dose of 25 kGy a well-accepted effective sterilising dose. It is generally believed that this dose provides an SAL 10^{-6}. Where it is not feasible to generate data on the radiation resistance of the natural microbial population present on the product items, a minimum sterilising dose of 25 kGy can be used.
- *Product loading pattern* — A loading pattern should be established for each type of product unit. Generally, this pattern should be designed to use the space within the irradiation container/carrier/ tote to the fullest extent possible within the weight limitation of the container. The loading pattern should also be designed to achieve a uniform distribution of density within the irradiation container, as feasible, in order to minimise dose variation.

- *Dose mapping* — Dose mapping is performed to identify the zone of minimum and maximum doses within the product load and to select a dose-monitoring location for use in routine processing.
- *Cycle timer setting* — The length of time that the product is being exposed to radiation is controlled by the cycle timer. The cycle timer setting provides the minimum required sterilising dose for a given Co-60 loading and depends on the overall bulk density of the products in the irradiation container. It must be determined for each product, load configuration and conveyor path.

5.4. Routine process control

In process control, several routine actions need to be established. A written process specification should be established, that describe the manner in which each product category should be handled before, during and after sterilisation.

Products awaiting sterilisation should be stored in a segregated area designated exclusively for non-sterile products. The use of colour change indicators to distinguish irradiated from non-irradiated product is optional. The selection of dosimeter, numbers and placement of dosimeter in the minimum zone is essential. It is often appropriate to monitor the maximum dose by placing dosimeters in the maximum dose zone.

The irradiation process should also be closely monitored. A hard copy of cycle time, conveyor operation, product arrangement within the irradiation container, and source position should be recorded.

Product unloaded from the irradiated container should be identified and stored in a segregated area designated exclusively for sterile products. The sterile products are ready to be released to the customer with proper documentation.

In the routine process control, the interruption of process, such as power breakdown, requires certain actions to be taken depending on whether the products are capable or not capable of supporting microbial growth. Radiation dose has cumulative effect on microorganisms.

Routine and preventive maintenance should be conducted to ensure the safe and reproducible operation of the irradiator and they should be recorded. These maintenance procedures do not affect the functional characteristics of the irradiator and, therefore, do not necessitate cycle revalidation.

5.5. Management and organisation

A radiation sterilisation plant, bears the responsibility of delivering the specific absorbed dose. The quality of the product is the responsibility of the manufacturer. Therefore, the plant staffing should be capable of ensuring safe operation of the irradiator, consistent compliance with GMP/GRP and other related international standards, and precise and efficient product processing. It is also imperative that the quality assurance functions be carried out independent of the production and operation functions. All staff should also be well trained in their respective tasks.

6. References

ALLEN, A.O. (1961). *The Chemistry of Water and Aqueous Solutions*, D. Van Nostrand Company, Inc., Princeton, New Jersey.

BIELSKI, B.H.J. and GEBICKI, J. (1970). In: *Advances in Radiation Chemistry*, Vol. 2, M. Burton and J.L. Magee, eds., Wiley Interscience, New York.

BURTON, M. (1969). *Chem. Eng. News* **46**, 86.

CHARLESBY, A. (1960). *Atomic Radiation and Polymers*, Pergamon Press, London.

COOPER, W.J., CURRY, R.D. and O'SHEA, K.E. (1998). *Environmental Applications of Ionizing Radiation*, John Wiley & Sons.

DRAGANIC, I.G. and DRAGANIC, I.D. (1971). *The Radiation Chemistry of Water*, Academic Press, New York.

DRAGANIC, I.G., NENADOVIC, M.T. and DRAGANIC, Z.D. (1969). *J. Phys. Chem.* **73**, 2564.

HUGHES, G. (1973). *Radiation Chemistry*, Oxford Chemistry Series.

IAEA-TECDOC-454 (1986). *Technical and Economic Comparison of Irradiation and Conventional Methods*.

IAEA-TECDOC-834 (1995). *Advanced Radiation Chemistry Research: Current Status*.

IAEA (1967). *Radiosterilization of Medical Products, Pharmaceuticals and Bioproducts*, IAEA Technical Report Series No. 72.

IAEA (1973). *Manual on Radiation Sterilization of Medical and Biological Materials*, IAEA Technical Report Series No. 149.

ISO 11137 (1995). Sterilization of Health Care Products — Requirements for Validation and Routine Control — Radiation Sterilization, International Standard.

MOZUMDER, A. and MAGEE, J.L. (1966). *Radiat. Res.* **28**, 203.

O'DONNELL, J.H. and SANGSTER, D.F. (1970). *Principles of Radiation Chemistry*, Edward Arnold, London.

PLESTER, D.W. (1967). The sterilization of plastics, *Trans J. Plastics Inst.*, p. 579.

SINGH, A. and SILVERMAN, J. (1992). *Radiation Processing of Polymers*, Hanser Publishers, Munich.

SPINKS, J.W.T. and WOODS, R.J. (1976). *An Introduction to Radiation Chemistry*, 2nd edn., John Wiley & Sons, New York.

SWALLOW, A.J. (1973). *Radiation Chemistry: An Introduction*, Longman, London.

THOMAS, J.K. (1969). In: *Advance in Radiation Chemistry*, Vol. 1, M. Burton and J.L. Magee, eds., Wiley Interscience, New York, p. 103.

Advances in Tissue Banking Vol. 5
© 2001 by World Scientific Publishing Co. Pte. Ltd.

19 EFFECT OF RADIATION ON MICROORGANISMS — MECHANISM OF RADIATION STERILISATION

NORIMAH YUSOF

Tissue Bank, Malaysian Institute for
Nuclear Technology Research (MINT)
Bangi, 43000 Kajang, Selangor, Malaysia

1. Introduction

Microorganisms embrace a wide range of primitive life forms. Most of them are unicellular, individually too small to be seen with the naked eye, therefore requiring a microscope to observe them. They are widely distributed in outdoor and indoor environments, on the human skin, in the mouth, the upper respiratory tract, large intestine, on equipment, in water and basically everywhere in a tissue bank.

Microorganisms are rarely harmful in their natural habitat but are likely to cause disease if they gain access to organs and tissues. They are responsible for most transmitted diseases. In tissue banking, we are concerned with epidemiology, i.e. how the organism is spread from one infected donor tissue to the recipient.

2. Types of Microorganisms

Microorganisms include bacteria, viruses, fungi (moulds and yeast), protozoa, some algae, and some forms of life that do not fit well into any of these groups. Sometimes they are called microbes or, in the layman term, germs. Table 1 provides some of distinguished characteristics of the five major groups of microorganisms (Gardner and Peel, 1986).

The first primitive microorganism is believed to have originated 3.5 billion years ago and subsequent evolution has resulted in a myriad of prokaryotic and eukaryotric cells (Volk and Wheeler, 1988). Prokaryotic cell is bounded by a plasma membrane but has no other separate membrane-bound organelles; most of them possessing a cell wall containing muramic acid. Eukaryotic cells possess a true nucleus that is separated from the cytoplasm by a well-defined two-layer nuclear membrane. The deoxyribose nucleic acid (DNA) and several proteins are organised into linear strands called chromosomes. The number of chromosomes is fixed according to species, such as one or two for certain fungi and 46 for human. Eukaryotic

Table 1. Distinguished characteristics of microorganisms.

Group	Affiliates	Growth Habits	Sources
Bacteria	Neither plants nor animals	Free-living or parasitic	Soil, water, organic materials, human, animal, plant
Viruses	Subcellular particles	Obligate intracellular parasites	Human, animal, plant or bacterial hosts
Fungi (moulds and yeast)	Some resemblance to plants, but not photosynthetic	Free-living or parasitic	Decaying organic matter, soil, fruit juice, plant, animal, human
Protozoa	Animals	Free-living or parasitic	Soil, water
Algae	Green plants	Free-living	Sea, fresh water, soil

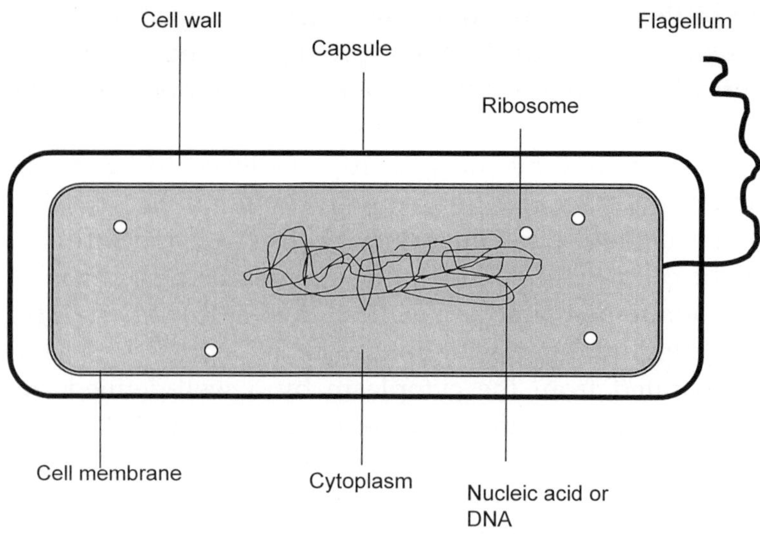

Fig. 1. Structure of a bacterial cell.

microorganisms comprise the fungi (mould and yeast) and the protozoa. Prokryotic microorganisms are categorised as bacteria and cyanobacteria. The single bacterial cells differ from those higher forms of life in that the nucleic acid or DNA is not confined within a membrane and does not break up into chromosomes during cell division (Fig. 1).

Viruses are not cells but consist primarily of nucleic acid surrounded by a protective coat. Viruses can replicate only when they are within a susceptible prokaryotic or eukaryotic cell.

Among microorganisms, bacteria are the most commonly found in/on medical products, including processed tissues. Fungi are next but in a smaller proportion, while viruses are of concern when dealing with body tissues.

3. Microbial Control

The principle of microbial control is to minimise or avoid the ravages of infectious diseases. Hygienic practices in procurement, processing and packaging can only minimise the microorganisms on processed tissues but there is still some probability of surviving microbes. Therefore, methods of killing microorganisms are developed, and they are directed towards the complete exclusion of all microorganisms.

Table 2. Comparison of sterilisation processes.

Considerations	Steam	ETO Gas	Radiation
Tissue materials	Damaged	None	Only at high dose
Interaction with products	Hydrolysis	Hydroxyethylation	Radiolysis
Parameters to control	Vacuum Pressure Temperature Time	ETO concentration Vacuum Pressure Temperature Humidity Time	Time
Reliability	Good	Good	Excellent
Post-sterilisation test	Desirable	Required	Not necessary
Quarantine	7 – 14 days	7 – 14 days	None
Post-sterilisation treatment	Dry	Aerate	None
Residues	None	Yes	None
Continuous operation	No	No	Yes
Environmental	Good	Poor	Good
Occupational safety	Good	Poor	Good
Economic	Good at low & high volume	Good at low & high volume	Good at high volume

Tissues are sterilised to make a recipient uninfected. Sterilisation is the process which renders the tissues sterile so as to achieve a high sterility assurance level.

Sterilisation methods vary considerably, depending on the materials to be treated and their usage. The main ones are physical and chemical sterilisation methods:

Physical treatment:

    Thermal   — dry heat, autoclave
    Non-thermal   — radiation, filtration

Chemical treatment:

                                — ethylene oxide gas

As for tissues, heat treatment will affect the physical, chemical as well as biological properties of tissues, whilst chemical treatment will leave behind chemical residues. In the Asia Pacific region, many tissue banks are using radiation sterilisation technology. Table 2 compares the three commonly used sterilisation processes at commercial scale.

4. Radiation Treatment

Two main types of radiations are employed for sterilisation, namely non-ionising and ionising. Ultraviolet ray is a non-ionising radiation, most effective at 253.7 nm wavelength. It is mainly used only for surface sterilisation as it has very low penetration. Ionising radiation includes those charged particles, such as high-energy electrons generated from accelerators, electromagnetic rays, such as gamma-rays emitted by radioisotopes cobalt-60 and caesium-137, and X-rays generated by machines. Ionising radiation is highly penetrating and readily passes through a product. The penetration depends on the energy of radiation and density of product. The high energy is sufficient to ionise or excise atoms but it is far below the level that could induce radioactivity in the treated material.

Radiation sterilisation means exposing tissue products containing certain level of microorganisms to a treatment by gamma-rays,

X-rays or accelerated electrons, all of which are ionising radiation. Ionising radiation kills all types of microorganisms through the ionisation process and it usually has enough energy for useful penetration into solids and liquids of the tissues. The treatment does not heat up tissue materials significantly and are widely used for industrial sterilisation of heat-sensitive medical and laboratory products. Therefore, it is suitable for sterilising tissues.

5. Effect of Ionising Radiation on Living Cells

The interaction of ionising radiation within a biological system can result from both direct and indirect effects.

5.1. Direct effect

The direct action of radiation involves the simple interaction between ionising radiation and critical biological molecules, which results in excitation, lesion and scission of polymeric structure. High-energy photons of ionising radiation or one active radical produced by the ionisation process can break and change the DNA strands. Studies on the macromolecules of DNA revealed that the possible changes occurring due to ionising radiation are: breaks in the sugar phosphate backbone of the individual polynucleotide strands (single-strand breaks), adjacent or near adjacent breaks in both polynucleotide strands (double-strand breaks), cross-linking (within single strand or between two strands/intermolecular) and base alterations. Extent of the damage depends upon the physical state of the DNA strands during the time of irradiation. The damages to DNA strand, if not repaired, will lead to inactivation of the ability of the cells to reproduce.

5.2. Indirect effect

The biological effects of radiation are basically due to biochemical changes within the organism. The presence of substantial quantities of water (70 to 90%) is normal in living microorganisms. Most of the absorbed energy of radiation will be taken up by the water molecules, which are most likely to be ionised. Interaction of ionising radiation with water molecules leads to production of short-lived free radicals and peroxy radicals. Consequently, these radiolytic products will interact with biological molecules including DNA, hence inactivating the reproduction process. This indirect effect of radiation normally occurs as an important part of the total chain reactions of ionising radiation, summarised as follows (Antoni, 1973; Coggle, 1973):

$$H_2O \Rightarrow H_2O^+ + e^-$$

$$e^- + H_2O \Rightarrow H_2O^-$$

These water ions decompose almost immediately while forming free radicals:

$$H_2O^+ \Rightarrow H^+ + OH^\bullet$$

$$H_2O^- \Rightarrow H^\bullet + OH^-$$

The free radicals ($H^\bullet$, $OH^\bullet$) will interact further

(i) among themselves (radical–radical reactions),

$$H^\bullet + H^\bullet \Rightarrow H_2$$

$$OH^\bullet + OH^\bullet \Rightarrow H_2O_2$$

$$H^\bullet + OH^\bullet \Rightarrow H_2O \qquad \text{water reconstitution}$$

(ii) with water molecules or with their own reaction products, or

$$H^\bullet + H_2O \Rightarrow H_2 + OH^\bullet$$

$$OH^\bullet + H_2O_2 \Rightarrow H_2O + HO_2^\bullet$$

$$HO_2^\bullet + HO_2^\bullet \Rightarrow H_2O_2 + O_2$$

$$HO_2^\bullet + OH^\bullet \Rightarrow H_2O + O_2$$

$$HO_2^\bullet + H_2O_2 \Rightarrow H_2O + OH^\bullet + O_2$$

$$HO_2^\bullet + H^\bullet \Rightarrow H_2O_2$$

(iii) with organic molecules, RH.

$$H^\bullet + RH \Rightarrow R^\bullet + H_2$$

$$OH^\bullet + RH \Rightarrow R^\bullet + H_2O$$

$$HO_2^\bullet + RH \Rightarrow R^\bullet + H_2O_2$$

$$HO_2^\bullet + RH \Rightarrow RO^\bullet + H_2O$$

The organic molecules, RH, also become directly ionised into free radicals as follows:

$$RH \Rightarrow R^\bullet + H^\bullet$$

Free radicals, $R^\bullet$ and $RO^\bullet$ (organic peroxide), react with biologically important molecules (such as proteins, enzymes, amino acids, metabolites, nucleic material, etc.) resulting in radio-biological damage. These chain reactions, which are called the indirect action of radiation, are generally held responsible for the radiation-induced effects. Therefore, indirect action involves aqueous free radicals known as radiolytic products which act as intermediaries in the transfer of radiation energy to biological molecules.

6. Radiation Damage

Radiation damage is mainly associated with the impairment of metabolic reactions and inability to reproduce. Unlike heat, radiation does not cause denaturation of protein. All microorganisms are affected by ionising radiation in a similar manner, but very much related to the nature of the organism and especially to its complexity. Much evidence showed that the damage occurs more in the (DNA) molecule compared to other critical sites, including membranes and lysosomes of the microorganism. The main biological target, DNA, controls the genetic constitution and reproductive process of the cell. DNA is the most vital cell constituent and it presents a relatively large volume in the microbial cell for absorption of radiation and a large surface for reaction with radiolytic products. The killing effect after irradiation is eventually due to loss of reproductive ability of microorganisms and cells.

The killing action of ionising radiation on microorganisms can be considered in three stages, each of extremely short duration: ionisation, radical formation and biochemical changes.

7. Repair of Damaged DNA

Some microorganisms have a great capability to repair damaged DNA molecules. *Micrococcus radiodurans* and *Micrococcus radiophilus* are more resistant than bacterial spores. Some strains of *Streptococcus faecium* are more resistant than any non-sporing bacteria. DNA strand breaks may be readily repaired by a polynucleotide ligase which can occur in the absence of any DNA synthesis or which would require post-irradiation protein synthesis (Idziak, 1973). The efficiency of a repair system is often reflected by a large increase in the dose of radiation for inactivation. However, the ability of cells to recover and grow after irradiation will not always reflect their resistance.

The amount of damage before death occurs also varies among the microorganisms. Death of the cell may result from about three double-strand breaks in *Escherichia coli* but 1400 may be required in *Micrococcus radiodurans*. Direct action may involve the addition of hydrogen atoms to the open bonds. Irradiated microorganisms are not killed immediately after a lethal dose has been absorbed. Death usually occurs during the first DNA replication.

Therefore, strand breaks alone could not be correlated with survival in microorganisms nor could the resistance of a radiation-resistant strain be correlated with a more effective repair system.

8. Factors Influencing Sensitivity to Radiation

The sensitivity or resistance of a microorganism to radiation depends on complexities of the biochemical and physiological state of the cell during irradiation time. It is also influenced by environmental conditions before, during and after irradiation (Ley, 1973; Russell, 1982).

8.1. Types and species

Microorganisms are more resistant to radiation than are higher forms of life. The correlation of radiation sensitivity is roughly inversely proportional to size. Viruses, the most minute living entities, are the most radiation resistant, some surviving at as high as 100 kGy (10 Mrad). Man, approximately at the other end of the size range and complexity, suffers death with only 5 Gy (500 rad).

The general order of increasing resistance is shown in Table 3 below.

Table 3. Radiation resistance of microorganisms.

Group	Organisms	Sterilising Dose (kGy)[*]
Sensitive	Vegetative bacteria (excluding some micrococci and streptococci).	0.5–10
	Animal viruses > 75 μm	
Moderately resistant	Moulds and yeasts	4–30
	Streptococcus faecium (suspended in buffer)	10–30
	Animal viruses 20–75 μm	
Resistant	Bacterial spores	10–50
	Bacillus pumilus	10–30
	Clostridium botulinum (some strains)	30
	Some viruses	10–30
	Streptococcus faecium (dried from serum broth)	10–45 / 30–40
	Animal viruses (except foot-and-mouth disease virus) < 20 μm	
Highly resistant	Moraxella (some strains)	~ 50
	Micrococcus radiodurans	55–70
	Bacillus spores (contrived mutants)	35–80
	Foot-and-mouth disease virus	~ 50
	Bacterial viruses	wide range

[*]Based on inactivation factor of 10^8 ($8D_{10}$).

The wide range of radiosensitivity may due to variation among genera, species and strains; but may also be attributed to variation in the conditions in which irradiation is carried out (Ley, 1973). Bacterial spores are usually more resistant than vegetative bacteria. The protection mechanism may be related to the spore core and the non-dividing stage. The particular phase of growth at the time of irradiation might account for the observed differences, e.g. high resistance is expected in the stationary phase and most sensitive in the dividing or vegetative stage. Viruses are moderately to highly resistant, depending on the DNA volume. Bacterial viruses are extremely resistant such as the "slow" viruses related to Creutzfeld-Jakob syndrome in man. The radio-resistance of *Micrococcus radiodurans* and *Streptococcus* sp. is associated to very efficient repair mechanisms.

The effect of radiation in fungi is slightly complicated since fungi possess more complex morphology, cytology and life cycles (Sommer, 1973). Spores, in the presence of moisture and favourable temperature, will germinate into tubes. In the presence of organic matters, these tubes develop further into hyphae and then mycelia which will again produce spores. Generally, a multicellular fungus has a greater resistance than single-celled fungus. If one cell is affected, other cells can still germinate. A multinuclear cell is more resistant than a unicellular one. Diploid cells are more resistant compared to haploid because of the presence of another set of chromosome. Spores at the germinating stage are increasingly sensitive to radiation. The radiation resistance of fungus spores is usually much less than the resistance of important spore-forming bacteria (Table 3). Radiation dose sufficient to inactivate bacterial contamination will normally eliminate fungal contamination.

Viruses vary from extremely simple systems comprising a relatively short single strand of nucleic acid with two to three proteins, which form the capsid, to those that contain a variety of proteins and some lipids (Pollard, 1973). Hence, the effect of ioni-sing radiation varies from virus to virus. Viruses have various properties, such as that of attachment, of injection, of coding a number of specific proteins and of lysis of a cell. Each of these properties reacts separately to ionising radiation. For instance, ionising radiation is used in the preparation of viral vaccines to kill the infectivity property of virus and not the antigenic property. Radiation penetrates well. It kills primarily the nucleic acid but not the protein antigen.

As a rule of thumb, the resistance of a species increases with decreasing size but this may not always true. In general, viruses are more resistant than bacterial spores. Bacterial spores are more resistant than vegetative forms, moulds and yeasts.

8.2. Oxygen

Oxygen enhances lethality when present during irradiation or if cells, irradiated under anoxic conditions, are exposed to oxygen immediately in the post-treatment. The resistance of microorganisms is usually increased two to five times if irradiated in anoxic conditions. The spores of *Bacillus pumilus* give a D_{10} value of 1.75 kGy when irradiated in air and 3.06 kGy in the absence of oxygen. If oxygen is present, it may react with e^- and $H^\bullet$ producing the perhydroxyl or superoxide radical ($HO_2^\bullet$), or with organic radicals giving peroxy species.

8.3. Moisture or water content

If tissues contain more water in its composition, the damage is more likely a consequence of indirect action. The amount of water will result in more radical formation due to radiolysis. The influence of moisture on microorganisms' susceptibility is interrelated with that of oxygen. The presence of oxygen may enhance radiation effect as oxygen reacts with free radicals such as $H^\bullet$ and e^-, leading to the production of hydroperoxy radicals ($HO_2^\bullet$) and hydrogen peroxide (H_2O_2), and with free organic radicals to produce organic peroxy radicals $RO_2^\bullet$ which will result in more radiation damage. Formation of free radicals increases the lethal effect of ionising radiation.

8.4. Temperature

An increase of the order of 10°C was reported to reduce D_{10} values by as much as 50%. Synergistic effect is observed under certain conditions when heat and irradiation are applied simultaneously, which is greater than the sum of the separate effects. Heating before or during irradiation may increase the sensitivity of fungus spores to radiation (Sommer, 1973). The combination of heat and radiation gives much more rapid loss of infectivity in virus than heat and radiation alone. Serum hepatitis virus can be treated at a moderate temperature of 45°C when in combination with radiation (Pollard, 1973).

When spores of *Clostridium botulinum* were irradiated in frozen phosphate buffer, there was a sharp increase in resistance. This is attributed to the reduction of indirect effect as the active radicals produced in water are immobilised. A 1.5-time increase is observed for *Salmonella typhimurium* when irradiated in the frozen state. The protective effect of low temperature is also observed in other vegetative organisms.

In general, the lower temperature before, during and after irradiation does not allow the proliferation of microorganisms while free radicals are not mobile in the frozen state. Therefore, microorganisms are more radio-resistant in frozen conditions.

8.5. Nutrient or organic substrates

Protection against radiation damage is conferred when irradiation is performed in dried serum broth, grease films, sucrose and other complex substrates. In a rich medium, microorganisms tend to be more resistant.

8.6. Chemical agents

Protective agents are chemicals which themselves reduce the lethal effect of radiation. Some chemicals, such as glycerol, aliphatic alcohols, thiourea, dimethyl sulphoxide and cysteine, protect bacteria against radiation damage. They possibly scavenge free radicals, thus blocking radiolysis or using up oxygen causing depletion during irradiation. Therefore, these chemicals act as protectors for microorganisms. On the other hand, other chemicals, including iodoacetic acid and potassium iodide, act as sensitisers, resulting in increase of single-strand breaks through reaction of iodine compound with radiolytic products of water or cell components. Compounds like phenylmercuric acetate react with the SH group and enhance the sensitivity of the cell. Some chemicals do influence the radiation effects after irradiation.

8.7. Dose rate

Dose-rate differences between gamma sources are too small to be of any significance with respect to bacterial inactivation. The large rate difference between gamma and electron beams could be significant. At very high dose rate, oxygen depletion occurs, resulting in more resistance. However, the dose rate used in commercial plants has no significant effect on the resistance.

9. Response to Radiation

The sensitivity of microorganisms to radiation is conveniently expressed as D_{10} (kGy), the dose required to reduce one log cycle or to kill 90% of the population. In practice, a number of equal-sized populations are exposed to different doses of radiation and the number of survivors counted. The counts, expressed as a fraction of the original number, are plotted linearly against the doses. The surviving fraction decreases against the dose, giving rise to an inactivation or dose response curve. It is convenient to plot the curve as a semi-logarithm plot. The inactivation curve can be linear, shouldered or exponential, as described earlier (Russell, 1982; Yusof, 1999).

The D_{10} is calculated as the gradient of the linear part of the curve, or as follows:

$$D_{10} = D/[\log N_o - \log N], \text{ where}$$
$$D = \text{the radiation dose (kGy)}$$
$$N_o = \text{the initial viable count}$$
$$N = \text{the viable count at dose D}$$

The D_{10} value is influenced by the type and species of micro-organism, cell cycle stage, oxygen, temperature during irradiation, water content, chemicals and nutrients, and to a certain extent, by the dose rate.

The formula can be used to determine the radiation sterilisation dose (D) when N_o (obtained from the bioburden test) and N (sterility assurance level or SAL is set by the manufacturer, usually 10^{-6}, i.e. the probability of getting one non-sterile product in a million) are given.

10. Discussion

DNA is a prime target of ionising radiation leading to the destruction of microorganisms. This target may be altered either directly by high-energy photons of ionising radiation or indirectly by the action of radicals produced by ionisation events. This can result in damages to the DNA strand and also to changes in the biochemical processes of important cell components. Unless the damages are repaired, the effect could be lethal, i.e. the microorganisms would not be able to reproduce.

Like other methods of sterilisation, the efficiency of radiation sterilisation is dependent on the number and type of contaminating organisms on the product presented to the treatment, and also upon the environmental conditions during the irradiation time. The ultimate objective in the application of sterilisation treatment is to avoid any risks of infection to patients in the use of tissue allografts. Therefore, every step involved in the production of high quality tissues including screening of donors, processing, packaging, storage, delivery and sterilisation, must be taken into account in order to achieve this objective. Inactivation of microorganisms by radiation sterilisation is only one of the many determining factors.

11. References

ANTONI, F. (1973). The effect of ionising radiation on some molecules of biological importance. In: *Manual on Radiation Sterilisation of Medical and Biological Materials*, IAEA Technical Reports Series No. 149, pp. 13–36.

COGGLE, J.E. (1973). *Biological Effects of Radiation*, Wykeham Science Series, London, p. 150.

GARDNER, J.F. and PEEL, M.M. (1986). *Introduction to Sterilisation and Disinfection*, Churchill Livingstone, Edinburgh, p. 183.

IDZIAK, E.S. (1973). Effects of radiation on microorganisms. *Int. J. Rad. Steril.* **1**, 45–49.

LEY, F.J. (1973). The effect of ionising radiation on bacteria. In: *Manual on Radiation Sterilisation of Medical and Biological Materials*, IAEA Technical Reports Series No. 149, pp. 37–63.

POLLARD, E.C. (1973). The effect of ionising radiation on viruses. In: *Manual on Radiation Sterilisation of Medical and Biological Materials*, IAEA Technical Reports Series No. 149, pp. 65–72.

RUSSELL, A.D. (1982). *The Destruction of Bacterial Spores*. Academic Press, London, pp. 110–151.

SOMMER, N. (1973). The effect of ionising radiation on fungi. In: *Manual on Radiation Sterilisation of Medical and Biological Materials*, IAEA Technical Reports Series No. 149, pp. 73–80.

VOLK, W.A. and WHEELER, M.F. (1988). *Basic Microbiology*, Harper & Row, New York, p. 687.

YUSOF, N. (1999). Quality system for the radiation sterilisation of tissue allografts. In: *Advances in Tissue Banking*, Vol. 1, G.O. Phillips, R. von Versen, D.M. Strong and A. Nather, eds., World Scientific, Singapore, pp. 261–321.

Advances in Tissue Banking Vol. 5

20 EFFECT OF IONISING RADIATION ON VIRUSES, PROTEINS AND PRIONS

N. HILMY and M. LINA

Batan Research Tissue Bank, Centre for Research and
Development of Isotopes and Radiation Technology
National Nuclear Energy Agency of Indonesia
Jalan Cinere Ps. Jumat
P.O. Box 7002, Jakarta 12070 JKSKL, Indonesia

1. Introduction

The possibility of transmission of infectious diseases by viruses, such
as HIV 1/2, hepatitis B/C (HBV and HCV), cytomegalovirus (CMC),
human T-lymphotropic virus 1 (HTLV-1), as well as by proteinaceous
infectious particle (prion), through transplantation of contaminated
allografts has been reviewed in many publications. The risk of the
disease transmission in musculoskeletal tissue allografts depends
upon the type of graft used and how it is processed. In general, the
risk can be eliminated through proper screening of the donor, proper
processing of tissues (by removing blood and bone marrow, freezing,
freeze drying) and then followed by radiation sterilisation (using
gamma-rays or particle electrons) of the finished product (Conrad
et al., 1993; Strong *et al.*, 1993; Thomford, 1993; Eastlund, 1996;
Dziedzic-Goclawska, 1997). Creutzfeld-Jacob disease (CJD) and rabies
have been transmitted through corneal transplant and dura mater
implant; Kuru disease had been shown to be transmissible by

injecting extracts of the diseased brains into the brains of healthy animals (Gajdusek *et al.*, 1972; Prusiner, 1991; Brown *et al.*, 1992).

It has been known that high-energy radiation of gamma-rays and electron beams has the ability to generate reactive species during interaction with matter. The process involves ionisation and excitation. Ionising radiation can affect the materials in two ways, i.e. direct and indirect. Direct effect usually means the interaction of radiation with molecules, causing ionisation or excitation and then causing damage in the molecules. Indirect effects usually refers to damage done to molecules by radiolytic products of irradiated water, oxygen or other materials in the medium. The major products of water radiolysis are free radicals (Taub, 1983; Arnikar, 1995).

In radiation microbiology, there are five types microorganisms that cause concern, i.e. viruses, vegetative bacterial cells, spores, yeasts and filamentous fungi (moulds). It has generally been found that in a model system, the smaller the cell the more radiation resistant it is. Therefore, viruses which are the smallest biological entities known, are also highly radiation resistant. The degree of resistance of these microbes to ionising radiation can be presented as follows: viruses > bacterial spores > vegetative bacterial cells > yeasts and moulds (Grecz *et al.*, 1983; Hilmy, 1998). Another generalisation is the law of Bergonie and Tribondeau which is, briefly, that cells which are reproductively active are more sensitive and cells that are no longer going to differentiate are less sensitive (Pollard, 1983). Although viruses are resistant to ionising radiation, it has been proven that radiation is a simple and efficient technique for inactivating a certain viral contamination (such as HIV and HCV) from bone and soft tissues allografts. Several reports described that a dose in the range of 30–40 kGy can be used to eliminate HIV from fresh-frozen patella ligament and freeze-dried bone grafts. However high doses (above the currently used sterilisation dose of 25 kGy) may evoke the degradation of important proteins of the musculoskeletal tissue allografts, such as collagen components, bone morphogenetic proteins (BMPs), as well as reduction of mechanical properties, although some of the changes caused are desirable, such as decreasing the immunogenicity of the grafts (Dziedzic-Goclawska *et al.*, 1991; Anderson *et al.*, 1992; Fideler *et al.*, 1994).

Many misconceptions involving the use of irradiation for sterilisation of allografts arise from the knowledge of therapeutic and accidental irradiation of animal and human *in vivo*. The effects of irradiation on tissues *in vivo* (in living organism) and on the same tissue *ex vivo* (outside the body) are very different. The radiation doses of 3 to 5 Gy can cause massive tissue damage in living human, but doses up to 10 kGy when used on a similar tissue *ex vivo* give no visible alteration on that tissue (Forsell, 1993; Strzelczyk, 1998).

This paper reviews the basic effects of radiation on proteins of tissues *ex vivo*, viruses and prions, and the possibility of reducing the damage of tissue allografts as well as eliminating contaminated viruses and prions from those tissues by radiation.

2. Effects of Radiation on Proteins of Tissue Grafts

Connective tissue is distributed throughout the body, in cartilage, ligaments, the matrix of bone, the pelvis of kidney, skin, etc. This connective tissue consists of mostly fibrous protein or collagen and collagen-like protein (the most abundant protein in the body, constituting 25 to 33% of the total proteins and therefore about 6% of the body weight), elastin and proteoglycans. Each tissue has a special type of collagen such as: collagen type I found in skin, bone and tendon; collagen type II found in cartilage; collagen type III found in foetal skin and blood vessel and collagen type IV found in basement membranes. Collagen consists of more than 20 kinds of amino acids, such as glycine, proline, alanine, etc. There are certain chemical and physical properties of collagen which also vary from tissue to tissue, such as the solubility, swelling and shrinkage temperature characteristics.

Elastin is another major protein of connective tissue. Its amino acid composition differs from that of collagen. Collagen is the principal protein of white connective tissue. Elastin is predominant in yellow tissue. The collagen content of human Achilles tendon is about 20 times of the elastin content, whereas in yellow ligamentum nuchae, the elastin content is about 5 times than that of collagen. Elastin is the predominant protein of elastic structures of several tissues, such as the wall of the big blood vessels. Proteoglycans contribute up to 30% of dry weight of the connective tissue and contain many different types of heteropolysaccharides (such as hyaluronic acids) which are linked to a polypeptide chain backbone and are found mostly in soft tissues such as skin, cartilage, heart valves and embryonic cartilage (Melvin *et al.*, 1968; Dereck, 1978). Based on their structure, proteoglycans are more sensitive to radiation as compared to collagen (Simic, 1983).

Bone is formed by osteoblasts which secrete organic substances composed of collagen, non-collagenous glycoproteins, phospho-proteins, mucopolysaccharides and lipids. These compounds are referred to as osteoid. The osteoid becomes embedded in the inter-cellular space to form an organic matrix. Calcium phosphate salt then precipitate around the organic matrix to become hydroxyapatite, which gives the bone its structural strength. The major constituent of the organic matrix is collagen, which accounts for 90 to 95% of the organic matrix. Osteoinduction is a unique property of bone tissue to stimulate new bone formation by differentiation of mesenchymal pluripotent progenitor cells. This property of bone is mediated by bone matrix which contains several bone morphogenetic proteins [BMP-2, BMP-4, BMP-5, BMP-6, osteogenin (MBP-3), osteoprotein (MBP-7) and transforming growth factor beta (TGF-β)]. Deficiency of BMP retards bone cell differentiation and accounts for the failure of fracture in post-menopausal women (Czitrom, 1994). BMPs were isolated by Urist *et al.* in 1969 and they contain mostly amino acids (more than 17 kinds) with molecular weight of around 17.5 KDa (Marshall *et al.*, 1983). Since proteins are macromolecules, they are one of the main target of radiation. The damage of BMPs will affect the quality of the irradiated bone grafts. Several publications described that gamma-rays from cobalt-60 source produce free radicals in the collagen phase of tissues that might be from direct or indirect effects of radiation. Most of those radicals are short-lived, but some radicals with extremely long lived have been identified in hydroxyapatite (Ostrowski *et al.*, 1980; Basril *et al.*, 1996). The major products of water radiolysis are free radicals $\bullet H$, e_{aq}^- (hydrated electron), $\bullet OH$ (hydroxyl radical), $\bullet HO_2$, positive ions H_2O^+ and molecular products H_2 and H_2O_2. The radicals are highly reactive chemical species and have a short life which is less that 10^{-11} seconds. The reaction of hydroxyl radicals with proteins of tissues as indirect radiation effects, leads to C–H bond abstraction, hydroxylation of aromatic, hetero-cyclic compounds as well as sulphur amino acid residues. The primary free radicals e_{aq}^-, and $\bullet OH$ are very reactive. Both of the radicals are very efficient in inactivating many enzymes, and they also produce cross-linkings and scissions in collagen components of tissues. If there are no other molecules, such as proteins and DNA, surrounding them, these radicals will disappear either in reaction with water or with other radiolytic products.

The presence of oxygen in tissues or in medium complicates the free radical reaction. One of the reaction is:

$$e_{aq}^- + O_2 \rightarrow O_2^-$$

$$\bullet H + O_2 \rightarrow \bullet HO_2$$

These radicals lead to formation of hydrogen peroxide, peroxide and hydroperoxydes, and will generate auto-oxidation reactions in wet tissues. The reactions will enhance radiation damage to tissues. On the other hand, irradiation at the frozen state (to immobilised water molecules and their radicals) will decrease the damage, but the temperature-dependent reduction of graft damage also concerns the inactivation of viruses. Reactivity of the radicals depends on the irradiation temperature, their reaction rate constants are higher at higher temperature. In the frozen state (solid water), the radicals are less mobile and less reactive. There is also a decrease in yield of the radicals as compared to the liquid state, such as liquid water, at room temperature. Radiation-induced damage of frozen biological specimen is tenfold lower than those of irradiation at room tempera-ture (Simic, 1983). Most of the fresh connective tissues have high water content, i.e. 30 to 80% w/w. Irradiation in the dry state (with water content of less than 8%) and absence of oxygen will reduce the damage. However, at a high dose of about 50 kGy, graft properties will be affected, caused by peptide-chain scission or cross-linking. The effect of various doses of ionising radiation on the osteoinductive properties of decalcified bone matrices (DBM) implanted hetero- topically was studied by Dziedzic-Goclawska *et al.* (1991). The results showed that lyophilised matrices irradiated at room temperature at doses of 35 to 50 kGy, were completely resorbed five weeks after implantation and did not induce osteogenesis, whereas the resorption of deep frozen ones irradiated with the same doses at $-72°C$ was slower and the small BMP molecules were not affected by radiation. However, the dose of 50 kGy affected the large molecule bone collagen, a carrier of BMPs. Wientroup *et al.* (1988) reported that a dose of 25 kGy did not destroy the bone induction properties of DBM and a dose of 30 to 50 kGy even enhanced bone induction. The interaction of radiation with connective tissues will produce cross-linkings and scissions in collagen components of tissues. Cross-linking will increase the mechanical properties of tissues. However, scissions will reduce those properties. The higher the dose of radia- tion given, the more adverse the effects would be on the tissues. At doses greater than 30 kGy, biomechanical properties of freeze-dried amnion membranes (such as tensile strength and elongation at break) and bone begin to be affected. The effects of these reactions can only be observed as the sum total of these effects, but not individually (Thomford, 1993; Hilmy, 1994). To reduce the damage, irradiation could be done in the frozen or dry state.

It can be summarised that the effects of radiation on tissue allografts can be controlled and these effects depend on:

— Irradiation dose (not more than 30 kGy)
— Type of the predominant proteins in tissues
— Water content of tissues (dry or wet state) and presence or absence of oxygen
— Temperature during irradiation (frozen or room temperature)

3. Effects of Radiation on Viruses

Virus is a subcellular organism with a parasitic intracellular life cycle and has no metabolic activity outside the host cell. Therefore, it cannot actually stay alive outside the host cell. In contrast to bacteria, yeasts and moulds, many of which may be beneficial or indifferent, it is characteristic of viruses that all are harmful. In biology, viruses are parasites at the cellular and molecular levels. The antibiotics and chemotherapeutic agents which inactivate bacteria are generally ineffective against viruses. Viruses are as a rule considerably more resistant to radiation than either bacteria or bacterial spores. A virus particle (virion) consists of a nucleic acid genome, either DNA or RNA but not both, and it is surrounded by a shell of protein which may also contain lipids and sugars. The function of the virion is to deliver the viral genome into a cell where it can replicate. The structure of most virus consists of the capsid (the protein structure surrounding the viral genome), the envelope that is a membrane derived from the host cell but with viral proteins embedded in it, and the genetic material (DNA or RNA) as the genome. Viral proteins are usually glycoproteins, with sugar groups attached to the polypeptides. All enveloped viruses have such proteins and, due to their nature and position on the surface of the virion, they are highly immunogenic. However, occasionally, viruses may carry ligase and endonuclease within their capsid. It is not yet clear if these enzymes play a role in radiation resistance of the viruses. Filoviruses (marburg and ebola haemorrhagic fever) are among the largest viruses. They have extremely long enveloped particles which although only 80 nm in width, can be 14 000 nm in length. The sizes of viruses range mostly from 20 nm to almost 14 000 nm. The proteins, as structural component and effectors, are responsible for the infection of cells, the production of the new (progeny) viruses, while the nucleic acids provide the viral genetic code required to produce proteins (Harper, 1994). Viruses can be subdivided by genome type as follows:

- double-stranded (ds) DNA, such as *Herpesviridae* (herpes simplex) and *Poxviridae* (chickenpox);
- single-stranded (ss) DNA such as *Parvoviridae* (B-19 infection);
- dsRNA such as *Reoviridae* (diarrhoea and colorado tick fever);
- ssRNA can be divided into positive-sense RNA such as *Picornaviridae* (common cold) and negative-sense RNA such as *Paramyxoviridae* (measles and mumps);

- viruses with RNA genome that use a DNA intermediate to produce the RNA genome, such as *Retroviridae* (AIDS, human T-cell leukaemia);
- viruses with DNA genome that use an RNA intermediate stage to produce the DNA genome, such *as Hepadnaviridae*.

Genomes (DNA and RNA) are the major targets for the biological effects of ionising radiation in killing the microbes. The main cause of virus inactivation is protein damage. The dose of radiation required to inactivate an infectious virus or its nucleic acid is much greater under direct than under indirect condition. The damage of the viral nucleic acid appears to be almost solely responsible for the loss of infectivity. The assumption that DNA is the most important target for radiation inactivation of microbes is based on its singularly important role in cell function (Redpath and Grossweiner, 1978). Sensitivity of the targets depends very much on their sizes. A large target is more sensitive to radiation compared to a smaller one. In general, a cell with a large nucleus and much DNA is more vulnerable than one with a small genome. Compared to genomes of bacteria, yeasts and moulds, viral genomes are very small. The size of the largest genome of virus (poxvirus) is about 3×10^2, bacteria (*E. coli*) is 10^5, yeast is 10^8, fruit fly is 10^9 and human is about 10^{10} kilobase pairs (kbp). The size of a single-stranded RNA genome of a picornavirus is only 7–8 kilobases (kb). That is the reason why viruses are more resistant to radiation compared to bacteria and yeasts (Fields and Knipe, 1990). Viruses with double-stranded (ds) DNA genomes often have among the largest of viral genomes and dsRNA genomes are mostly small genomes. The single-stranded (ss) genomes are smaller than the double-stranded genomes. The radiation resistance of different Virus groups shows considerable differences. Viruses with single-stranded genomes are about ten times more sensitive than viruses with double-stranded genomes although the genomes are smaller. Viruses with large genomes may be five times more sensitive than viruses with small genomes. However, their resistance may vary as much as tenfold, depending on a number of factors, particularly the concentration of oxygen (O_2), the organic materials in the suspending substrate, the temperature, the pH (which is unfavourable to microbes) during irradiation and the degree of dehydration. Ionising radiation can affect the DNA and RNA in two ways, i.e. (a) directly — the interaction of radiation with molecules causing the ionisation or excitation and producing damage in the molecules; and (b) indirectly — damage done to the molecules by toxic radiation products (free radicals) of water (H_2O) or O_2, or other materials (such as free radicals from irradiated protein) in the medium. Those radicals are •H, •OH, •O_2, e_{aq}^- and others. It is assumed that the various radicals produced by the ionising radiation of water are considered as toxic agents to viruses. The hydroxyl radicals (•OH) and oxygen radicals (•O_2) are among the most reactive in causing chromosome aberrations, such as the single- and double-strand breaks of the DNA or RNA which in turn cause the death of the viruses (Grecz *et al.*, 1983). The bases and amino acids which form the components of nucleic acids and proteins are reactive to products of radiation. Irradiation at the frozen state (-70 to $-80°C$) where water is immobilised, as well as in organic substrate, such as in a high concentration of protein, will increase the radiation resistance of viruses. In contrast, radiation in wet condition at room temperature will increase the sensitivity of viruses compared to radiation in dry state (Sullivan *et al.*, 1971). The action of those free radicals consists of random cleavage of internucleotide phosphate-ester bonds and then a decrease in molecular weight. The rupture of cross-linking hydrogen bonds, such as the adenine–thiamine pair of bases, occur more rapidly than those linking the guanine–cytosine pair (Cox *et al.*, 1955).

Ionising radiation under indirect conditions in poliovirus inactivation causes large alterations in protein capsids, such as cleavage of proteins, some aggregations, cross-link formations (occur among proteins or between proteins and nucleic acids), and release of viral RNA from virions. Capsid protein damage result in the inability of some virions to recognise receptors on the surface membrane of the host cells. Therefore, they will lose their abilities to bind to the host cells. Glycoproteins are the components sensitive to radiation and •OH radicals are the major damaging species acting on glycoproteins in the membrane, resulting in the inactivation of viral functions.

Although strand breakage has still been reported as an important cause of radiation inactivation of single-stranded nucleic acid, the combination of base damage and intrastrand cross-link formation is also important. The alteration is lethal because the viruses cannot reproduce after damage of their nucleic acids (Michaels *et al.*, 1978).

HBV, a member of the hepadnavirus from *Hepadnaviridae* family, possesses a double-stranded circular DNA genome that uses an RNA intermediate. The genome is 3.2 kilobase pairs (kb) containing promoters that drive the synthesis of viral transcripts (Chisari *et al.*, 1997). There is no data on the sensitivity of Hepatitis B virus to ionising radiation. However, this virus is known to be resistant to heat sterilisation. Since it has a small genome (only 3.2 kb) and a double-stranded DNA, it is assumed to be resistant to ionising radiation.

HCV is a positive single-stranded RNA virus and has a lipid envelope. The virus is related to the *Flaviviridae* family (Houghton, 1996). Both viruses (HBV and HCV) can cause liver disease. Based on the fact that it has a genome with a single-stranded RNA, it is assumed that this virus is also sensitive to radiation. Conrad *et al.* (1995) described that an irradiation dose of 17 kGy can eliminate this virus from grafts.

Human immunodeficiency virus (HIV) types 1 and 2 are members of the subfamily *Lentiviridae* of the *Retroviridae* family. Both of them can cause immune deficiency but HIV-1 infection appears to be more virulent. The viruses contain a single-stranded RNA genome and RNA-dependent DNA polymerase. The genome of HIV is 9.7 kb (O'Brien *et al.*, 1996). Since it has a single-stranded genome, it is assumed that this virus is also sensitive to radiation. Some results show that the irradiation dose needed to reduce the viral load by $1 \log_{10}$ (D_{10} value) of the HIV depends on the medium and the temperature during irradiation which is between 4 to 6 kGy. The generally accepted concentration levels for people infected with HIV virus who developed AIDS is 10^2–10^3 infectious particles per ml blood. Therefore, the sterilisation doses for HIV are 30–40 kGy (at the sterility assurance level/SAL of 10^{-6}). Many D_{10} values of viruses exceed 5 kGy, and some of them, such as foot-and-mouth disease, have D_{10} values of 13 kGy when irradiated at frozen state. The effects of radiation on microorganisms, including viruses, are exponential. The radiation sterilisation dose used depends on the viral bioburden (Conway *et al.*, 1990; Conway and Thomford, 1992). A radiation dose of 29.5 kGy leads to a depletion of the enveloped DNA-virus pseudorabies of more than $5 \log_{10}$ stages irradiated in frozen bone (Pruss *et al.*, 1999). Poliovirus is a member of the *Picornaviridae* family and has a single-stranded RNA genome. D_{10} value of the virus in high-protein medium as 4.8–5.0 kGy (Grecz, 1983; Ward, 1980). The same author also revealed that the D_{10} value of herpes simplex virus in the same medium was 4.3 kGy. Herpes simplex virus is a member of the *Herpesviridae* family which has double-strand DNA.

According to Megumi *et al.* (1993), Sendai virus as a single-stranded RNA virus, related to *Orthomyxoviridae* family, has D_{10} value of around 0.5 kGy.

4. Effects of Radiation on Prions

Unlike virus, a prion is an infectious protein, produced by modifying the structure of a specific prion protein (PrP) which is found on nerve cell membranes. It consists of more than 250 kind of amino acids. The gene for PrP is present in most mammals. The prions are completely without nucleic acid and they have no genetic information. The term prion was introduced by Prusiner (1982), to distinguish the protein-aceous infectious particles that cause scrapie in sheep, bovine spongi-form encephalopathy (BSE) in cow, fatal neuro-degenerative diseases in humans, such as Creutzfeldt-Jacob disease (CJD), Gerstmann-Straussler-Scheinker (GSS), fatal familial insomnia (FFI) and Kuru, from both viroids and viruses. Collectively, these diseases are known as transmissible spongiform encephalopathies (TSE). In the beginning, the prion hypothesis postulates that the diseases are caused by an unconventional infectious agent, described as a slow virus and then as a self-replicated protein and more recently as a small proteinaceous infectious particle (prion), i.e. a normal protein (PrP^c) which adopts an abnormal converted form or the disease-associated form which is known as PrP^{Sc}. The sequence of amino acids in PrP^c and PrP^{Sc} is identical. The PrP^{Sc} protein is catalytic and self-propagating and it resists inactivation by agents which destroy nucleic acid. It also contains an essential modified isoform of a cellular protein (Prusiner, 1996).

The process of the diseases begins when one molecule of prion or PrP^{Sc} contacts a normal prion protein molecule (PrP^c) and then induces it to refold into a PrP^{Sc} molecule in an exponential process. That means one PrP^{Sc} can convert more PrP^c into PrP^{Sc}, causing disease by the loss of normal PrP^c function. The accumulation of prions will reach a certain dangerous level which can then induce the disease (Prusiner, 1991).

The most common form of prion disease in human being is sporadic CJD. Less than 1% of CJD cases are infectious and most of these appear to be iatrogenic. Between 10 and 15% of prion disease cases are inherited. The remaining are sporadic. Kuru was once the most common cause of death among New Guinea women but has virtually disappeared with the cessation of ritualistic cannibalism (Alper, 1979). PrP^{CJD} has been found in the brains of most patients who died of prion disease. The term PrP^{CJD} is preferred by some investigators when referring to the abnormal isoform of human PrP in human brain. PrP^{Sc} is always used after human CJD prions passage into an experimental animal. At present, prions have gained wide recognition as extraordinary protein agents that cause a number of infectious, genetic and spontaneous disorders (Prusiner, 1995). Prions are very resistant to endogenous protease, that would normally destroy the protein, to temperatures above 100°C, to formalin, to extremes of pH, to non-polar organic solvents, to years of burying. It is able to pass through 0.1 μm filters (Brown *et al.*, 1982). Infectivity of prions can be destroyed by 0.1 to 1N NaOH for one hour at room temperature, or one hour in 0.5% solution of sodium hypo-chlorite as well as 30 to 60 minutes at 130°C (Brown *et al.*, 1984). Prion (PrP^{Sc}) is a protease-resistant polypeptide with molecule weight (MW) of 27–30 kDa (kilodalton), designated as PrP 27–30. It is in-soluble in non-denaturing detergent. PrP^c with MW of 33–35 kDa, designated as PrP 33–35, is protease-sensitive and soluble in non-denaturing detergent. It is assumed that reduction in protein size from 33–35 kDa to 27–30 kDa, increases the resistancy of prions. Compared to the molecular weight of very small virus-like particles associated with fibrils in hamsters, i.e. 750 kDa, the size of prions are very small.

The effects of gamma-rays and UV light on prions have been reported by several investigators. Since prion is a very small modified protein (PrP^{Sc}) without any nucleic acid component which can be degraded by ionising radiations, it is resistant to ultraviolet and gamma radiation which break down the nucleic acid. Irradiation dose of 25 kGy could not eliminate prions from lyophilised dura mater (Center for Disease Control, 1987).

5. References

ALPER, M. (1979). Epidemiology and ecology of kuru. In: *Slow Transmissible Diseases of the Nervous System*, Vol. I, S.B. Prusiber and W.J. Hadlow, eds., Academic Press, New York, pp. 67–90.

ANDERSON, M.J. (1992). Compressive mechanical properties of human cancellous bone after gamma irradiation. *J. Bone Joint Surg.* **74**, 749.

BROWN, P., ROHWER, R.G., GAJDUSEK, D.C. (1984). Sodium hydroxide decontamination of Creutzfeldt-Jacob disease virus. *New Engl. J. Med.* **310**, 727.

BROWN, P., GIBBS, C.J., AMYX, H.L., KINGSBURY, D.T., ROHWER, R.G., SULIMA, M.P. and GAJDUSEK, D.C. (1982). Chemical disinfections of Creutzfeldt-Jacob disease virus. *New Engl. J. Med.* **306**, 1279.

BROWN, P., PREECE, M.A. and WILL, R.G. (1992). Friendly fire in medicine: Hormones, homografts, and Creutzfeldt-Jacob disease. *Lancet* **340**, 24–27.

BASRIL, A., JAMIL, A., SUTJIPTO, S. and HILMY, N. (1996). Radicals formation of irradiated lyophilized cancellous bovine and human bone. Presented at the *6th APASTB and First World Congress of Tissue Bank*, 2–5 October, Gold Coast, Australia.

CENTER FOR DISEASE CONTROL (1987). Up date: Creutzfeldt Jacob disease in a patient receiving a cadaveric dura mater graft. *JAMA* **258**, 309–310.

CHISARI, F.V. and FERRARI, C. (1997). Viral hepatitis. In: *Viral Pathogenesis*, N. Nathanson, R. Ahmed, F.G. Scarano, D.E. Griffin, K.V. Holmes, F.A. Murphy and H.L. Robinson, eds., Lippincott-Raven Publisher, Philadelphia, pp. 745–747.

CONRAD, E.U., GRETCH, D., OBERMEYER, K., MOOGK, M., SAYERS, M., WILSON, J. and STRONG, D.M. (1995). The transmission of Hepatitis C virus through tissue transplantation. *J. Bone Joint Surg.* **77-A**, 214–224.

COX, R.A., OVEREND, W.G., PEACOXKE, A.R. and WILSON, S. (1955). Effect of gamma–rays on solution of sodium dioxyribonucleate. *Nature* **12**, 919–921.

CZITROM, A.A. (1994). Biology of bone grafting and principles of bone banking. In: *The Pediatric Spine, Principle and Practice*, S.L. Weinstein, ed., Raven Press, New York.

DERECK, J.J., MACNOW, A., MICHAEL, L.B., AMSTRONG, T. (1978). *Principle of Biochemistry*, McGraw Hill Inc., USA.

DZIEDZIC-GOCLAWSKA, A. and STACHOWICZ, W. (1997). Sterilization of tissue allografts. In: *Advances in Tissue Banking*, G.O. Phillips, R. von Versen, D.M. Strong, A. Nather, eds., World Scientific, Singapore, pp. 261–321.

DZIEDZIC-GOCLAWSKA, A., OSTROWSKI, K., STACHOWICKZ, W., MICHALIK, J. and GRZESIK, W. (1991). Effect of radiation sterilization on osteoinductive properties and the rate of remodeling of bone implants preserved by lyophilization and deep freezing. *Clin. Orthop. Rel. Res.* **272**, 30–37.

DZIEDZIC-GOCLAWSKA, A., WASILEWSKA, M., KAMINSKI, A. and MAROWSKA, J. (1996). The effect of radiation sterilization conditions on solubility *in vitro* of bone matrix collagen as a carrier of bone morphogenetic proteins. *Proc. 5th Int. Conf. Tissue Banking*, EATB, Berlin.

EASTLUD, T. (1996). Infectious hazards of bone allograft transplantation: Reducing the risk. In: *Orthopaedic Allograft Surgery*, A.A. Czitrom and H. Winkler, eds., Springer, New York, pp. 10–28.

FIDELER, B.M., VANGSNESS, C.T., MOORE, T., LI, Z. and RASHEED, S. (1994). Effects of gamma irradiation on human immunodeficiency virus. *J. Bone Joint Surg.* **76-A**, 1032–1035.

FIELDS, B.N. and KNIPE, D.M. (1990). *Virology*, 2nd edn., Raven Press, New York.

FORSELL, J.H. (1993). Irradiation of musculoskeletal tissues. In: *Musculoskeletal Tissue Banking*, W.W. Tomford, ed., Raven Press, New York, pp. 149–80.

GAJDUSEK, D.C., GIBBS, C.J., ROGERS, N.G., BASNIGHT and HOOK, S.J. (1972). Persistence of viruses of kuru and CJD in tissue cultures of brain cells. *Nature* **235**, 104–105.

GRECZ, N., ROWLEY, D.B. and MATSUYAMA, A. (1983). The action of radiation on Bacteria and Viruses, In: *Preservation of Food by Ionizing Radiation*, Vol. II, A.S. Josephson and M.S. Peterson, eds., CRC Press Inc., Boca Raton, Florida, pp. 168–209.

HARPER, D.R. (1994). *Molecular Virology*. BIOS Scientific Publisher Ltd., Oxford, pp. 1–48.

HILMY, N. (1998). Benefits of ionizing radiation to increase hygienic quality of medical devices, pharmaceutical products and their raw materials, food products and their environment. *Quart. J. Indonesian Nuclear Soc.* **1**, 69–80.

HILMY, N., BASRIL., A. and FEBRIDA, A. (1994). The effects of procurement, packaging materials, storage and irradiation dose on physical properties of lyophilized amniotic membranes. *Proc. IAEA Project Formulation Meeting of Radiation Sterilization of Tissue Grafts*, Manila.

HOUGHTON, M. (1996). Hepatitis C virus. In: *Fields Virology*. B.N. Fields, D.M. Knipe and P.M. Howley, eds., Lippincott-Raven Publisher, Philadelphia, pp. 1035–1057.

MARSHALL, R.,URIST, M.R., DE LANGE, G.A. (1983). Bone cell differentiation and growth factors. *Science*, **220**, pp. 680–686.

MEGUMI, T., FUJITA, S.I., IWAI, Y. and ITO, T. (1993). The effect of gamma-ray-induced radicals on activities and membrane structure of sendai virus in aqueous solutions. *Radiat. Res.* **134**, 129–133.

MELVIN, J.G. and STEPHEN, M.K. (1968). The organization and structure of bone and the mechanism of calcification. In: *A Treatise on Collagen*, Vol. II, B.S. Gould and G.N. Ramachandran, eds., Academic Press, London.

MICHAELS, H.B. and HUNT, J.W. (1978). A model for radiation damage in cells by direct effect and by indirect effect: A radiation chemistry approach. *Radiat. Res.* **74**, 23–24.

O'BRIEN, W.A. and POMERANTZ, R.J. (1996). HIV infection and associated disease. In: *Viral Pathogenesis*, N. Nathanson, R. Ahmed, F.G. Scarano, D.E. Griffin, K.V. Holmes, F.A. Murphy and H.L. Robinson, eds., Lippincott-Raven Publisher, Philadelphia, pp. 815–836.

OSTROWSKI, K., DZIEDZIC-GOCLAWSKA, A. and STACHOWICZ, W. (1980). Stable radiation-induced paramagnetic entities in tissue mineral and their use in calcified tissue research. In: *Free Radicals in Biology*, Vol. IV, W. Pryor, ed., Academic Press, New York, pp. 321–344.

POLLARD, E.C. (1983). Effects of radiation at the cellular and tissue level. In: *Preservation of Food by Ionizing Radiation*, Vol. II, A.S.

Josephson and M.S. Peterson, eds., CRC Press Inc., Boca Raton, Florida, pp. 220–242.

PRUSINER, S.B. (1982). Novel proteinaceous infectious particles cause scrapie. *Science* **216**, 136–144.

PRUSINER, S.B. (1993). Molecular biology of prion diseases. *Science* **252**, 1515–1522.

PRUSINER, S.B. (1995). Prion disease. *Sci. Am.* **272**, 48–57.

PRUSINER, S.B. (1996). Prions. In: *Fields Virology*, D.M. Fields and D.M. Knipe, eds., Lippincott-Raven, Philadelphia, pp. 2901–2949.

PRUSS, A., VON VERSEN, R., MOENIG, H.J., KIESEWETTER, H., PAULI, G. (1999). Irradiation sterilization in tissue banking-validation of the procedure using pseudorabies virus as a model. To be published.

REDPATH, B.J.L. and GROSSWEINER, L.I. (1978). Radiation inactivation of T7 phage. *Radiat. Res.* **73**, 51–74.

SIMIC, M.G. (1983). Radiation Chemistry of Water Soluble Food. In: *Preservation of Food by Ionizing Radiation*, Vol. II, A.S. Josephson and M.S. Peterson, eds., CRC Press Inc., Boca Raton, Florida, pp. 1–70.

STRONG, D.M. and MACKENZIE, A.P. (1993). Freeze-drying of tissue. In: *Musculoskeletal Tissue Banking*, W.W. Tomford, ed., Raven Press, New York, pp. 181–208.

STRZELCZYK, J. (1998). Radiogenic health effects, communicating risks to the general public. *Proc. 8th Annual National Radiology Emergency Preparedness Conference*, Hyannis, Massachusetts, USA.

SULLIVAN, R., FASSOLITIS, A.C., LARKIN, E.P., READ, R.B. and PEELER, J.T. (1971). Inactivation of thirty viruses by gamma radiation. *Appl. Microbiol.* **22**, 62.

TAUB, I.A. (1983). Reaction mechanisms, irradiation parameters and product formation. In: *Preservation of Food by Ionizing Radiation*,

Vol. II, A.S. Josephson and M.S. Peterson, eds., CRC Press Inc., Boca Raton, Florida, pp. 125–166.

TOMFORD, W.W. (1993). Disease transmission, sterilization and clinical use of musculoskeletal tissue allografts. In: *Musculoskeletal Tissue Banking*, W.W. Tomford, ed., Raven Press, New York, pp. 209–230.

URIST, M.R. (1969). Bone morphogenetic protein, bone regeneration, heterotopic ossification and the bone marrow consortium. In: *Bone and Mineral Research*, W.A. Peck, ed., Elsevier Science Publisher, pp. 57–112.

WARD, R. (1980). Mechanism of poliovirus inactivation by direct and indirect effects of ionizing radiation. *Radiat. Res.* **83**, pp. 330–344.

WIENTROUB, S. and REDDI, A.H. (1988). Influence of irradiation on osteoinductive potential of demineralized bone matrix. *Calcif. Tissue Int.* **42**, 255–260.

SECTION VI:

BIOLOGY OF HEALING OF ALLOGRAFTS

Advances in Tissue Banking Vol. 5

21 THE SCIENTIFIC BASIS OF WOUND HEALING

KEITH MOORE

Clinical Research Laboratory
Wound Management Division
Smith & Nephew Medical Limited
Imperial House, Imperial Way
Newport, South Wales NP10 8UH, UK

1. Introduction

Because of the potential life-threatening nature of open wounds and the problems associated with consequential sepsis in the pre-antibiotic era, mankind has tried many empirical interventions to assist healing. Honey has been widely used and is still undergoing investigation as a wound treatment. Using our present knowledge of cell biology and modern analytical techniques, honey can be demonstrated to exert antibacterial effects by osmotic lysis and generation of hydrogen peroxide and may even modulate cell function at the wound site. Other more exotic treatments such as application of dove's dung have thankfully fallen into disuse. The inflammatory response was noted by the ancient Egyptians who identified infected wounds as requiring different treatment from those not producing pus. The Greek Celsus identified the cardinal signs of inflammation as rubor, tumour, calor and dolour (redness, swelling, heat and pain).

With the development of antiseptic techniques and an understanding of the causes of infection in the 19th century, the treatment of wounds advanced dramatically. At the same time, advances in the fields of cell biology and histopathology allowed development of an understanding of the cellular basis of wound healing. Metchnikoff, studying the tissue response to acute injury, described the migration of microphages (neutrophils) and macrophages to the site of injury. One hundred years later, we now believe these events to be crucial to the regulation of the healing response.

Wound healing research is a diverse field drawing on many disciplines. Increasing knowledge of the cellular and molecular processes involved allows development of an integrated description of the many-fold cellular processes and control mechanisms that allow for efficient repair after acute tissue injury.

2. Dermal Healing

The skin can be considered as an organ of considerable elasticity and tensile strength that provides a barrier to the external environment. Its prime function is to prevent the ingress of bacteria and viruses and to maintain internal homeostasis. This barrier function is provided by the external layer of keratinocytes which form the epidermis (Fig. 1). Tensile strength and elasticity are provided by

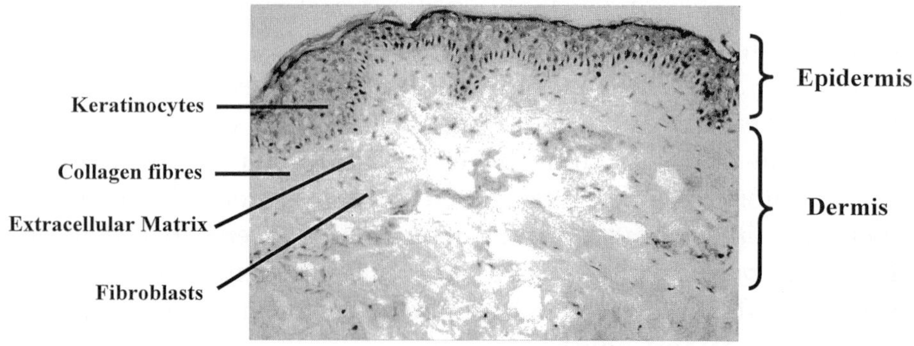

Fig. 1. Normal skin.

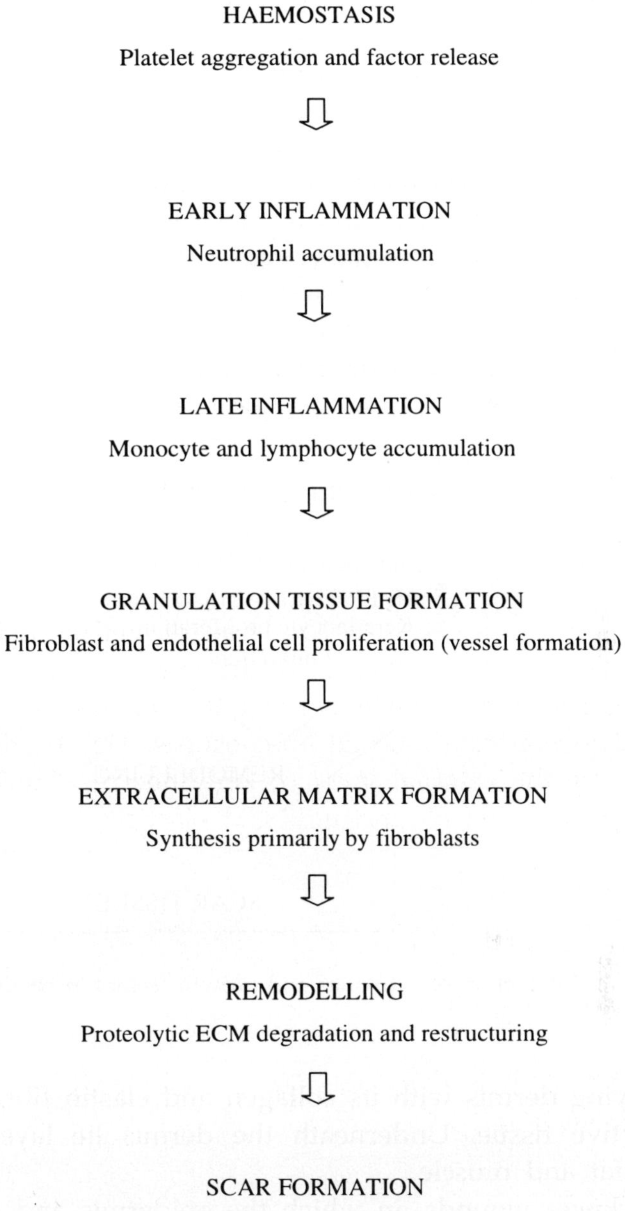

HAEMOSTASIS

Platelet aggregation and factor release

⇩

EARLY INFLAMMATION

Neutrophil accumulation

⇩

LATE INFLAMMATION

Monocyte and lymphocyte accumulation

⇩

GRANULATION TISSUE FORMATION

Fibroblast and endothelial cell proliferation (vessel formation)

⇩

EXTRACELLULAR MATRIX FORMATION

Synthesis primarily by fibroblasts

⇩

REMODELLING

Proteolytic ECM degradation and restructuring

⇩

SCAR FORMATION

Fig. 2. The healing sequence.

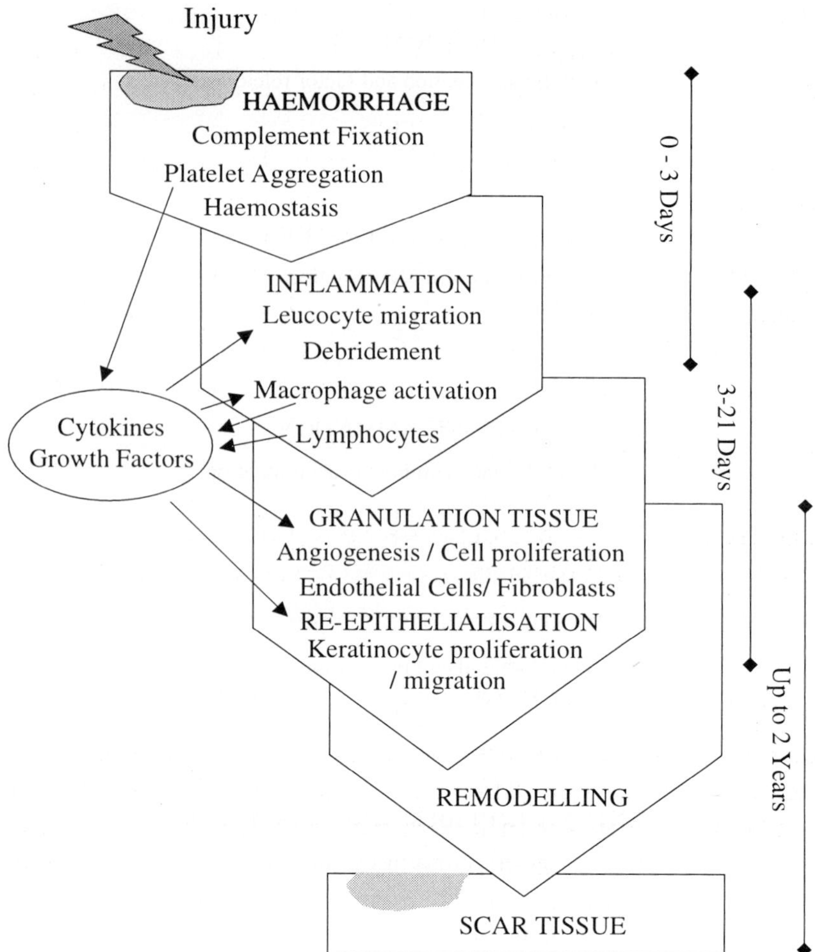

Fig. 3. Interaction of cytokines and growth factors in healing.

the underlying dermis with its collagen and elastin fibrils forming the connective tissue. Underneath the dermis lie layers of sub-cutaneous fat and muscle.

Full thickness wounds, in which the epidermis and dermis are removed down to the fat layer by traumatic injury or surgery, can heal by either primary or secondary intention. Suturing of the wound will draw the edges together and is described as primary healing. Secondary healing occurs where the wound is left open and temporary barrier function is provided by a sterile dressing in modern clinical practice. The wound space is filled by newly synthesised granulation tissue, the wound edges are drawn together by wound contraction and the surface of the wound covered by keratinocytes migrating from the intact epidermis at the wound margin. The cellular basis of healing by secondary intention will be considered in this review.

Wound healing is a complex-ordered biological process that can be divided into a number of distinct phases which follow a logical sequence (Fig. 2).

The sequential phases overlap, and at each phase, different cell types play key roles. Progression between phases and cell function during each phase is considered to be regulated by locally synthesised and secreted growth factors and cytokines (Blistein-Willinger, 1991) (Fig. 3).

3. Cytokines and Growth Factors in Healing

Cytokines and growth factors are polypeptide molecules that regulate migration, proliferation, differentiation and metabolism of mammalian cells. They may act in a paracrine manner on cells adjacent to the secreting cell, as autocrine factors on the secreting cell and also as endocrine factors bound to carrier proteins. A diverse range of these factors have been identified in wound interstitial fluid and a number have been identified as potentially playing a key role in regulating healing. Platelet-derived growth factor (PDGF) and transforming growth factor (TGF) are released by platelets and are important in initiating healing. The inflammatory phase of healing is modulated by cytokines such as tumour necrosis factor alpha (TNFα), interleukin-1 (IL-1), interleukin-4 (IL-4) and the peptide chemokine interleukin-8 (IL-8). The sequential phases of granulation tissue formation, re-epithelialisation and extracellular matrix formation are regulated by fibroblast growth factors, transforming growth factors and epidermal growth factor, amongst many others.

3.1. Platelet-derived growth factor

PDGF is a family of three isoforms, composed of dimers of the PDGF-A or PDGF-B chains, which have overlapping but distinct biological properties generated by interaction with two types of receptor. It is produced by platelets, macrophages, endothelial cells and keratinocytes. Release of PDGF by platelets is important in initiating healing. It stimulates chemotaxis of fibroblasts, neutrophils and macrophages. Once these cells are attracted to the wound site, PDGF can then activate macrophages and induce proliferation of fibroblasts. Additionally, it can stimulate the production of the extracellular matrix components fibronectin and hyaluronan, although not as effectively as other factors such as TGFβ.

Recombinant PDGF has been evaluated in several clinical trials to treat non-healing chronic wounds and has been demonstrated to be of benefit in treatment of wounds where healing is impaired by diabetes (Brown and Breeden, 1994).

3.2. Transforming growth factor

The three isoforms of TGFβ (β1, β2 and β3) have a broad range of activity within healing. TGFβ1 is the most abundant in all tissues and is the form found in platelets. All cells involved in healing can produce and/or respond to TGFβ.

Release of TGFβ by platelets at the same time as PDGF is important in initiating healing as, at low concentrations, it is chemotactic for monocytes, lymphocytes and fibroblasts. Its role in angiogenesis is controversial as, in some experimental systems, it stimulates endothelial cell proliferation and tubule formation, whilst in others, it is inhibitory. Its actions may therefore be contextual and concentration dependent.

TGFβ plays a central role in regulating the maturation and strength of wounds. It regulates many matrix proteins, including collagen, proteoglycans, fibronectin, matrix-degrading proteases and their inhibitors. Topical application of TGFβ increases the strength of experimental incisional wounds (Mustoe *et al.*, 1987). Manipulation of the TGFβ isoforms during healing can modify scarring. Antibody neutralisation of TGFβ1 and β2 or increasing TGFβ3 concentrations by exogenous application decreases post-surgical scarring (Shah *et al.*, 1995).

3.3. Fibroblast growth factor

Although at least ten fibroblast growth factor (FGF) family members are known, FGF-1 (acidic FGF or aFGF) and FGF-2 (basic FGF or bFGF) are most widely characterised with respect to wound healing. They are weakly soluble with a strong affinity for heparan sulphate, leading to them being bound in the wound extracellular matrix. FGF-2 has been detected at the wound site early in healing and its rapid appearance after injury suggests that pre-existing tissue FGF-2 may be important in healing rather than that synthesised *de novo* by inflammatory macrophages. It stimulates angiogenesis, leading to accelerated re-epithelialisation after experimental application (Mustoe *et al.*, 1991).

3.4. Epidermal growth factor

Epidermal growth factor (EGF) is a small molecule which exhibits homology with regions of the TGFα molecule. It is produced by macrophages and epidermal cells with the keratinocyte and fibroblast as targets. Its primary role is to stimulate keratinocytes to migrate across the wound provisional matrix and induce epidermal regeneration (Brown *et al.*, 1991)

3.5. Cytokines

The term cytokine generally refers to molecules such as the interleukins, which have initially been investigated for their role in regulation of the immune response. Because of the inflammatory response that is associated with wounded tissue, they also have a potential role to play in the regulation of healing either directly by their effect on the structural cells in wounded tissue, such as fibroblasts, endothelial cells or keratinocytes, or indirectly by their modulation of growth factor production by macrophages.

IL-1 and TNFα are both pro-inflammatory cytokines that will induce expression of adhesion molecules such as ICAM-1 and E-selectin by endothelial cells, allowing leukocytes to adhere to the lumen of capillaries and extravasate into the wound site. These cytokines activate macrophages and initiate production of growth factors required for healing and more pro-inflammatory mediators to prolong the inflammatory response. Overproduction of TNFα may lead to a persisting chronic inflammatory response that is involved in the pathogenesis of chronic wounds. However, there is a requirement for TNFα to allow normal healing (Lee *et al.*, 1999) and induction of a transient TNFα response may re-initiate healing in non-healing chronic wounds (Moore, 1999).

In order for monocytes to differentiate into activated macrophages, they need to pass through a priming stage of differentiation. During this stage, they are programmed for responsiveness to subsequent stimuli by exposure to the cytokine micro-environment. For example, interferon-γ will give a positive priming signal, whilst exposure to interleukin-4 acts to down-regulate the inflammatory response by inhibition of priming.

3.6. Other factors

Many other factors are likely to be involved in the regulation of healing. There include vascular endothelial cell growth factor (VEGF), insulin-like growth factor (IGF-1), and granulocyte monocyte colony-stimulating factor (GM-CSF).

4. Haemostasis

Blood coagulation at the injury site is essential to prevent blood loss but it is also important in initiating the healing sequence. When platelets are released from damaged vessels, exposure to the connective tissue and activation by interaction with collagen induce aggregation and release of the contents of their alpha-granules. These contain a number of bioactive molecules, including fibrinogen, Von Willebrand factor VIII and thrombokinase which triggers coagulation to form a fibrin clot. Platelet-derived growth factor, TGFα and TGFβ are also released and are important in initiating healing. Both PDGF and TGFβ are multifunctional with respect to healing and play roles in recruitment of cells to the wound site and subsequent modulation of cell activity. Both are chemotactic for fibroblasts and will induce their migration from dermis at the wound margin into the fibrin clot which plugs the wound site. Additionally, PDGF is chemotactic for blood neutrophils and monocytes and thus helps initiate an inflammatory response, which is the second phase of healing.

5. Inflammation

The wound inflammatory response can be divided into an early inflammation predominated by a neutrophil infiltrate and a late inflammation which is characterised by a mononuclear cell infiltrate of macrophages and lymphocytes.

A number of neutrophil chemo-attractants are generated at the site of injury. These include proteolytic degradation products of fibrinogen and fibrin, complement components C3a and C5a, platelet factor 4 and PDGF from platelets. Their release induces a rapid increase in neutrophil number at the wound site within hours of injury. The neutrophils are activated during chemotaxis and produce elastase and collagenase to facilitate extravasation and migration. In normal healing, the role of neutrophils is restricted to destruction of bacteria contaminating the wound site. The bacteria are phagocytosed and contained within phagosomes where they are killed by reactive oxygen species, such as superoxide, hydroxyl free radicals and hydrogen peroxide. In the absence of wound infection, the number of neutrophils rapidly decreases, and they play no role in subsequent healing events.

At the same time as initiation of neutrophil chemotaxis, monocytes and lymphocytes are attracted to the wound site by factors such as PDGF. Responding to the tissue environment, monocytes differentiate into macrophages. Within the immune response, these cells are scavenger cells that phagocytose and kill bacteria that have been opsonised by binding specific antibody and complement fixation products present within serum exuding through the wound tissue. Concomitantly, macrophages will also phagocytose cell debris, senescent neutrophils and devitalised tissue. This latter function is described as debridement. In evolutionary terms, the macrophage is present at the wound site as a component of the primitive innate immune response which pre-dates the aquired immune response. However, as a consequence of the role played in the immune system, the macrophage demonstrates an exquisite responsiveness to its micro-environment. This is manifested by the ability to synthesise and release a large number of bioactive molecules, many of which may interact in the healing process (Table 1).

The ability to release these molecules gives rise to the concept that the macrophage plays a pivotal role in regulation of healing (Clark, 1996). This is supported by the demonstration that depletion of macrophages from the wound site inhibits healing (Liebovich

Table 1. Macrophage-derived cytokines and growth factors involved in regulation of wound healing.

Interleukin-1
Interleukin-6
Interleukin-8
Tumour necrosis factor alpha
Transforming growth factor beta
Epidermal growth factor
Fibroblast growth factor
Platelet-derived growth factor
Granulocyte-monocyte growth factor
Vascular endothelial cell growth factor

and Ross, 1975), that defective healing in aged mice can be restored by transfer of macrophages from young mice (Danon *et al.*, 1989) and that the proliferation of fibroblasts and endothelial cells during granulation tissue formation follows on from the increase in macrophages during the late inflammatory phase of healing.

Lymphocytes form the other component of the late inflammatory infiltrate. These are predominantly T-lymphocytes although B-lymphocytes have also been observed in human wound tissue. Murine experiments have indicated that systemic depletion of T-lymphocytes by administration of an anti-CD3 monoclonal antibody can impair healing (Barbul, 1990). T-lymphocytes can be divided into two major subsets of $CD4^+$ T_{helper} cells and $CD8^+$ $T_{cytotoxic/suppressor}$ cells. These functional definitions are derived from their roles played in the immune response. However, they also appear to be relevant to healing as depletion of $CD8^+$ T-lymphocytes enhances murine wound healing and $CD4^+$ T-lymphocytes promote healing in an *in vitro* rat epitenon healing model. Further support for this subpopulation dichotomy is given by the observation in humans that within one week of surgery, wound tissue contains a raised level of $CD4^+$ cells as compared to the increased number of $CD8^+$ cells found immediately prior to wound closure when the rate of granulation tissue formation and re-epithelialisation is decreasing (Boyce *et al.*, 2000).

6. Granulation Tissue Formation

Granulation tissue is formed during what is often referred to as the proliferation phase of healing. During the inflammatory phase, many chemotactic and mitogenic factors are released and these initially attract fibroblasts and endothelial cells into the wound site and then stimulate them to proliferate. Granulation tissue was so called by early clinicians because, under examination by magnifying glass, it has a granular appearance. Healthy granulation tissue appears red because of the presence of a high density of blood vessels. It is a fragile tissue composed of a matrix of fibrin, fibronectin, glycosaminoglycans with proliferating endothelial cells and fibroblasts mixed with a population of inflammatory macrophages and lymphocytes.

Fibroblasts that migrate from the adjacent epidermis proliferate under the influence of mitogenic factors such as FGF, IGF-1 and PDGF. They then undergo phenotypic modulation to form a specialised subset of fibroblasts known as myofibroblasts (Darby *et al.*, 1990) which align into arrays parallel with the wound surface. The myofibroblast has contractile features and is thought to exert a cytoskeleton-dependent tension on the granulation tissue and draw the wound edges together by contraction. After wound closure, the myofibroblast is removed by apoptosis and wound tension decreases (Desmouliere *et al.*, 1995).

The formation of new blood vessels (angiogenesis) is essential to provide a blood supply to the metabolically-active healing wound. Following injury, haemostasis and inflammation, induction of angiogenesis are an early event. Under the influence of mitotic factors, such as FGF from tissue origins and VEGF from macrophages, which upregulate production in response to hypoxia, endothelial cells in the walls of vessels at the wound margin proliferate and form capillary buds. The endothelial cells are activated by exposure to βFGF, TGFβ1, IL-1 or TNFα and secrete proteases which allow them to dissect through the wound matrix and migrate into the granulation tissue in response to chemotactic stimuli provided by higher concentrations of PDGF and βFGF. Functional wound bed capillaries are formed by endothelial cell–cell and cell–matrix interactions involving the intercellular adhesion molecule PECAM-1 and β1 and β3 integrins as substrate adhesion molecules.

7. Re-Epithelialisation

Re-epithelialisation is initiated after approximately 24 hours and before the late inflammatory response has peaked. Keratinocytes from the wound margin epidermis migrate over a provisional matrix in the wound bed composed primarily of fibrin and fibronectin. At this stage, keratinocytes have not initiated the proliferation seen later in healing. If the wound is not a full thickness wound through to the subcutaneous fat, then keratinocytes associated with hair follicles will migrate over the matrix and establish beds of proliferating cells. The only source of keratinocytes in a full thickness non-sutured wound is the wound margin and this leads to delayed re-epithelialisation as compared to the partial thickness wound. At this early stage of re-epithelialisation, keratinocytes can also contribute to the inflammatory cell response by secreting GM-CSF, IL-1, TNFα and TGFβ.

Subsequently, keratinocytes at the wound margin initiate proliferation to give the characteristic thickening of the wound margin epidermis that can be observed histologically. These cells then migrate over the developing matrix formed by the granulation tissue. In wounds left open to the air, a layer of eschar (scab) composed of dried wound exudate and dead cells forms over the granulation tissue. While providing some protection to the wound, this also acts as a barrier to keratinocyte migration so that they have to dissect underneath the eschar to form the neoepidermis. Prevention of eschar formation by maintaining an optimally moist wound environment (Winter, 1962) accelerates re-epithelialisation. This observation has led to development of the current generation of wound dressing materials, which by virtue of their water vapour permeability characteristics, prevent wound drying yet allow the passage of water vapour to prevent wound moisture saturation and consequent tissue maceration.

In normal intact skin, the epidermis is attached to the basement membrane. During healing, the basement membrane is removed by injury and keratinocytes have to use the wound provisional matrix as a substratum over which to migrate. This matrix is rich in fibronectin which localises in the upper layer of the granulation tissue to form a surface over which keratinocytes can migrate. Keratinocytes express two cell surface receptors for fibronectin — the $\alpha_3\beta_1$ and $\alpha_5\beta_1$ integrins. The $\alpha_5\beta_1$ integrin is more specific for fibronectin, and blocking the receptor with an Arg-Gly-D-Asp (RGD) acid peptide, inhibits migration (Kim *et al.*, 1992).

Intact normal skin is characterised by a basement membrane at the dermal–epidermal junction, and in order to restore skin integrity, the migrated keratinocytes have to re-establish attachment. This process is to some extent controlled by TGFβ which can upregulate synthesis of attachment molecules, such as $\alpha_6\beta_4$ integrin, and basement membrane components, such as collagen type IV. The basement membrane also contains anchoring structures, such as type VII fibrils, and their synthesis is upregulated by TGFβ, TNFα and IL-1, which can be produced locally by keratinocytes and macrophages.

8. The Extracellular Matrix

Collagen is the major protein component of the extracellular matrix (ECM) of skin and composes 60–80% of its dry weight. Wound ECM is composed of a mixture of collagen and elastin fibrils interspersed with glycosaminoglycans, long unbranched poly-saccharides and proteoglycans, glycosaminoglycans combined with protein. Whilst the ECM fulfills an important structural role it also plays a bioregulatory role, in modifying the behaviour of cells that come into contact with it and also by acting as a reservoir of bound growth factors and enzymes.

Collagens are composed of three alpha chains which have a common repeating Gly–X–Y motif that allows folding into a triple helix. Thirty-two distinct alpha chains are known, allowing the existence of at least 19 different collagen types in vertebrates. Of these, only seven are found in significant quantities in skin. These are collagens I, III, V, XII and XIV which form structural fibrils, collagen VI which forms microfilaments, collagen V which forms reticular fibres and collagen VII which forms fibrils anchoring the epidermis to the dermis.

Collagen is synthesised primarily by wound fibroblasts. It is released at the ribosome as a three-chain molecule which then undergoes post-translational modification to form procollagen. These modifications include prolyl and lysyl hydroxylation and glucosyslation, and galactosylation of lysyl and hydroxylysyl residues (Kivirikko and Myllyla, 1985). The trimeric molecule is then secreted into the extracellular space where mature collagen is formed by the proteolytic cleavage of procollagen peptides. The collagen molecules are then able to associate into fibrils which are stabilised by intermolecular cross-link formation. The cross linkages aquire greater stability as the healing process continues.

Collagen synthesis is regulated by the coordinated actions of a number of cytokines. TGF-β1 mRNA co-expresses with collagen α1 mRNA early in healing, and IL-4 and low concentrations of IL-1 stimulate production of collagen I by fibroblasts *in vitro*. Counter regulation has been demonstrated by high concentrations of IL-1, interferon-γ and TNFα (Eckes *et al.*, 1996).

The other major ECM components are the proteoglycans. These are protein–carbohydrate complexes characterised by their glycosaminoglycan (GAG) component. GAGs are highly charged sulphated and carboxylated polyanionic linear polysaccharides. Those most commonly present within the ECM are hyaluronan, chondroitin sulphate, dermatan sulphate, heparan sulphate and keratan sulphate.

Hyaluronan (HA), previously known as hyaluronic acid, consists of alternating glucuronic acid and N-acetylglucosamine units. Each repeating disaccharide unit has one carboxyl, four hydroxyl and an acetamido group. It differs from the other major GAGs in that it does not possess any sulphate groups and is not covalently linked to proteins to form proteoglycans, although it can non-covalently bind proteins and cell surface receptors, such as the CD44 molecule. It is synthesised by fibroblasts and is a major component of wound ECM, being highly hydrated and conferring viscosity to tissues and fluids.

HA is a component of normal skin and is present throughout the entire healing process. It has the potential to modulate cell function by its physico-chemical properties, by acting as a hygroscopic osmotic buffer, by its visco-elasticity, its chemical properties, such as free-radical scavenging, antioxidant effects and the ability to exclude enzymes from the local cellular environment. Additionally, it may interact directly with cells via the RHAMM receptor (receptor for HA mediated motility), the CD44 receptor and the ICAM-1 (inter-cellular adhesion molecule 1) receptor. Receptor interaction may be via a ligand-receptor-type interaction (CD44) or via a receptor blockade (ICAM-1).

HA has the potential to interact in each phase of healing. During the inflammatory phase of healing, wound tissue is rich in HA. It may play multiple roles promoting inflammation early in healing by enhancing leucocyte infiltration and also moderating the inflammatory response as healing progresses towards granulation tissue formation.

Granulation tissue is also rich in HA and here, its role includes facilitation of cell migration (fibroblasts and endothelial cells) into the provisional matrix. Although HA has not been demonstrated to be mitogenic, its oligosaccharide derivatives do stimulate endothelial cell proliferation (West and Kumar, 1989).

HA is present in high concentrations in the basal layer of the epidermis in normal skin and co-localises with the CD44 receptor expressed by keratinocytes migrating over the provisional matrix of wound granulation tissue. Suppression of CD44 expression and consequential decreased HA binding result in defective inflammatory responses, decreased skin elasticity and impaired healing.

In contrast to wounds in the adult, foetal wounding is characterised by a lack of fibrotic scarring. The HA content of foetal wounds remains high for longer periods than in adult wounds. Whilst it is attractive to confer a causal relationship between these two observations, many other differences exist between the foetal and adult wounds. For instance, the foetal wound is a sterile environment with a relatively lower capacity for generation of the early inflammatory phase of healing. However, applied HA has been demonstrated to induce scarless healing of adult tympanic membranes.

9. Remodelling and Scarring

Collagen is constantly being degraded and resynthesised even in normal intact skin. Following injury, its rate of synthesis increases dramatically along with an increase in degradation. Collagen synthesis decreases to normal levels by day 21 after wounding.

Remodelling of the collagen fibres by degradation and resynthesis allows the wound to gain strength by re-orientation of collagen fibres. The resulting scar is less cellular than normal skin and never achieves the same tensile strength as uninjured skin.

Collagen degradation requires specific enzymes known as collagenases. These are members of the matrix metalloproteinase (MMP) family. MMPs are produced by a number of cell types, including, macrophages, fibroblasts and keratinocytes. Their production is inducible and regulated by cytokines, growth factors, hormones and contact with ECM components. Pro-inflammatory cytokines such as TNFα and IL-1 appear to be major inductive factors whilst TGF-β inhibits procollagenase production and induces synthesis of specific inhibitors of MMPs known as TIMPs (tissue inhibitors of metalloproteinases).

Remodelling can continue for up to two years after injury as the healed wound becomes covered with mature tissue. The relative weakness of the scar compared to normal skin is a consequence of the collagen fibre bundle orientation and abnormal molecular cross-linking. The fibres in normal skin are relatively randomly ordered whilst in scar tissue, more of the fibres run in parallel. Where there are large areas of scarring, such as those following burn wounds, scar tissue tends to contract abnormally so that normal function may be lost.

10. References

BARBUL, A. (1990). Immune aspects of wound repair. *Clin. Plas. Surg.* **17**, 433–442.

BLISTEIN-WILLINGER, E. (1991). The role of growth factors in wound healing. *Skin Pharmacol.* **4**, 175–182.

BOYCE, D.E., JONES, W.D., RUGE, F., HARDING, K.G. and MOORE, K. (2000). The role of T lymphocytes in human dermal wound healing. *Br. J. Dermatol.* **143**, 59–65.

BROWN, G.L., NANNEY, L.B., GRIFFEN, J., CRAMER, A.B., YANCEY, J.M., CURTSINGER, L.J., HOLTZIN, C., SCHULTZ, G.S., JURKEWICZ, M.J. and LYNCH, B. (1991). Stimulation of wound healing by topical treatment with epidermal growth factor. *New Engl. J. Med.* **321**, 76–80.

BROWN, R.L., BREEDEN, M.P. and GREENHALGH, P. (1994). PDGF and TGF-alpha act synergistically to improve wound healing in the genetically diabetic mouse. *J. Surg. Res.* **56**, 562–570.

CLARK, R.A.F. (1996). Wound repair: Overview and general considerations. In: *The Molecular and Cellular Biology of Wound Repair*, 2nd edn., R.A.F. Clark ed., Plenum Press, New York and London, pp. 3–50.

DANON, D., KOWATCH, M.A. and ROTH, G.S. (1989). Promotion of wound repair in old mice by local injection of macrophages. *Proc. Natl. Acad. Sci.* **86**, 2018–2020.

DARBY, I., SKALLI, O. and GABBIANI, G. (1990). Alpha-smooth muscle actin is transiently expressed by myofibroblasts during experimental wound healing. *Lab. Invest.* **63**, 21–29.

DESMOULIERE, A., REDARD, M., DARBY, I. and GABBIANI, G. (1995). Apoptosis mediates the decrease in cellularity during the transition between granulation tissue and scar. *Am. J. Path.* **146**, 56–66.

ECKES, B., AUMAILLEY, M. and KRIEG, T. (1996). Collagens and re-establishment of dermal integrity. In: *The Molecular and Cellular Biology of Wound Repair*, 2nd edn., R.A.F. Clark ed., Plenum Press, New York and London, pp. 493–512.

KIM, J.P., ZHANG, K., CHEN, J.D., WYNN, K.C., KRAMER, R.H. and WOODLEY, D.T. (1992). Mechanisms of human keratinocyte migration on fibronectin: Unique role of RGD site and integrins. *J. Cell. Physiol.* **151**, 443–450.

KIVIRIKKO, K.I. and MYLLYLA, R. (1985). Posttranslational processing of procollagens. *Ann. NY Acad. Sci.* **460**, 187–201.

LEE, R.H., EFRON, D.T., TANTRY, U., STUELTEN, C., MOLDAWER, L.L. and BARBUL, A. (1999). Inhibition of TNF attenuates wound healing. *Bull. Eur. Tissue Repair Soc.* **6**, 990.

LIEBOVICH, S.J. and ROSS, R. (1975). The role of the macrophage in wound repair. A study with hydrocortisone and anti-macrophage serum. *Am. J. Path.* **78**, 71–100.

MOORE, K. (1999). Cell biology of chronic wounds, the role of inflammation. *J. Wound Care* **8**, 345–348.

MUSTOE, T.A., PIERCE, G.F., THOMASON, A., GRAAMATES, P., SPORN, B. and DUEL, T.F. (1987). Accelerated healing of incisional wounds in rats induced by transforming growth factor –beta. *Science* **237**, 1333–1336.

MUSTOE, T.A., PIERCE, G.F., MORISHIMA, C. and DUEL, T.F. (1991). Growth factor induced tissue repair through direct and inductive activities in a rabbit dermal ulcer model. *J. Clin. Invest.* **8**, 694–703.

SHAH, M., FOREMAN, D.M. and FERGUSON, M.W.J. (1995). Neutralisation of TGFβ1 or TGFβ2 or exogenous addition of TGFβ3 to cutaneous rat wounds reduces scarring. *J. Cell. Sci.* **108**, 15–17.

WEST, D.C. and KUMAR, S. (1989). The effect of hyaluronate and its oligosaccharides on endothelial cell proliferation and monolayer integrity. *Exp. Cell Res.* **183**, 179–196.

WINTER, G.D. (1962). Formation of scab and rate of re-epithelialisation of superficial wounds in the skin of the young domestic pig. *Nature* **193**, 293–294.

Advances in Tissue Banking Vol. 5
© 2001 by World Scientific Publishing Co. Pte. Ltd.

22 HEALING OF SKIN AND AMNION GRAFTS

JAN KOLLER

Ruzinov General Hospital
Centre for Burns and Reconstructive Surgery
Centre Tissue Bank, Ruzinovka 6, 82606 Bratislava
Slovak Republic

Abstract

Growth, regeneration and repair are the processes by which new tissues are formed. Normal post-natal wound healing consists of a combination of regeneration and repair. The process requires the coordinated completion of a variety of cellular activities, including phagocytosis, chemotaxis, mitogenesis, and the synthesis of collagen and extracellular matrix components. Some of the processes, which are involved in the wound healing mechanisms, also participate in the healing of skin grafts and amnion. For better understanding of how the grafts can be incorporated into the host, the basic principles of the wound healing processes will first be discussed.

1. Pathophysiology of the Wound Healing

There are four general types of wound healing: primary, delayed primary, secondary, and the healing that occurs in partial-thickness wounds.

Wound healing consists of a continuous sequence of signals and responses in which epithelial, endothelial and inflammatory cells, platelets and fibroblasts briefly come together outside of their usual domains, interact, restore a semblance of their discipline, and having done so, resume their functions (Hunt, 1990).

The classical (descriptive) theory of wound healing comprises four stages (Mathes, 1987):

(i)   Inflammatory stage: interruption of tissue continuity triggers a sequence of events that constitute the acute inflammatory response.
(ii) Migratory stage: a variety of cells like neutrophils, lymphocytes, macrophages and fibroblasts migrate to the site of injury to remove necrotic debris, to protect against infection, to produce mediators for regulation of the processes and cell functions.
(iii) Proliferative stage: includes fibroblast multiplication, extra-cellular deposition of collagen and connective tissue matrix, formation of granulation tissue, and finally, epithelialisation and scar formation.
(v)   Maturation stage: starts gradually as fibroplasia proceeds further. This stage reflects the body's attempt to achieve the best scar to resist tension and shearing forces.

According to the final result, two basic types of healing processes can be recognised:

Regeneration: complete restoration of shape and function, i.e. healing "ad integrum".
Repair: incomplete restoration of shape and function — the end result is scar.

2. Components of the Healing Process (Hunt, 1990)

Although wound repair can be divided into four stages, most processes occur closely in sequence and no clear-cut boundaries exist. Where one stage and between one stage and another. The components of the healing process, are as follows: coagulation and inflammation, fibroplasia, matrix deposition, angiogenesis, epithelialisation, contraction, and remodelling.

Not all wounds are the same. Wounds inflicted by defferent methods in defferent sites and depths recruit different components. For instance, partial-thickness wounds heal largely by epithelialisation. Deeper wounds enlist more angiogenesis, matrix synthesis and contraction. Epithelialisation plays no role in closed fracture healing, and so forth. Many factors can influence the healing process.

3. The Importance of the Injury

The injury itself has considerable effect on the form of subsequent repair. For instance, a clean incision with immediate anatomic closure requires minimal synthesis of new tissue and the wound is sealed from external environment within 24 to 48 hours. Major burns influence wound healing by local and systemic mechanism. Locally, deep and full thickness burns result in massive destruction of cells and connective tissue matrix. In extensive burns, many organs and systems are affected in a characteristic fashion, resulting in the "burn syndrome". This results in primary delay in wound healing, which may be further hindered by subsequent malnutrition and infection (Smahel, 1993).

4. Overview of Wound Healing Processes (Table 1)

4.1. Coagulation and inflammation

Damage to the capillary walls due to injury causes adhesion and activation of platelets. Activated platelets initiate two important processes: — coagulation
         — release of growth factors.

Healing begins with coagulation. Coagulation includes a cascade of processes where factors from platelets and plasma interact together with a final result of fibrinogen polymerisation and clot formation.

Table 1. Overview of the wound healing processes.

Time	Event	Cells	Cell products	Effect
0 h	Coagulation	Platelets (Plt)	PDGF, TGFβ Plt Factor IV	Plt aggregation, degranulation, clot formation, permeability, cells attraction
0–48 h	Early inflammation	Neutrophils (N)	Enzymes, free radicals	N margination, diapedesis, ingestion of foreign particles, killing bacteria
48–72 h	Late Inflammation	Macrophages (MF)	Variety of growth factors	Phagocytosis, initiation and regulation of the whole process
>72 h	Fibroplasia Matrix deposition	Fibroblasts (F)	Growth factors collagens, GAGs, matrix proteins	Filling the wound Space for vascular ingrowth Granulation tissue formation Strengthening the wound
	Angiogeneseis	Endothelial Platelets Fibroblasts	Endothelial GF TGFβ, PDGF bFGF, TNFα	Proliferation of endothelial cells New vessels formation
	Epithelialisation	Keratinocytes	bFGF, KGF, EGF, keratin	Mitosis and migration of epithelial cells from the wound margins
>5 days	Contraction	Contractile fibroblasts	??	Drawing the periphery of the wound to its centre, reduction of wound area scar formation
>3 weeks	Remodelling	Fibroblasts	Collagenases	Flattening of the scars, reduction of scar vasculature, scar softening

Abbreviations: PDGF — platelet-derived growth factor, TGF — transforming growth factor, GAG — glycosaminoglycan, GF — growth factor, bFGF — basic fibroblast growth factor, EGF — epidermal growth factor, KGF — keratinocyte growth factor, TNF — tumour necrosis factor.

Activated platelets release into the wound a number of growth factors and other products which then attract and activate fibroblasts and macrophages. The end-product of coagulation pathways is fibrin, which is derived from Factor I, also known as fibrinogen. Fibrin is essential for early wound healing because it provides the matrix into which cells can migrate. The clot, consisting of fibrin and fibronectin, traps platelets, blood-borne cells, and plasma proteins.

The inflammation process (Peacock, 1984) is initiated by tissue injury and starts immediately afterwards. It peaks for one to two days, being replaced gradually on the fifth to seventh day by the repair activity proper. Early vascular changes allow the exudation of protein-rich plasma and the migration of leukocytes into the wound space. Inflammatory cells accumulate in the next few days and thereafter control repair. The first cells which migrate early into the damaged tissues are granulocytes (neutrophils). They release a variety of intracellular products and kill bacteria. Macrophages are the next cells after granulocytes to collect in wounds. Macrophages are the key cells of wound healing. Macrophages release growth factors and other products on stimulation. Lymphocytes infiltrate the wound as third-line cells in later phases of the inflammatory process. They are clearly equipped to influence repair, and they are capable of producing lymphokines. Their role is not yet fully understood. The effect of mast cells seem to be minor. Endothelial cells serve as a selective permeability barrier, their monolayer arrangement results in a non-thrombogenic surface. Finally, they are active in the synthesis and secretion of products that inhibit haemostasis and thrombosis in the normal state (Mathes, 1987).

By the end of this phase, inflammation has provided the wound spaces with cells essential for debridement of the injured tissue, elimination of bacteria and mediation of repair.

4.2. Fibroplasia

This is also referred to as the proliferative phase of repair. Fibroplasia is characterised by migration of fibroblasts into the wound area after 72 hours, and the formation of capillary blood vessels.

These events are more florid in open wounds and result in excessive granulation tissue formation. The major source of matrix proteins which restore the continuity of injured tissues are fibroblasts (Martin, 1981). Fibroplasia is enhanced by inflammation.

4.3. Matrix deposition

The major components of extracellular matrix are collagen and proteoglycans. Both are synthesised by fibroblasts. Collagen is the ultimate product of fibroblasts and its presence results in the development of wound strength. The type of collagen deposited in the wound site differs with time. Elastin is the second major fibrous protein in connective tissue. Elastin lost with time is not replaced to any significant extent. The failure to deposit elastin in scar tissue results in stiffness, a major indicator of the imperfect quality of repair.

4.4. Angiogenesis

New capillaries are formed by endothelial cells (ETCs) growing into the wound. Neovascularisation is induced by at least two classes of angiogenic factors: those that stimulate only migration of ETCs and those that stimulate both migration and mitosis (Hunt, 1990).

4.5. Epithelialisation

It is the final stage of wound closure — a turn-off signal. Epithelial cells advance over receptive surfaces by "flowing". The first cell advances, anchors and stops movement. A cell from behind advances over it, anchors, and is subsequently overridden by other cells, which advance over both. Mitotic activity, the source of the new cells, is in the periphery of the wound, or at other sources, like hair follicles, etc. Epithelial cells move most rapidly in moist environments. They secrete lytic enzymes, which can cleave a space through tissue and eschar for movement. Epithelialisation can be accelerated by growth factors such as TGFβ, EGF, PDGF, IGF-I (insulin-like GF), alone or in combination (Brown 1989; Malcherek, 1993). The resulting scar epithelium has no appendages, is characteristically thin and fragile, and lacks its previous attachments to the underlying dermis (rete pegs).

4.6. Contraction

New collagen in the wound is organised and draws the periphery towards the centre of the wound, under forces developed by resident fibroblasts. Gabbiani (1971) used the term "myofibroblasts" for fibroblasts with the characteristics of both a fibroblast and a smooth muscle cell, capable of causing wound contraction. Contraction is not limited to the full thickness burn wound only. The second degree burn wound, which involves only the partial thickness of the skin, also contracts during healing.

4.7. Remodelling

All wounds remodel themselves over many months after healing is complete. Collagen turns over rapidly in wounds, most rapidly in inflamed wounds. Inflammatory cells produce a variety of enzymes which degrade collagen. The rate of lysis in severe wound infections can be so great, that if collagen synthesis fails, even well healing wounds lose mass and may break open.

5. Growth Factors and Cytokines

The proliferation and activity of mammalian cells are regulated largely by extracellular agents — growth factors and cytokines. While a universally accepted definition does not exist, growth factors can be defined as polypeptides, that stimulate cell proliferation through binding to specific high-affinity cell membrane receptors. The interaction of growth factors with the specific surface receptors delivers in turn intracellular signals, ultimately leading to DNA synthesis and cell division (Herndon, 1992).

A wide variety of cell types, including lymphocytes, macrophages, platelets, fibroblasts, endothelial cells and keratinocytes produce hormone-like factors called cytokines. Many of the cytokines exert multiple biological effects and regulate immunologic host response by serving as intercellular messengers that modulate cell functions.

Distinct surface receptors for many growth factors have been identified. Binding of growth factor receptors initiates a cascade of events that transmit intracellular signals to nuclear DNA, where transcription leads to the production of target proteins.

It is proposed that growth factors mediate the entry of cells which participate in wound healing process into the wound, activate them, and inhibit their action as healing progresses through its various phases (Herndon, 1992). The final level of control in the growth factor response to tissue repair comes by way of growth factor and growth factor receptor (GFR) interaction. As a result, a cell in the wound expressing multiple GFRs receives coordinated control through cell surface "cross talk" between receptors.

So far, many factors are known which can retard the healing rate. In contrast, very few factors have been proved to accelerate the healing process.

Wound healing disturbances can be systemic or local (Robson, 1988). Systemic disturbances at this point can be diagnosed but not necessarily treated. In the future, these disturbances may be reversed with a specific drug. On the other side, local factors responsible for most of the disturbances in wound healing are often under the control of the physician. These can be diagnosed and frequently corrected.

There is a variety of local factors which can influence healing, such as timing and type of repair, bacterial colonisation of the wound, physical factors (negative pressure, ultrasound, electric current, etc.), oxygen, growth factors and cytokines (Table 2). Substantial effect on wound healing process was observed with the use of biological skin substitutes like amnion, skin xenografts and allografts (Herndon, 1992; Wang, 1996; 1997; Spence, 1997). Some of them, e.g. amnion and xenografts, act as a wound-covering material or biological dressing, whereas skin allografts are capable

Table 2. Factors influencing healing.

Type of injury — clean surgical wounds heal with minimal response
                — major burns elicit maximum response

Location of wound — degree of perfusion
                  — degree of contamination
                  — element of motion

Age — older age groups

Nutrition — hypoproteinaemia
          — malnutrition
          — deficiency of: vitamins
                           microelements

Concomitant diseases — diabetes
                     — vascular diseases

Bacterial colonisation of the wound
Growth factors and cytokines
Physical factors — negative pressure, ultrasound, electric current
Oxygen
Wound dressing/covering materials
Drugs — corticosteroids
      — BAPN (beta amino propionitril)

of temporary healing, meaning incorporation into the host and establishing vascular connections between the host bed and graft vasculature.

6. Healing of Skin Grafts

Skin grafts are portions of skin which are detached from their original positions and transferred to a host bed. The process of transferring grafts is called *grafting or transplantation.*

Skin grafts consist of epidermis and dermis. The dermal component is important because the epidermis is avascular and healing is assured by establishing connection between the host bed and graft vasculatures. These grafts are commonly referred to as *dermo-epidermal grafts*.

6.1. Types of skin grafts

Skin autograft (*isograft*) is a graft transferred from a donor to a recipient site in the same individual.

Skin allograft (*homograft*) is a graft transplanted between genetically disparate individuals of the same species.

Skin xenografts (*heterografts*) are grafts transplanted between individuals of different species.

6.2. Autografts

Autologous skin grafts can be partial (split) or full thickness. In *split-thickness grafts* only a part of the dermis is included, whereas in *full-thickness grafts*, the entire dermis is included. Both require a recipient bed that is well vascularised and free of devitalised tissue and bacterial contamination ($< 10^5$ microorganisms per g of tissue). Haemostasis at the recipient site is important as haematoma beneath the graft is a common cause of graft failure. The transplanted skin derives its initial nutrition via serum from the recipient site, the graft then gains blood supply from the recipient bed by ingrowth of blood vessels. At this stage, the graft is susceptible to mechanical shearing and should be protected by immobilisation.

The full-thickness skin graft was the first skin graft described. It gives an excellent cosmetic result with limited graft contraction but has the disadvantage of less reliable graft "take". The amount of full-thickness skin graft available is also limited if primary closure of donor site is to be achieved. In cases in which large areas are to be covered with a full-thickness graft, as in resurfacing a face after burns, the donor area can be increased by pre-operative tissue expansion or the donor area can be covered with a split-thickness skin graft.

Autologous split-thickness skin grafting as first described by Thiersch is the most commonly practised form of tissue transplantation in plastic surgery today. The graft can be taken at different thicknesses, depending on the level at which it is harvested through the dermis. It has the advantages of large available donor areas and better graft "take", but is prone to increased graft contraction and hypertrophic scarring, especially in children. Expansion of the split-thickness skin graft by meshing with expansion ratios from 1:1.5 to 1:9 can be useful and sometimes essential in extensive burns.

Donor sites for split-thickness skin graft may be limited in patients with extensive burns. This lack of available tissue has spurred the development of alternatives to conventional skin graft. One method involves growing autologous keratinocytes in culture with the ability to expand the available tissue 10 000-fold. This technique has been applied in the treatment of large thermal injuries (Rheinwald, 1975). Cultured autologous keratinocytes have also been used to treat leg ulcers and other benign conditions. There are reported disadvantages with the use of cultured keratinocytes. This technique is more susceptible to bacterial contamination than split-thickness grafts and its "take" has been reported to be less reliable than meshed graft. After healing, cultured autograft has been found to blister spontaneously, to be more prone to minor trauma, and to contract more in comparison to split-thickness skin graft. These effects are purported to be related to a poorly developed dermo-epidermal junction. Increased "take" has been reported in recipient beds of early granulation tissue and/or allogeneic dermal support rather than chronic granulating wounds (Heck, 1985).

The lack of a dermal component in these autografts was overcome by a combination of cultured autologous keratinocytes and allogeneic dermis (after removal of the more antigenic epidermis) (Hickerson, 1994). The technique has had favourable reports in patients with extensive burns but the problem of dermal antigenicity remains. An acellular or "artificial skin" consisting of dermal components, collagen and a glycosaminoglycan, overlaid with a Silastic sheet was developed to combat this antigenic problem (Burke, 1981). A disadvantage of this approach is the need to skin graft the "dermis" after removal of the outer Silastic dressing. Development of a skin substitute containing allogeneic or xenogeneic structural proteins and ground substance seeded with autologous cells has also been described: This comprised cultured autologous fibroblasts populating the "dermis" and cultured autologous keratinocytes covering the "dermis" (Hansbrough, 1992).

6.3. Mode of survival (take) of skin grafts

The survival of skin autografts is permanent, whereas the survival of skin allografts is only temporary until rejection occurs. The fate of amnion grafts and skin xenografts are different and will be described later.

6.4. The phases of skin graft survival

At the time of surgical excision (removal, harvesting) of the skin graft from its donor site, the grafts are completely detached from the surrounding skin and subjacent tissue layer. The circulation, lymphatic drainage and nerve continuity are therefore abruptly terminated. The survival of the graft is dependent on how rapidly it can aquire a new blood supply for nutrition and disposal of metabolic products.

6.4.1. The phase of serum imbibition

In the meantime, between transplantation and revascularisation the survival of the graft appears to be ensured by the absorption of fluids very similar to plasma from the host bed. This early process of fluid nourishment was termed *"plasmatic circulation"*. The sequence of events is as follows: The blood vessels of a freshly cut skin graft are collapsed and empty as a result of the spasm of vessels after their separation from the donor site vasculature. As early as eight hours after grafting, a faint pink tint in the graft can be noted. Within 24 hours after transplantation, the graft vessels are again dilated, although they contain only a few haemic elements. By 48 hours, the vessels are more distended and contain large numbers of erythrocytes. The exudate which accumulates between the graft and the host tissues consists of plasma, erythrocytes and polymorphonuclear leucocytes. This can explain the rapid colour change observed within hours after transplantation. The fibrinogen from the plasma precipitates and forms fibrin on the surface of the host bed. In addition to fibrin, the initial bond (so-called fibro-elastic bond) of the graft with the host bed is assured by "binding proteins", such as fibronectin and integrins. In summary, the "phase of serum imbibition" is a period during which the graft vessels fill with a fibrinogen-free fluid and cells from the host bed (Converse, 1956; 1977). There is no real "plasmatic circulation" because the fluid absorbed by the graft is passively trapped within the graft.

However, this mechanism can assure the nutrition of the graft only for a short time until the establishment of vascular connection occurs. It is not capable of maintaining the graft survival in the long term in case the graft fails to become succesfully vascularised.

6.4.2. Revascularisation of the skin grafts

This can occur by one or a combination of three mechanisms:

(i) Direct connection of the graft and host vessels referred to as "inosculation" (Converse, 1975)
(ii) Ingrowth of vessels from the host bed into endothelial channels of the graft itself
(iii) Ingrowth of host vessels into the graft dermis creating new endothelial channels

Immediately after application, the blood vessels of the graft are less filled with the host bed fluid. On the day after grafting, many vessels show distention and rapid filling with static blood. On the second day, the vessel distention continues but blood circulation has not commenced. A sluggish flow of blood occurs in the graft

Table 3. Skin graft vascularization.

Time	Event	Clinical Appearance
24 hours	absorption of wound bed fluids, dilation of vessels, fibroelastic bond of graft to graft bed (fibrin and fibronectin)	pink hue, can be lifted easily
48 hours	so-called "plasmatic circulation", vessels are more distended	pale, fixed by fibroelastic bond
Days 2–5	starting vascular ingrowth by connection of venous site of capillaries, sluggish blood flow, start of fibrotisation	livid appearance, sluggish refill fenomenon
Days 6–7	completion of vascularisation, collagen fibres proliferation	cherry-red hue, intensive, good capillary refill
Days 7 >	firmer bond, partly by collagen, gap closure, increased blood flow	cherry-red hue, more pale, detaching more difficult, bleeding if lifted
Days 14 >	firm fibrous bond, cessation of blood flow	firm, almost impossible to lift, normal appearance

vasculature on the third and fourth day and continues to improve until the fifth or sixth day. During the next few days, the blood vessels return to normal calibre and circulation in all autografts. The process of graft vascularisation is completed on the sixth or seventh day (Table 3).

6.5. Allografts

Skin allograft was the first "organ" transplant achieved. It formed the foundation of modern transplant immunology. However, skin is strongly antigenic and is subject to rejection even in the presence of surviving organ allografts in the same experimental animal. Rejection of allogeneic tissue occurs through cellular and humoral immunologic responses. These responses are generated when the host defence system detects certain antigens expressed on the donor cell surface. These antigens are referred to as major histocompatibility complex (MHC) antigens.

The revascularisation process in allografts is identical to autografts only until the onset of the allograft rejection. Early symptoms of rejection are increased distention of the vascular system, followed by sluggish circulation and clumped elements. Complete obstruction of the blood flow and vascular disruption in most of the skin allografts occur usually between seven to ten post-operative days in immunologically non-compromised individuals. The immuno-compromised state of patients after a major burn usually delays rejection of allografts for several weeks.

The use of skin allografts has been found to be beneficial in large burns with or without concurrent skin autografts. In cases where the allografts are used alone, it is not advisable to leave them in place until they become rejected. They must be removed or changed before rejection occurs. Modified allograft rejection was observed in some of the so-called "combined" grafting techniques. The Mowlem-Jackson technique (Jackson, 1954) used alternate placement of narrow auto- and allograft stripes on the wound. As both the grafts healed, the rejection was starting in the allograft epidermis, which was gradually replaced by the neighbouring autograft epidermis with the result of a healed wound. The same basic principle was modified later in the 1970s by the Chinese (Burns Unit, 1973) who reported the use of large sheets of allografts with chess-like tiny holes where small pieces of autografts were placed. The allografts provided favourable wound conditions for the spread and growth of the autograft skin islands, with the autograft epidermis gradually replacing the rejected allograft epidermis, while the allograft dermis stayed in place and was not rejected. The mechanism decribed above was called "sandwich phenomenon".

The mechanism of healing in combined grafting techniques in humans was studied histologically by Omi and co-workers (1996). They found that at five days after transplantation, variable numbers of lymphocytes and neutrophils were scattered throughout the graft with fibrin strands at the borders between grafted and recipient tissues. At two weeks after transplantation, the allografted epidermis was completely sequestrated and gradually replaced by autologous epidermal cells. At three weeks after transplantation, the new epidermis of recipient origin became acanthotic and covered the remaining allografted dermis, which appeared basophilic and contained an increasing number of fibroblasts and capillaries. At four weeks after transplantation, the capillaries tended to be arranged perpendicularly to the epidermal surface. Fibroblasts migrated through the gaps in the basement membrane where they appeared to participate in the formation of new connective tissue elements. In this phase, the connective tissue elements from the allograft skin became indistinguishable in areas subjacent to the new epidermis of recipient origin.

In the USA, the technique was modified by using a double meshgraft technique which they called "sandwich grafting" (Alexander, 1981). Widely meshed (1:6–1:9) autografts were placed on the wound surfaces and covered by allografts meshed 2:1 with similar results after healing.

Cultured allogeneic keratinocytes have also been used as a temporary covering. Such grafts can be grown in culture preemptively for burn treatment but are susceptible to rejection in addition to the problems associated with cultured autografts.

6.6. Xenografts

It has been generally held that the survival time of xenografts is too restricted to permit a re-establishment of blood circulation. In animal xenografting experiments (mouse to rat, rabbit to rat, pig to rat or rabbit), it was shown that blood flow in the xenografts was initiated usually on the fourth day after transplantation, attained the maximal rate soon therafter, and suddenly ceased on or around the sixth day (Toranto, 1974). The vasculature of the xenograft was not newly formed, but the original graft vascular system established direct connection with that of the host. In the human host, it was unable to distinguish between xenograft vascularisation and invasion of the graft–host interface by granulation tissue formation. At 14 days, there was no evidence of vascularisation or viability of any xenografts. In human burn recipients of skin xenografts from pigs (McGabe, 1973), an initial non-immune, inflammatory cellular response during the first week was followed by an increasingly immunocompetent cellular reaction that peaked at 30 days. Anti-pigskin humoral factors could not be detected. There was no clinical manifestation of any host sensitisation.

The most commonly used xenografts are grafts from the skin of domestic pigs. Porcine xenograft has been used as a temporary dressing in both superficial burns without excision, and in deep excised burns as a temporary skin substitute. Xenografts were also used in the sandwich grafting technique for covering of microskin grafts or largely meshed autografts in large burns (Sheng, 1992; Wang, 1997). The application of xenogeneic dermis has also been found valuable in preparing a wound for sub-sequent grafting by stimulation of granulation tissue formation. Porcine skin xenografts are not suitable for temporary biological dressing of skin graft donor sites because the porcine collagen can be incorporated in the subepithelial area of the donor sites, leading to donor site inflammation and delay in repair. The acellular artificial skin described by Yannas and associates (1980) uses a bovine collagen "dermis", which recipient fibroblasts repopulate.

Other animal skins used for grafting were from calves, frogs and sheep.

7. Amnion Grafts

Although application of amnion grafts is referred to as grafting, in fact, amnion (which is avascular), regardless of its method of processing (fresh, fresh-frozen, freeze-dried, glycerol-preserved), can never establish vascular connections between the host and the graft. Amnion on the wound surface behaves as a biological dressing with all its beneficial properties (Panakova, 1997). Due to its thinness, pliability and elasticity, amnion adheres very well to the wound surface initially. Several hours following the application, the adherence is reinforced by fibroelastic bonding mechanism as in other types of grafts. Amnion is translucent. Therefore, the progress of wound healing can be observed directly through the membrane. The beneficial effects of amnion include pain reduction, slight reduction of evaporative water loss, stimulation of tissue growth and enhancement of epithelialisation (Koller, 1998). It has also been found to control bacterial proliferation in the healthy wound bed. However, in full-thickness and infected wounds, it disintegrates rapidly (within 48 hours), requiring frequent re-applications.

8. Summary

Healing of wounds and grafts is a unique process of biological events, where many mechanisms participate. They include cells from both the host and the graft which are regulated by a variety of extrinsic and intrinsic factors. Extensive research is going on in this field, and every day, new factors and mechanisms are discovered. For practical use, it is more important to understand the basic principles of the healing process with their possible applications for clinical and laboratory practice.

9. References

ALEXANDER, J.W., MACMILLAN, B.G., LAW, E. and KITTUR, D.S. (1981). Treatment of severe burns with widely meshed skin autograft and meshed skin allograft overlay. *J. Trauma* **21**, 433–438.

BROWN, G.L., NANNEY, L.B., GRIFFEN J. *et al.* (1989). Enhancement of wound healing by topical treatment with epidermal growth factor. *New Engl. J. Med.* **321**, 76–79.

BURKE, J.F., YANNAS, I.V., QUINBY, W.C. Jr. *et al.* (1981). Successful use of a physiologically acceptable artificial skin in the treatment of extensive burn injury. *Ann. Surg.* **194**, 413–428.

BURNS UNIT (First Affiliated Hospital of Number 245 Unit, Chinese PLA) (1973). A review of the management of extensive third-degree burns in 14 successive years. *Chinese Med. J.* **11**, 148.

CONVERSE, J.M., MCCARTHY, J.G., BRAUER, R.O. and BALLANTYNE, D.L. (1977). Transplantation of skin grafts and flaps. In: *Recontructive Plastic Surgery*, J.M. Converse, ed., W.B. Saunders Co., Philadelphia, pp. 157–191.

CONVERSE, J.M. and RAPAPORT, F.T. (1956). The vascularization of skin autografts and homografts: An experimental study in man. *Ann. Surg.* **143**, 306.

CONVERSE, J.M., ŠMAHEL, J., BALLANTYNE, D.L. and HARPER, A.D. (1975). Inosculation of vessels of skin graft and host bed. A fortuitous encounter. *Br. J. Plast. Surg.* **28**, 282.

GABBIANI, G., RYAN, G.B. and MAJNO, G. (1971). Presence of modified fibroblasts in granulation tissue and their possible role in wound contraction. *Experientia* **27**, 549–550.

HANSBROUGH, J.F., COOPER, M.L., COHEN, R., SPIELVOGEL, R., GREENLEAF, G. and BARTEL, R.L. (1992). Evaluation of a biodegradable matrix containing cultured human fibroblasts as a dermal replacement beneath meshed skin grafts on athymic mice. *Surgery* **111**, 438–446.

HECK, E.L., SERGSTRASSER, P.R. and BAXTER, C.R. (1985). Composite skin graft: frozen dermal allograft support of the engraftment and expansion of autologous epidermis. *J. Trauma* **25**, 106–111.

HERNDON, D.N. (1992). Perspectives in the use of allograft. *J. Burn Care Rehab.* **18**, S6–S9.

HERNDON, D.N., HAYWARD, P.G., RUTAN, R.L. and BARROW, R.E. (1992). Growth hormones and factors in surgical patients. *Adv. Surg.* **25**, 65–97.

HICKERSON, W.L., COMPTON, C., FLETCHALL, S. and SMITH, L.R. (1994). Cultured epidermal autografts and allodermis combination for permanent burn wound coverage. *Burns* **20**(Suppl. 1), S52–S56.

HUNT, T.K. (1990). Basic principles of wound healing. *J. Trauma* **30**(Suppl. 12), S123–S128.

JACKSON, D. (1954). A clinical study of the use of skin homografts for burns. *Br. J. Plast. Surg.* **7**, 26.

KOLLER, J. and PANÁKOVÁ, E. (1998). Experience in the use of foetal membranes for the treatment of burns and other skin defects. In: *Advances in Tissue Banking*, Vol. 2, G.O. Phillips, D.M. Strong, R. von Versen and A. Nather, eds., World Scientific, Singapore, pp. 353–359.

MALCHEREK, P., SCHULTZ, G., WINGREN, U. and FRANZÉN, L. (1993). Effect of epidermal growth factor on cell proliferation in normal and wounded connective tissue. *Wound Repair Regeneration* **1**, 63–68.

MARTIN, G.R., KLEINMAN, H.K., GAUSS-MULLER, V. *et al.* (1981). Regulation of tissue structure and repair by collagen and fibronectin. In: *The Surgical Wound*, P. Dineen and G. Hildich Smith, eds., Philadelphia, Lea & Febiger, p. 110.

MATHES, S.J. and ABOULJOUD, M. (1987). Wound healing. In: *Clinical Surgery*, J.H. Davis, ed., C.V. Mosby, St. Louis, Washington D.C., Toronto, pp. 461–504.

MCCABE, W.P., REBUCK, J.W., KELLY, A.P. and DITMARS, S.M. (1973). Cellular immune response of humans to pigskin. *Plast. Reconstr. Surg.* **55**, 181.

OMI, T., KAWANAMI, O., MATSUDA, K. *et al.* (1996). Histological characteristics of the healing process of frozen skin allograft used in the treatment of burns. *Burns* **22**, 206.

PANÁKOVÁ, E. and KOLLER, J. (1997). Utilisation of foetal membranes in the treatment of burns and other skin defects. In: *Advances in Tissue Banking*, G.O. Phillips, D.M. Strong, R. von Versen and A. Nather, eds., Vol. 1, World Scientific, Singapore, pp. 165–181.

PEACOCK, E.E. Jr. (1984). Inflammation and cellular response to injury. In: *Wound Healing*, 3rd edn., W.B. Saunders, Philadelphia.

RHEINWALD, J.G. and GREEN, H. (1975). Serial cultivation of strains of human keratinocytes: The formation of keratinizing colonies from single cells. *Cell* **6**, 337–343.

ROBSON, M.C. (1988). Disturbances in wound healing. *Ann. Emergency Med.* **17**, 1274–1278.

SMAHEL, J. (1993). The problem of dehydration and healing of burn wounds. *Burns* **19**, 511–512.

SHENG-DE, G. (1992). Skin substitutes. In: *Modern Treatment of Burns*, F. Zhi-yang, S. Zhi-yong, L. Ngao and G. Sheng-de, eds., Springer, Berlin Heidelberg, pp. 253–260.

SPENCE, R.J. and WONG, L. (1997). The enhancement of wound healing with human skin allograft. *Surg. Clin. N. Am.* **77**, 731–745.

TORANTO, I.R., SALYER, K.E. and MYERS, M.B. (1974). Vascularization of porcine skin heterografts. *Plast. Reconstr. Surg.* **54**, 195.

WANG, H.J., WAN, H.L., YANG, T.S. *et al.* (1996). Acceleration of skin graft healing by growth factors. *Burns* **22**, 10.

WANG, H.J., CHEN, T.M. and CHENG, T.Y. (1997). Use of a porcine dermis template to enhance widely expanded mesh autologous split-thickness skin graft growth: Preliminary report. *J. Trauma* **42**, 177–182.

YANNAS, I.V. and BURKE, J.F. (1980). Design of artificial skin I. Basic design principles. *J. Biomed. Mat. Res.* **14**, 65–81.

23 THE ROLE OF BMP IN BONE INCORPORATION

KENNETH M.C. CHEUNG and KEITH D.K. LUK

Department of Orthopaedic Surgery
The University of Hong Kong
The Duchess of Kent Children's Hospital
12 Sandy Bay Road, Hong Kong

1. Growth Factors in Bone

Growth factors are low molecular weight polypeptides that are generally synthesised by specific tissues and act as local regulators of cell function. Their action is elicited by binding to specific transmembrane receptors on the cell surface of target cells, and acting via protein kinases, activates the transcription of a gene into mRNA, which is then translated into proteins to be used within the cell or exported.

Bone morphogenetic proteins (BMPs) are one of a number of growth factors identified in bone. Other factors include insulin-like growth factor I and II (IGF-I and IGF-II), transforming growth factor beta (TGF-β), platelet-derived growth factor (PDGF) and basic and acidic fibroblast growth factors (bFGF and aFGF) (Solheim, 1998).

Most of the knowledge about the effect of growth factors on osteogenic cells are derived from studies on cultures of osteoblast-like cells from embryonic bone tissues of mouse or rat, or from osteosarcoma cell lines. Less is known about the physiological roles of each of the growth factors, timing of their expression, and how they normally interact to help promote bone growth and healing. It is also worth bearing in mind that current animal and clinical studies on BMPs are using doses far in excess of that seen physiologically.

2. Bone Morphogenetic Proteins

Of all the bone growth factors described, BMPs have been the most developed for clinical use. This is mainly because of its powerful ability to induce bone formation in even non-bony tissues (heterotopic/ectopic bone formation).

The solubilisation and extraction of BMP was first realised in 1979 by Urist and co-workers (Urist, 1979). To date, some 15 BMPs have been identified. They are labelled from BMP-1 to BMP-15. All except BMP-1 are part of the TGF-β superfamily. Their effects are wide ranging and they are known to play a crucial role in cell growth and differentiation into a variety of cell types, including osteoblasts. They are also important in skeletal and extra-skeletal organogenesis (Solheim, 1998).

BMP-2, BMP-3, BMP-4, BMP-6 and BMP-7 are able to convert the differentiation pathway of different pluripotent mesenchymal cell lines into an osteoblastic lineage and form bone (Ahrens *et al.*, 1993; Yamaguchi *et al.*, 1996). BMP-7 can make different pluripotent mesenchymal cell lines differentiate into both chondroblasts or osteoblasts, depending on the stage and potential of the target cell (Asahina *et al.*, 1996).

When bone is injured, such as by fracture or by surgical excision, a local population of pluripotent progenitor cells is activated by growth and/or differentiating factors. The local cells are determined osteoprogenitor cells (i.e. bone-forming cells) that reside in the cambial layers of the periosteum and endosteum. Additionally, inducible osteoprogenitor cells, such as pericytes, arrive at the injury site three to five days after bone injury by passing through developing capillary sprouts (Schmitt *et al.*, 1999). Pericytes may become osteoblasts following interactions with endogenous BMP, which are released in response to bone injury.

This conversion of both the determined and the inducible osteoprogenitor cells to mineralising osteoblasts is a key event for bone regeneration, a process that is known to be mediated by BMPs. They initiate bone formation in a sequential cascade on the basis of concentration-dependent thresholds (Reddi, 1994). It is this ability of BMPs to cause uncommitted and committed pluripotent progenitor cells to differentiate into bone-forming cells that makes them potentially a powerful therapeutic substance, as bone formation can be induced even at sites remote from bone.

3. Studies on BMP-2 and BMP-7

BMP-2 and BMP-7 (the latter is also known as osteogenic protein-1 or OP-1) are now manufactured by recombinant DNA technology, and are available for clinical use in certain countries. Both have undergone quite extensive evaluation in animal and more recently human studies. The majority of reports on their use to induce bone growth have been favourable.

3.1. Restoration of large diaphyseal segmental bone defects

Critical-sized segmental defects were created in the long bones of animals. These defects are of such size that would not allow for spontaneous healing without additional intervention, such as bone grafting. Addition of BMP-2 or BMP-7 without bone grafting to these defects resulted in regeneration of bone that is fully functional, both biologically and biomechanically. These results have been demonstrated in rabbits, dogs and non-human primates, and demonstrate the ability of BMPs to induce new bone formation (Wang *et al.*, 1990; Yasko *et al.*, 1992; Wang, 1993; Cook *et al.*, 1994a; 1994b; 1995b; Cook and Rueger, 1996; Zegzula *et al.*, 1997; Cook, 1999).

3.2. Accelerated healing in non-critical size defects

Based on the encouraging early results, researchers started applying BMP to clinically relevant animal models. In a study on fracture repair, addition of BMP-7 to the fracture site helped to accelerate the repair process. New bone formed significantly faster and restored strength and stiffness earlier than in non-treated controls (Cook, 1999). Similar findings were made in another study using BMP-2 in a rabbit model with mechanically unstable fractures (Bax *et al.*, 1999). The fractures injected with BMP-2 healed in 21 days as compared with controls of 28 days. However, the authors found in mechanically stable fractures, there was no difference between the two groups. They argued that mechanical factors influence the size of the callus of normally healing fractures. Although BMP-2 accelerated the rate of development of the callus and cortical union, it did not affect the amounts of bone and cartilage produced. Thus, under stable mechanical conditions when little callus is produced, the rate of fracture healing may not be significantly improved.

3.3. Enhanced allograft incorporation

Little work has been done to look at the potential of BMP to enhance bone fusion in patients requiring allograft reconstruction. The majority of reports is in relation to the use of demineralised bone matrix as a carrier for BMP (Schwartz *et al.*, 1998), which appears to be useful. One report (Cook, 1999) suggested that the addition of BMP-7 dramatically improved the biological activity of both morsellised autograft and allograft, resulting in greater new bone formation and earlier graft incorporation. There are no published reports in the literature which deals specifically with the use of BMP to promote allograft union in reconstructive surgery after tumour excision.

3.4. Promotion of spine fusion

Studies have demonstrated that BMP-2 significantly enhances posterolateral spinal fusion in both canine and non-human primate models (Cook *et al*, 1994a; Sandhu *et al.*, 1995; Fischgrund *et al.*, 1997; Helm *et al.*, 1997). This success has prompted the development of an endoscopic posterolateral fusion technique, which will minimise the morbidity of paraspinal muscle denervation and devascularisation seen with open posterolateral fusions. This minimally invasive technique is based on the application of BMP to the transverse processes under endoscopic guidance, and also aims to eliminate the problem of graft donor site morbidity (Boden *et al.*, 1996; 1999). However, the carrier used to deliver the BMP was found to be important. A soft collagen sponge is not a good carrier for posterolateral spinal fusion because the paraspinal muscles may squeeze the BMP out of the sponge (Martin-GJ *et al.*, 1999). This could be dangerous because the application of BMP to exposed dura can result in new bone formation and spinal stenosis (Paramore *et al.*, 1999). A hydroxyapatite-tricalcium-phosphate carrier appears to be as effective a carrier as collagen sponge, and avoids the problems of lack of structural stability.

Our own experience with the use of BMP-7 in a non-human primate posterolateral fusion model is similar to those reported by others (Cheung *et al.*, 1999). The fusion rate in the BMP group was 100% on histological assessment compared to only 33% in the control group with autogenous graft alone. However, mechanical testing showed no significance difference between the two groups. We felt that it is important to respect both the biology and the mechanics of the spine in order to achieve a solid fusion, such that BMP is viewed as a substance to enhance bone fusion, and not something that can replace current fusion techniques.

Other authors have assessed the use of BMP-2 in enhancing anterior spinal fusion with equal success, either placed inside a cage (Boden *et al.*, 1998; Takahashi *et al.*, 1999) or within an allograft bone dowel (Hecht *et al.*, 1999). In the report by Hecht and co-workers in which the allograft bone dowels were filled with BMP-2 soaked in a collagen I sponge, histological analysis revealed complete resorption of the allograft by six months, an observation not seen when the allograft bone dowels were filled with autogenous bone graft from the iliac crest (Hecht *et al.*, 1999).

3.5. Enhanced stabilisation of implanted devices

The use of BMP-7 may provide a means of obtaining earlier host bone to prosthesis integration by encouraging bony ingrowth into the implant (Cook *et al.*, 1995; Cook and Rueger, 1996). However, there has been no work on the use of BMP at the implant–allograft junction in cases of limb salvage surgery, although parallel work in spinal fusion models using allograft bone suggests that there may be enhanced replacement of the allograft bone with autogenous bone (Hecht *et al.*, 1999).

3.6. Clinical studies on BMP

Based on the encouraging results of the animal studies, a number of clinical studies have been started, although many of these trials are on-going, preliminary reports.

Studies using partially purified, naturally occurring human BMP in the management of refractory femoral fracture non-unions have been reported with good results. The fractures healed in an average of 4.7 months after surgery. However, these were uncontrolled studies and the good results may be due to the aggressive surgical technique rather than the BMP (Johnson *et al.*, 1990; 1992).

BMP-7 has been evaluated in the treatment of human tibial fracture non-union (Cook, 1999). In a prospective randomised study of 30 patients with 31 tibial non-unions, all patients were treated by reamed intramedullary nail fixation and either BMP-7 or autogenous bone graft added to the fracture site. The results suggested that BMP-7 used alone with a collagen I carrier is as effective as autogenous bone graft in the healing of these fractures. In both groups, the fractures took nine months to achieve radiographic union. The authors claim that although BMP-7 was not superior to autogenous bone graft in its effects, it has the advantage of avoiding the need to obtain autogenous graft and therefore bone graft donor site morbidity.

Two studies looked at the effect of BMP in human bone defects. The first examined the dose-response relationship of BMP-2 carried on a fibrillar collagen vehicle in a defect created in the anterior iliac crest after donor bone harvesting. The control group consisted of a sham operation in which the collagen sponge has not been soaked in BMP-2. Early observations by computed tomography suggested bone formation in the iliac crest site along the BMP-2 and collagen implant. In a similar controlled study using BMP-7, patients undergoing high tibial osteotomy had BMP-7 added to a critically-sized fibular defect. All patients except one showed formation of new bone from six weeks onwards (Geesink *et al.*, 1999).

BMP-2 has been used as a substitute for bone graft in the spine in anterior lumbar interbody fusions (Boden *et al.*, 1998). The BMP was soaked in a collagen sponge and placed inside a threaded titanium interbody fusion cage. New bone formation within the cage and bridging across the vertebral segments could be demonstrated by computed tomography. Bone formation anterior, posterior and lateral to the cages was also noted.

4. Clinical Applications of BMP

The availability of recombinant BMP-2 and BMP-7 has opened up many possibilities in their use in clinical practice. Although these two proteins are somewhat structurally and functionally different, both appear to have the ability to induce new bone formation. There are no studies directly comparing their bone-forming ability against each other. Recombinant BMP-2 and BMP-7 (OP-1) may be useful in enhancing bone formation in fracture repair, joint replacement surgery, spinal fusion and tumour reconstruction.

There are still some issues that need to be addressed before widespread clinical use can be recommended, and their effectiveness in humans ascertained. Firstly, the dose used is far in excess of that found physiologically (Boyne *et al.*, 1997; Cook, 1999). Whether this has any long-term sequelae is not known. Secondly, the optimal timing of administration is not known. The current proteins have a very short half-life. Bone formation is a process that takes weeks to months. The most ideal time to administer the protein may not be at the beginning. Thirdly, the optimal carrier is still under investigation. Multiple carriers have been tried, including polylactic acid, demineralised bone matrix, hydroxyapatite, collagen sponges, etc. Unfortunately, these delivery vehicles are limited by factors relating to biodegradability, inflammatory reactions, immunologic rejection, disease transmission and an inability to provide sustained release. Fourthly, in the animal models, the adjacent host bone were well vascularised and with an intact soft tissue envelope. The models do not simulate the poor conditions that are often encountered clinically. For example, fracture non-unions are often associated with poor bone stock, compromised vascularity and extensive scar tissue that can inhibit bone repair. In such a poor environment, a single exposure to an exogenous growth factor may be insufficient to stimulate an adequate osteoinductive response.

5. Gene Therapy

An alternative approach in dealing with some of the problems outlined in the previous section would be to create a system of local-sustained release of BMP at more physiological doses. This may be achievable using a gene therapy approach.

Human gene transfer can be performed with the use of either an *ex vivo* or an *in vivo* gene transfer strategy. With the *in vivo* method, also known as direct gene transfer, viruses carrying the BMP cDNA are directly injected into the host tissue. They will infect the host cells and cause the host cells to start producing BMP. A number of different viral vectors have been used. These include retroviruses, adeno-associated viruses, lentiviruses and herpes viruses. Most of the studies on BMP have used adenoviruses, because of their high transduction rates, high BMP production titres, and ability to infect both replicating and non-replicating cells (Alden *et al.*, 1999;

Musgrave *et al.*, 1999). Moreover, they do not integrate their DNA into the host cell genome. Therefore, the adenoviral genome is not passed onto daughter cells. This, in combination with the immune response, leads to eventual loss of the adenoviral vector and only a transient transgene expression with only a transient production of BMP. While this virus may not be useful for conditions that may require long-term production of proteins (e.g. cystic fibrosis), it is sufficient for the purpose of bone regeneration, which requires only production of the protein in the intermediate term. The major disadvantage of the adenoviral vectors is their high immunogenicity in the host. How this may affect the duration of production of proteins and its effect on the host is still under investigation. In one study comparing the use of direct gene transfer in a BMP-2 expressing adenoviral vector in immunocompetent and immuno-deficient mice, the latter produced more bone than the former. This suggests that the host immune response does play a significant role in the longevity of the transfected cells, and therefore does affect the amount of new bone formation (Musgrave *et al.*, 1999).

In the *ex vivo* method, the cDNA coding for the BMP gene is first transferred to cells in tissue culture using a viral vector. These genetically modified cells are then locally implanted where an effect is required. In a rat model, Lieberman and co-workers (1999) infected their bone marrow cells with an adenoviral vector expressing BMP-2. These marrow cells were then re-introduced to a critical-sized defect in the femur. This was compared to another group in which the BMP-2 protein was directly added to a similarly created critical-sized defect. The fusion rates in both groups were the same, but the bone production was more profuse and robust in the femur treated with BMP-2-producing bone marrow cells than those treated with BMP-2 protein alone. This difference can only be due to the kinetics of protein release or to the use of the rat bone marrow cells as a carrier, or both. The authors suggest that as gene therapy allows for a continuous release of BMP-2 after implantation of the transfected cells, the osteoinductive stimulus is prolonged and resulted in better bone formation (Lieberman *et al.*, 1999). In another study using a retroviral vector to introduce BMP-7 to rabbit periosteal cells, subsequent replantation also resulted in healing of critical-sized cranial defects (Breitbart *et al.*, 1999).

6. The Future

While research into bone induction using BMP has made remarkable progress over a relatively short period of time, a lot still remains unknown. The molecular mechanisms by which BMP acts, the optimal carrier for the protein, the dosage and effectiveness in humans, long-term effects of using non-physiological doses, advantages of gene therapy approaches, and the possibility of administering multiple growth factors have yet to be resclued.

As the behaviour of BMP becomes better understood, the role of bone morphogenetic proteins in bone induction and incorporation will no doubt expand. This will lead to a rethinking of surgical principles, as current techniques used to achieve long-term stability while waiting for bone formation may no longer be relevant or important.

7. References

AHRENS, M., ANKENBAUER, T., SCHRODER, D., HOLLNAGEL, A., MAYER, H. and GROSS, G. (1993). Expression of human bone morphogenetic proteins-2 or -4 in murine mesenchymal progenitor C3H10T1/2 cells induces differentiation into distinct mesenchymal cell lineages. *DNA Cell Biol.* **12**, 871–880.

ALDEN, T.D., PITTMAN, D.D., BERES, E.J., HANKINS, G.R., KALLMES, D.F., WISOTSKY, B.M., KERNS, K.M. and HELM, G.A. (1999). Percutaneous spinal fusion using bone morphogenetic protein-2 gene therapy. *J. Neurosurg.* **90**, 109–114.

ASAHINA, I., SAMPATH, T.K. and Hauschka, P.V. (1996). Human osteogenic protein-1 induces chondroblastic, osteoblastic, and/or adipocytic differentiation of clonal murine target cells. *Exp. Cell Res.* **222**, 38–47.

BAX, B.E., WOZNEY, J.M. and ASHHURST, D.E. (1999). Bone morphogenetic protein-2 increases the rate of callus formation after fracture of the rabbit tibia. *Calcif. Tissue Int.* **65**, 83–89.

BODEN, S.D., MARTIN-G.J., J., HORTON, W.C., TRUSS, T.L. and SANDHU, H.S. (1998). Laparoscopic anterior spinal arthrodesis with rhBMP-2 in a titanium interbody threaded cage. *J. Spinal Disord.* **11**, 95–101.

BODEN, S.D., MARTIN-G.J., J., MORONE, M.A., UGBO, J.L. and MOSKOVITZ, P.A. (1999). Posterolateral lumbar intertransverse process spine arthrodesis with recombinant human bone morphogenetic protein 2/hydroxyapatite-tricalcium phosphate after laminectomy in the nonhuman primate. *Spine* **24**, 1179–1185.

BODEN, S.D., MOSKOVITZ, P.A., MORONE, M.A. and TORIBITAKE, Y. (1996). Video-assisted lateral intertransverse process arthrodesis. Validation of a new minimally invasive lumbar spinal fusion technique in the rabbit and nonhuman primate (rhesus) models. *Spine* **21**, 2689–2697.

BOYNE, P.J., MARX, R.E., NEVINS, M., TRIPLETT, G., LAZARO, E., LILLY, L.C., ALDER, M. and NUMMIKOSKI, P. (1997). A feasibility study evaluating rhBMP-2/absorbable collagen sponge for maxillary sinus floor augmentation. *Int. J. Periodont. Restorative Dent.* **17**, 11–25.

BREITBART, A.S., GRANDE, D.A., MASON, J.M., BARCIA, M., JAMES, T. and GRANT, R.T. (1999). Gene-enhanced tissue engineering: applications for bone healing using cultured periosteal cells transduced retrovirally with the BMP-7 gene. *Ann. Plast. Surg.* **42**, 488–495.

CHEUNG, K.M.C., LEONG, J.C.Y., LIU, S.L., LI, C.H., LU, W., LUK, K.D.K. and WALSH, W. (1999). Augmentation of intertransverse spinal fusion in primates using OP-1. *Int. Lumbar Spine Soc. Meeting,* Kona, Hawaii, June 21–25 (Abstract).

COOK, S.D. (1999). Preclinical and clinical evaluation of osteogenic protein-1 (BMP-7) in bony sites [see comments]. *Orthopedics* **22**, 669–671.

COOK, S.D., BAFFES, G.C., WOLFE, M.W., SAMPATH, T.K. and RUEGER, D.C. (1994a). Recombinant human bone morphogenetic protein-7 induces healing in a canine long-bone segmental defect model. *Clin. Orthop.* 302–312.

COOK, S.D., BAFFES, G.C., WOLFE, M.W., SAMPATH, T.K., RUEGER, D.C. and WHITECLOUD, T.S. (1994b). The effect of recombinant human osteogenic protein-1 on healing of large segmental bone defects. *J. Bone Joint Surg. [Am]* **76**, 827–838.

COOK, S.D., DALTON, J.E., TAN, E.H., WHITECLOUD, T.S. and RUEGER, D.C. (1994c). *In vivo* evaluation of recombinant human osteogenic protein (rhOP-1) implants as a bone graft substitute for spinal fusions. *Spine* **19**, 1655–1663.

COOK, S.D. and RUEGER, D.C. (1996). Osteogenic protein-1: biology and applications. *Clin. Orthop.* 29–38.

COOK, S.D., SALKELD, S.L. and RUEGER, D.C. (1995a). Evaluation of recombinant human osteogenic protein-1 (rhOP-1) placed with dental implants in fresh extraction sites. *J. Oral Implantol.* **21**, 281–289.

COOK, S.D., WOLFE, M.W., SALKELD, S.L. and RUEGER, D.C. (1995b). Effect of recombinant human osteogenic protein-1 on healing of segmental defects in non-human primates. *J. Bone Joint Surg. [Am]* **77**, 734–750.

FISCHGRUND, J.S., JAMES, S.B., CHABOT, M.C., HANKIN, R., HERKOWITZ, H.N., WOZNEY, J.M. and SHIRKHODA, A. (1997). Augmentation of autograft using rhBMP-2 and different carrier media in the canine spinal fusion model. *J. Spinal Disord.* **10**, 467–472.

GEESINK, R.G., HOEFNAGELS, N.H. and BULSTRA, S.K. (1999). Osteogenic activity of OP-1 bone morphogenetic protein (BMP-7) in a human fibular defect. *J. Bone Joint Surg. [Br]* **81**, 710–718.

HECHT, B.P., FISCHGRUND, J.S., HERKOWITZ, H.N., PENMAN, L., TOTH, J.M. and SHIRKHODA, A. (1999). The use of recombinant human bone morphogenetic protein 2 (rhBMP-2) to promote spinal fusion in a nonhuman primate anterior interbody fusion model. *Spine* **24**, 629–636.

HELM, G.A., SHEEHAN, J.M., SHEEHAN, J.P., JANE-JA, J., DIPIERRO, C.G., SIMMONS, N.E., GILLIES, G.T., KALLMES, D.F. and SWEENEY, T.M. (1997). Utilization of type I collagen gel, demineralized bone matrix, and bone morphogenetic protein-2 to enhance autologous bone lumbar spinal fusion [see comments]. *J. Neurosurg.* **86**, 9–100.

JOHNSON, E.E., URIST, M.R. and FINERMAN, G.A. (1990). Distal metaphyseal tibial nonunion. Deformity and bone loss treated by open reduction, internal fixation, and human bone morphogenetic protein (hBMP). *Clin. Orthop.* 234–240.

JOHNSON, E.E., URIST, M.R. and FINERMAN, G.A. (1992). Resistant nonunions and partial or complete segmental defects of long bones. Treatment with implants of a composite of human bone morphogenetic protein (BMP) and autolyzed, antigen-extracted, allogeneic (AAA) bone. *Clin. Orthop.* 229–237.

LIEBERMAN, J.R., DALUISKI, A., STEVENSON, S., WU, L., MCALLISTER, P., LEE, Y.P., KABO, J.M., FINERMAN, G.A., BERK, A.J. and WITTE, O.N. (1999). The effect of regional gene therapy with bone morphogenetic protein-2-producing bone-marrow cells on the repair of segmental femoral defects in rats. *J. Bone Joint Surg. [Am]* **81**, 905–917.

MARTIN-G.J., J., BODEN, S.D., MARONE, M.A. and MOSKOVITZ, P.A. (1999). Posterolateral intertransverse process spinal arthrodesis with rhBMP-2 in a nonhuman primate: Important lessons learned regarding dose, carrier, and safety. *J. Spinal Disord.* **12**, 179–186.

MUSGRAVE, D.S., BOSCH, P., GHIVIZZANI, S., ROBBINS, P.D., EVANS, C.H. and HUARD, J. (1999). Adenovirus-mediated direct gene therapy with bone morphogenetic protein-2 produces bone. *Bone* **24**, 541–547.

PARAMORE, C.G., LAURYSSEN, C., RAUZZINO, M.J., WADLINGTON, V.R., PALMER, C.A., BRIX, A., CARTNER, S.C. and Hadley, M.N. (1999). The safety of OP-1 for lumbar fusion with decompression — A canine study. *Neurosurgery* **44**, 1151–1155.

REDDI, A.H. (1994). Bone and cartilage differentiation. *Curr. Opin. Genet. Dev.* **4**, 737–744.

SANDHU, H.S., KANIM, L.E., KABO, J.M., TOTH, J.M., ZEEGAN, E.N., LIU, D., SEEGER, L.L. and DAWSON, E.G. (1995). Evaluation of rhBMP-2 with an OPLA carrier in a canine posterolateral (transverse process) spinal fusion model. *Spine* **20**, 2669–2682.

SCHMITT, J.M., HWANG, K., WINN, S.R. and HOLLINGER, J.O. (1999). Bone morphogenetic proteins: an update on basic biology and clinical relevance. *J. Orthop. Res.* **17**, 269–278.

SCHWARTZ, Z., SOMERS, A., MELLONIG, J.T., CARNES-D.L., J., Wozney, J.M., DEAN, D.D., COCHRAN, D.L. and BOYAN, B.D. (1998). Addition of human recombinant bone morphogenetic protein-2 to inactive commercial human demineralized freeze-dried bone allograft makes an effective composite bone inductive implant material. *J. Periodontol.* **69**, 1337–1345.

SOLHEIM, E. (1998). Growth factors in bone. *Int. Orthop.* **22**, 410–416.

TAKAHASHI, T., TOMINAGA, T., WATABE, N., YOKOBORI-A.T., J., SASADA, H. and YOSHIMOTO, T. (1999). Use of porous hydro-xyapatite graft containing recombinant human bone morphoge-netic protein-2 for cervical fusion in a caprine model. *J. Neurosurg.* **90**, 224–230.

URIST, M.R. and MIKULSKI, A.J. (1979). A soluble bone morphogenetic protein extracted from bone matrix with a mixed aqueous and nonaqueous solvent. *Proc. Soc. Exp. Biol. Med.* **162**, 48–53.

WANG, E.A. (1993). Bone morphogenetic proteins (BMPs): Therapeutic potential in healing bony defects. *Trends Biotechnol.* **11**, 379–383.

WANG, E.A., ROSEN, V., D'ALESSANDRO, J.S., BAUDUY, M., CORDES, P., HARADA, T., ISRAEL, D.I., HEWICK, R.M., KERNS, K.M., LAPAN, P., *et al.* (1990). Recombinant human bone morphogenetic protein induces bone formation. *Proc. Natl. Acad. Sci. USA* **87**, 2220–2224.

YAMAGUCHI, A., ISHIZUYA, T., KINTOU, N., WADA, Y., KATAGIRI, T., WOZNEY, J.M., ROSEN, V. and YOSHIKI, S. (1996). Effects of BMP-2, BMP-4, and BMP-6 on osteoblastic differentiation of bone marrow-derived stromal cell lines, ST2 and MC3T3-G2/PA6. *Biochem. Biophys. Res. Commun.* **220**, 36–371.

YASKO, A.W., LANE, J.M., FELLINGER, E.J., ROSEN, V., WOZNEY, J.M. and WANG, E.A. (1992). The healing of segmental bone defects, induced by recombinant human bone morphogenetic protein (rhBMP-2). A radiographic, histological, and biomechanical study in rats [published erratum appears in *J. Bone Joint Surg. [Am]* **74**(7), 1111]. *J. Bone Joint Surg. [Am]* **74**, 659–670.

ZEGZULA, H.D., BUCK, D.C., BREKKE, J., WOZNEY, J.M. and HOLLINGER, J.O. (1997). Bone formation with use of rhBMP-2 (recombinant human bone morphogenetic protein-2). *J. Bone Joint Surg. [Am]* **79**, 1778–1790.

Advances in Tissue Banking Vol. 5

24 BIOLOGY OF HEALING OF LARGE DEEP-FROZEN CORTICAL BONE ALLOGRAFTS

A. NATHER

NUH Tissue Bank
National University Hospital
Lower Kent Ridge Road
Singapore 119074

1. Introduction

Bridging large bone defects is one of the most challenging problems in orthopaedic and maxillofacial surgery. Options available include vascularised bone transplants (Weiland and Daniel, 1979), non-vascularised bone autografts (Enneking *et al.*, 1980), prostheses (Sim *et al.*, 1987; Natarajan, 1998), ceramics (Yamamuro, 1990) and bone allografts (Mankin *et al.*, 1996).

The disadvantage of using vascularised bone transplant as the option is that the highly specialised technical expertise required is not always available. Furthermore, the demanding surgical technique requires prolonged operating time which is also not always readily available. Besides, in some situations such as in the femur, the bone transplanted — the fibula (Pho, 1981) is not always large enough to match the large defect in a much bigger bone to provide for immediate biomechanical stability.

With non-vascularised bone autografts, the size and amount of bone graft available is limited. Furthermore, it is often associated with considerable donor site morbidity (Montgomery *et al.*, 1990) — in particular, donor site pain and donor site infection.

With modular prostheses, cost is the main limiting factor. With hip and shoulder modular prostheses, the average costs range from US$10 000 to $15 000 per prosthesis. With elbow modular prostheses, the costs are slightly cheaper being about US$7000. With custom-made prostheses (Sim *et al.*, 1987), the same prohibitive cost factor remains. In addition, there is the additional problem of meeting transportation costs and coping with the delay factor of one to two weeks to allow for the fabrication of the individually tailored prostheses.

Ceramics also incur large costs — about US$10 000 to $15 000. It is also not readily available locally, though it is commercially available in Japan (Yamamuro, 1990).

On the other hand, allografts present as a very favourable option, provided there is a good tissue bank locally to provide bone allografts of high quality. There is no limitation as to the number and size of the bone grafts that could be provided. The local costs are very cheap compared to the expensive costs incurred with using prostheses and ceramics. For example, in Singapore, the cost of a whole femur allograft is only about US$800. The option of using an allograft is therefore about 13 to 19 times cheaper in term of costs compared to using prostheses.

It is not surprising therefore that in the Asia Pacific region, where cost considerations are very important, bone allografts become the option of choice. There is an increasingly large demand for bone allografts in the region. This in turn is responsible for the increasing mumber of new tissue banks that are being set up in the region within the last decade.

2. Biological Reconstruction Using Bone Allografts

In using bone allografts for intercalary reconstruction of bone, or for bone reconstruction where joint function is sacrificed (resection-arthrodesis) in the lower limb because the biomechanical demand is high and weight-bearing function is required, deep-frozen cortical bone allografts must be used. Freeze-dried cortical bone allografts are too weak and should not be used. In the case of bone reconstruction where joint function is to be preserved, cryopreserved, osteoarticular allografts are the only allografts that could be used.

Where articular cartilage transplantation is not required, the deep-frozen bones could either be used without irradiation — "sterile procured" and relying totally on the sterility of the procurement technique for safety or they could be used after gamma irradiation to a dose of 25 KGy. Irradiation not only further sterilises the bones procured but also destroys the immunogenicity of the allograft (Dziedzic-Goclawska *et al.*, 1991; Fideler *et al.*, 1994) and inactivates hepatitis C virus (Conrad *et al.*, 1995). For these reasons, deep-frozen gamma-irradiated bones are recommended for use by the author in such circumstances.

The author is of the opinion that the best method for reconstructing a bone defect is by using bone itself. Long-term problems of loosening of the prostheses or ceramics requiring revision surgery could be obviated. For this reason, biological reconstruction is the best option especially for children. For successful reconstruction of biological reconstruction using bone allografts, one must first understand the biology of healing of massive, deep-frozen, cortical bone allografts (Nather, 1990a).

3. Terminology For Bone Transplantation

Before one can understand easily the biology of healing of large bone allografts, it is important to review the meaning of various types of transplants, such as autograft, allograft and xenograft and also to review the meaning of the various biological healing processes occurring in bone transplantation, such as "creeping substitution", osteoconduction, osteoinduction and osteogenesis.

AUTOGRAFT
is the tissue removed from one portion of the skeleton and transferred to another location in the same individual. AUTOGENIC is the adjective replacing the term autogenous or autologous.

ALLOGRAFT
is the tissue transplanted between genetically non-identical members of the same species. It replaces the previous term homograft. ALLOGENEIC is the adjective replacing the previous term homogenous.

XENOGRAFT
is the tissue transplanted between members of different species. It replaces the previous term heterograft. XENOGENEIC is the adjective replacing the previous term heterogenous.

"CREEPING SUBSTITUTION" comes from a Germanic phrase — "ersatz schleichender". It refers to the invasion of new bone tissue along channels made by invasive blood vessels or along pre-existing Haversian or Volkmann's channels in the transplanted bone. The process is referred to as "resorption and apposition" by Axhausen.

OSTEOCONDUCTION
refers to the ingrowth from the recipient bed into the graft of capillaries, perivascular tissue and osteoprogenitor cells. The grafts act as inert scaffolds for the ingrowth of this host tissue.

OSTEOINDUCTION
is the mechanism in which new bone is formed by the active recruitment of

host pluripotential cells that differentiate into chondroblasts and osteoblasts. It is accomplished by diffusion of osteogenic bone matrix proteins referred to as bone morphogenetic proteins (BMPs) from demineralised bone matrix.

OSTEOGENESIS is the formation of new bone from surviving cells within a bone graft — namely the cells from the inner cambium layer of periosteum that survive autogenous transplantation. It does not occur with allograft transplantation.

4. Biological Healing of Bone Transplants

There are two important issues in the biological healing of bone transplants:

(i) Union of host–graft junctions — fracture healing of host–graft junctions by formation of osteoid callus. This is very important since non-union of host–graft junction can lead to graft resorption.
(ii) Graft incorporation — healing of the graft itself by resorption activity, new bone formation and "callus encasement" (Dell *et al.*, 1985; Nather *et al.*, 1990b).

5. Non-Vascularised Cortical Bone Autograft Transplantation

Nather *et al.* (1990b) showed that in the tibia of adult cats, union of a large cortical graft (two-thirds of the diaphysis) — a 4 cm segment occurred by eight weeks (Fig. 1). Revascularisation, resorption activity, new bone formation and "callus encasement" took place readily (Fig. 2) with increased new bone formation occurring with time as quantitated by the bone resorption index, new bone formation

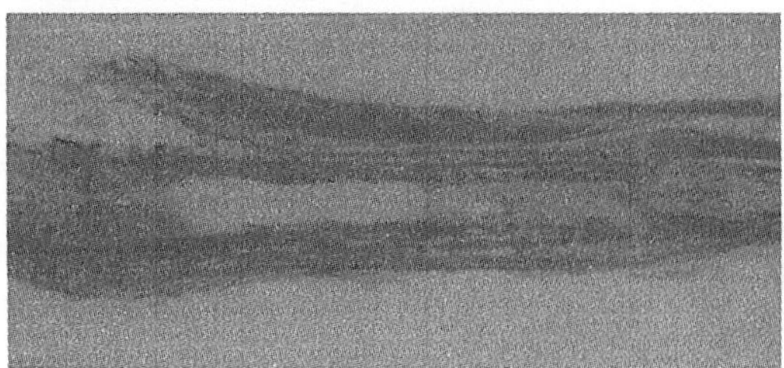

Fig. 1. Histological section of an autograft specimen (D_6) at eight weeks with osteoid callus at both host–autograft junctions. Several resorption cavities could be seen in both cortices of the autograft.

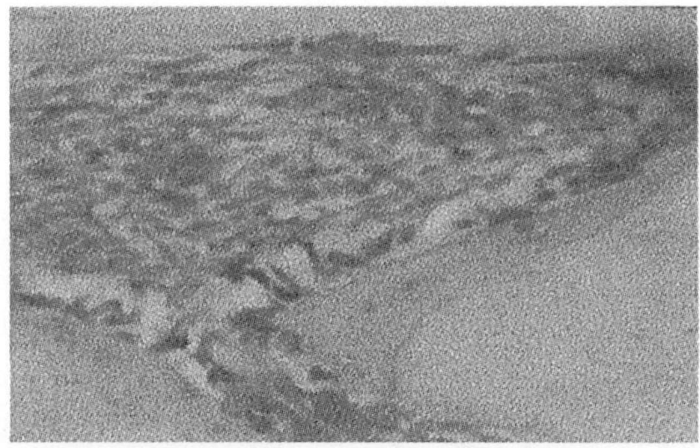

Fig. 2. Higher power magnification of a resorption cavity (40×) in the same autograft specimen (D_6) showing new bone formation lining the cavity. Osteoblasts could be seen in the new bone being laid down.

index and "callus encasement" index. Bone resorption reached a peak of 13% at 12 weeks and then dipped to 6.5% at 16 weeks (Fig. 3). New bone formation steadily increased with time up to 16 weeks reaching 4.3% (Fig. 4). "Callus encasement" appeared from two weeks onwards and reached a value of 8% at 16 weeks (Fig. 5).

Revascularisation was first seen at two weeks (Fig. 6). By six weeks, the entire segment became revascularised (Nather *et al.*, 1990c). The revascularisation index gradually increased till six weeks

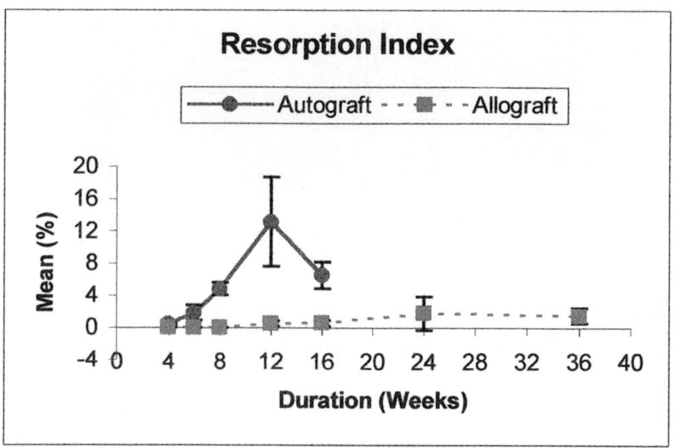

Fig. 3. Resorption index of autografts and allografts in adult cats.

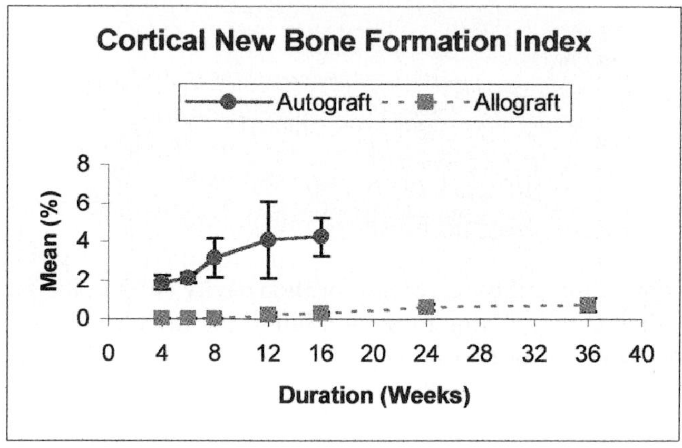

Fig. 4. Cortical new bone formation index of autografts and allografts in adult cats.

with a value of 0.14 mm/sq mm. It reached a plateau at 8, 12 and 16 weeks (Fig. 7).

Excision of the periosteum did not produce any difference to the healing of the autografts compared to controls. Obliteration of the medullary canal using a silastic rod also produced no differences. However, when the muscle bed was isolated from the autograft

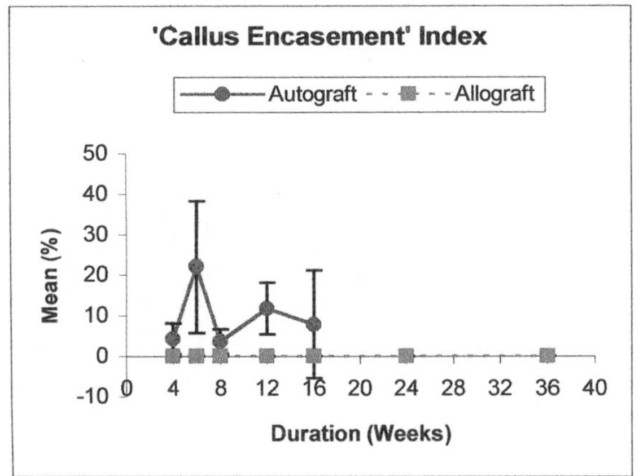

Fig 5. "Callus encasement index" of autografts and allografts in adult cats.

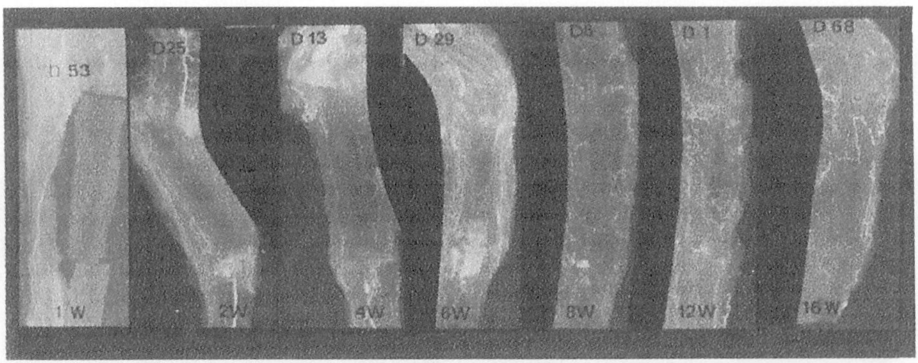

Fig. 6. Microangiograms of non-vascularised autograft specimens. Revascularisation started at two weeks. By six weeks, the entire autograft specimen has become revascularised.

(Fig. 8), the reparative processes were markedly impaired (Nather *et al.*, 1990b). This showed that the muscle bed contributed significantly towards the healing of the non-vascularised, large, cortical autograft segment.

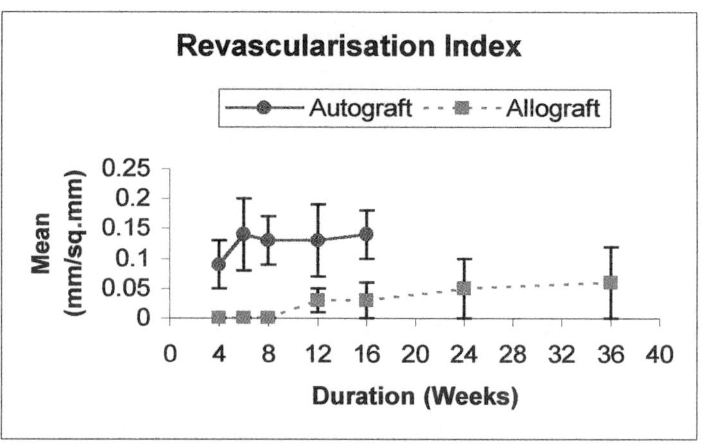

Fig. 7. Graph showing revascularisation index of non-vascularised autografts.

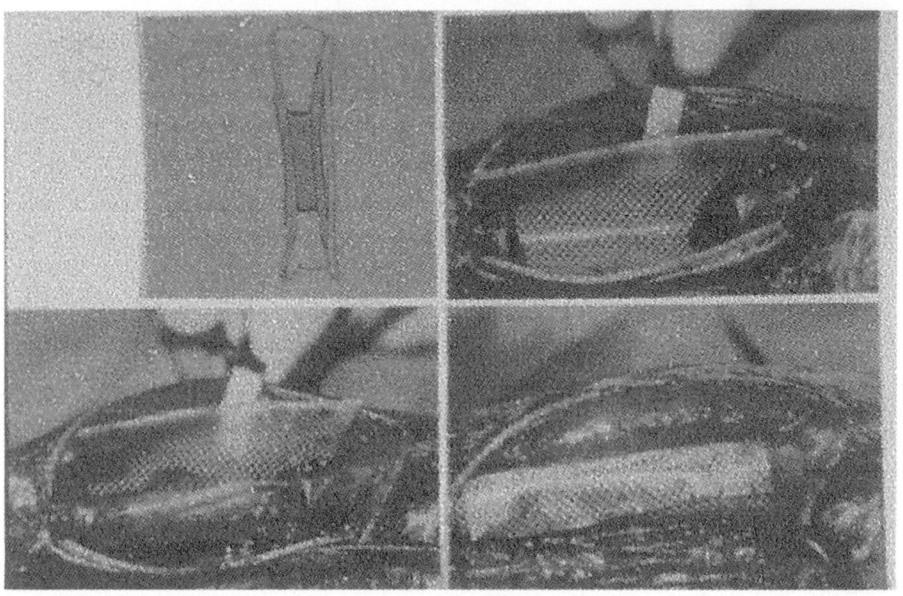

Fig. 8. Silastic sheath isolating the large cortical autograft from the surrounding muscle bed.

6. Soil-Seed Theory

Nather proposed the "Soil-seed theory": When the soil is good, any seed planted in it will grow. The soil is the vascular muscle bed. The seed could be a vascularised autograft (the best seed) or a non-vascularised autograft (the next best seed) or an allograft or even a xenograft (the poorest seed).

7. Vascularised Autograft Transplantation

With the transplantation of a vascularised autograft, the process of resorption — apposition does not occur. The bone transplanted with its blood supply re-anastomosed maintains total viability of its living cells — the osteocytes (Ostrup and Frederickson, 1974).

8. Deep-Frozen Cortical Allograft Transplantation

Nather (1990) reported the healing of deep-frozen cortical allografts using the same experimental model — the tibia of adult cats. The tibia of adult cats is chosen as the experimental model because, compared to dogs and rabbits, the tibia and fibula in the cat most closely resemble that of man. In the dog (D) as in the rabbit (R), the fibula is a separate bone only in the upper portion, being fused to the tibia in the lower portion. The fibula in the dog is therefore not fully weight-bearing. The canine fibular model usually employed for bone transplantation studies (Enneking *et al.*, 1975) is less ideal than the feline tibial model (Nather, 1990b; 1990d) since the tibia in the cat is fully weight-bearing (Fig. 9). A total of 24 adult cats were employed, four cats for each observation period of 1, 2, 3, 4, 6 and 9 months. The parameters studied included revascularisation, fracture union, resorption activity, new bone formation activity and "callus encasement" activity.

The allografts in adult cats were procured under sterile conditions, and with the periosteum stripped off, were stored using a sterile double-jar technique (Fig. 10) in an electrical freezer at −80°C. For standardisation, all allografts were deep-frozen for at least one month

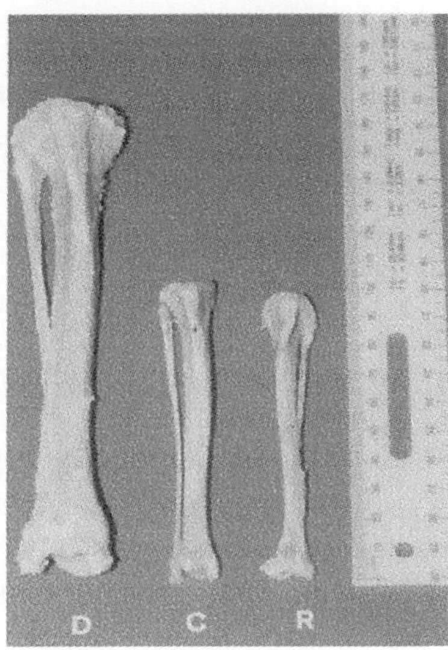

Fig. 9. The feline tibia (C) is fully weight-bearing as in man compared to the fibula in the dog (D) or in the rabbit (R) which is not fully weight-bearing.

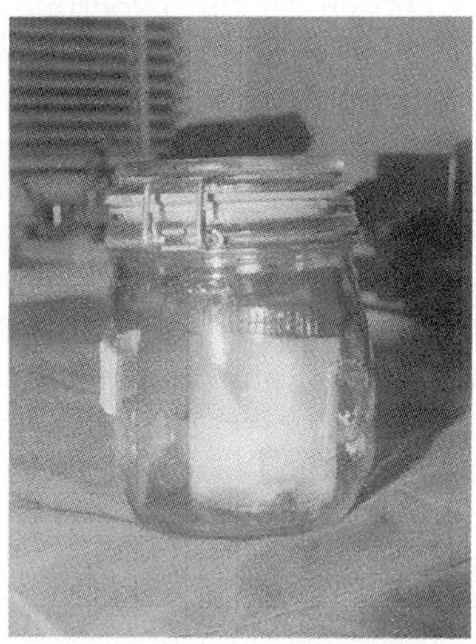

Fig. 10. Sterile double jar. Inner bottle containing the sterile cat tibial allograft procured devoid of its periosteum.

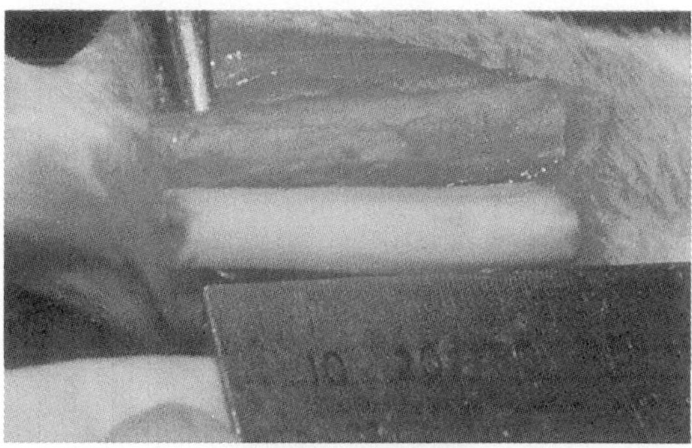

Fig. 11. Allograft devoid of periosteum (white bone in lower part of picture) used to reconstruct the defect resulting from excising a large bone segment (upper part of picture) in the recipient tibia.

before use. This processing by deep-freezing is important to reduce the immunogenicity of the deep-frozen allograft considerably. By deep-freezing, within five to seven days, the cells in the marrow (the most immunogenic component of the graft) would die. By two weeks, all living cells within the allograft would be dead, rendering the allograft with little if any residual antigenicity.

At transplantation, the deep-frozen allograft was used to reconstruct the large bone defect (4 cm) created by excising a large segment (two-thirds of the tibial diaphysis) of the tibia in the recipient cat (Fig. 11). Internal fixation was performed using an intramedullary rod — 2.3 mm in diameter (Fig. 12).

Microangiography was performed using barium sulphate perfusion. The cannula is inserted into the lower abdominal aorta for perfusion of both lower limbs with barium sulphate before the cat is sacrificed. The leg specimen is then retrieved. A central 2 mm thick longitudinal slice is cut from the decalcified specimen. This longitudinal slice is then subjected to soft X-rays using a Watson Mobilix 60 Mobile X-ray Unit at an exposure of 43 kilovolts and 60 millamperes for two seconds at a fixed target-to-film distance of 50 cm using special Du Pont Cronex NDT 55 non-screen films according to the technique described by Nather *et al.* (1990c). Upon

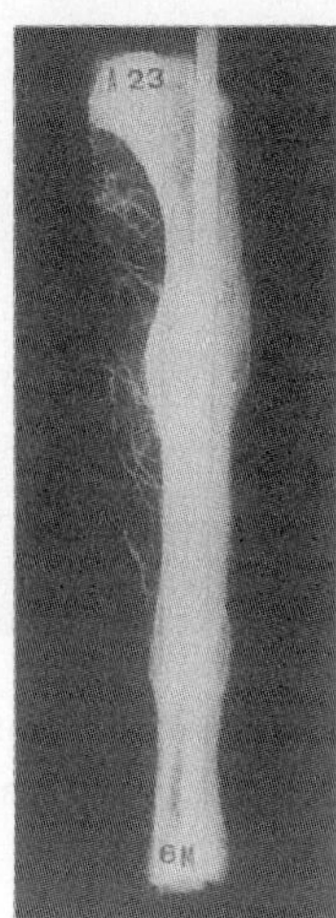

Fig. 12. Radiograph of allograft specimen at six months (A23) showing the intramedullary rod fixation. Good callus formation could be seen at both host–allograft junctions.

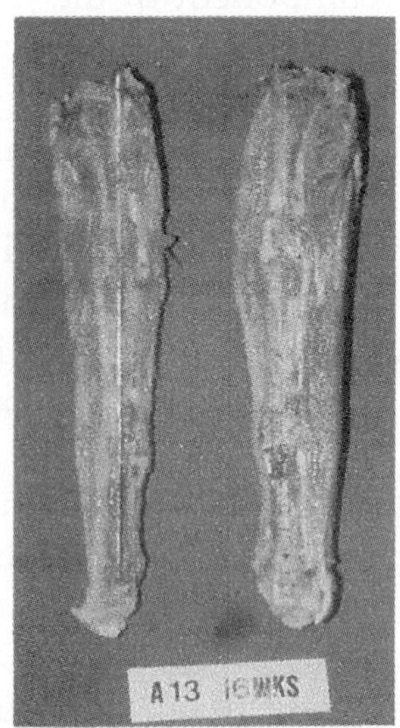

Fig. 13. Gross appearance of allograft specimen at 16 weeks (A13). Intramedullary rod used for fixation readily seen on left side of picture. Solid callus visible at both host–allograft junctions.

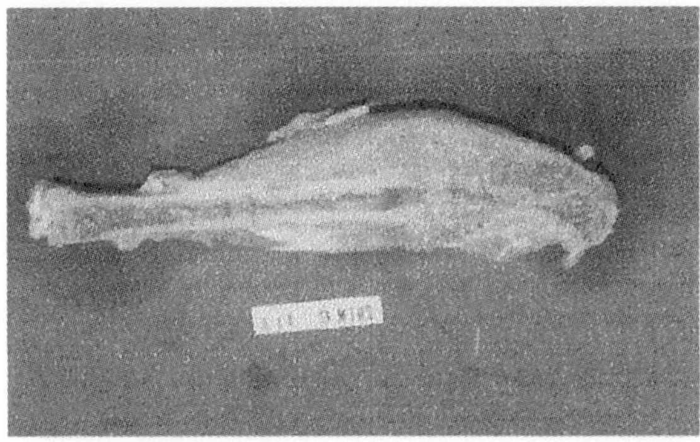

Fig. 14. Gross appearance of allograft specimen at nine months (A11). Solid union seen at both host–allograft junctions.

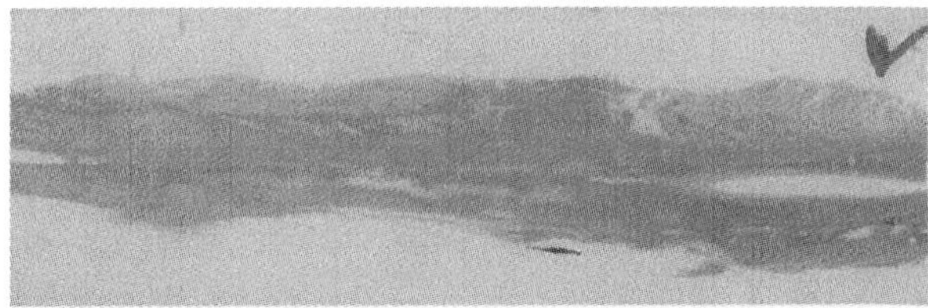

Fig. 15. Histological section of allograft at 12 weeks (A14) showing bridging of both host–allograft junctions by osteoid callus. Both cortices of allograft showed few and tiny resorption cavities only. No "callus encasement" could be seen around the allograft.

completion of the microangiography, histology was performed using the same longitudinal 2 mm decalcified strip embedded in paraffin wax. Longitudinal sections of 10 microns were cut for staining with haematoxylin and eosin.

Macroscopically, solid union could be seen at both host–allograft junctions from 12 weeks onwards (Nather, 1990a), as seen in Figs. 13 and 14.

Microscopically, callus could be seen in the allograft specimens from about four weeks onwards. Histologically, this callus was mainly cartilaginous in nature. It is only from 12 weeks onwards that osseous callus was seen in all specimens (Fig. 15). Allografts

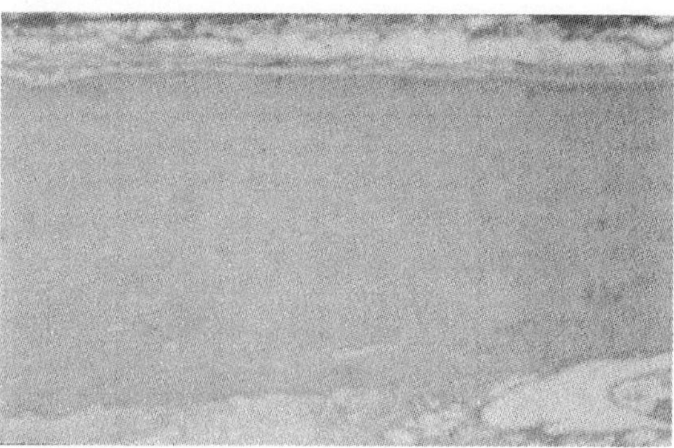

Fig. 16. Higher magnification (10×) of histological section of allograft at nine months (A15). Only few and very small resorption cavities were visible in the cortex.

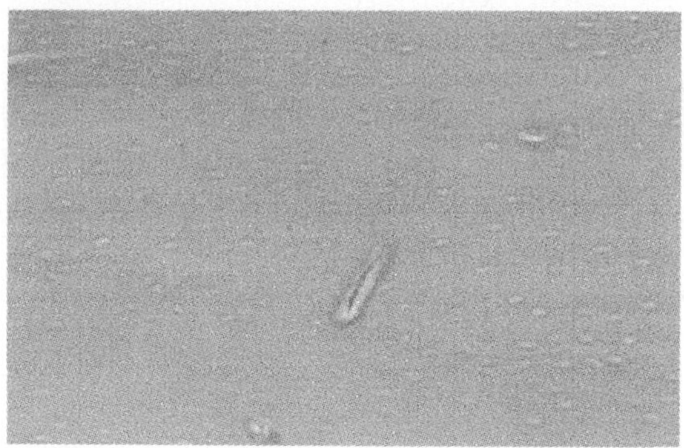

Fig. 17. Higher magnification (20×) of same histological section of allograft at nine months (A15) showing the presence of "ghost cells". No osteoblast could be seen to occupy the empty lacunae.

took a longer time to achieve osseous union (12 weeks) at host–graft junctions, as compared to autografts (8 weeks).

Microscopically, no resorption cavity was seen in all allografts at 4, 6 and 8 weeks. Only very small and few resorption cavities appeared in the peripheral part of the cortex subjacent to the periosteal surface at 12 and 16 weeks. Even at six and nine months, only a few, small resorption cavities could be seen (Figs. 16 and 17) in the peripheral part of the cortex on the periosteal side. No periosteum was reformed. No resorption cavity was seen in the inner cortex adjacent to the endosteal surface. The resorption index measured only 0.48% at 12 weeks and was less than 2% even at nine months (Fig. 3). The resorption activity occurring in allografts was markedly lower than that occurring in autografts (statistically significant).

Likewise, no new bone formation could be seen at 4, 6 and 8 weeks. Minimal new bone formation could be seen at 12 and 16 weeks. Even at six and nine months, the amount of new bone formation taking place was again very little (Nather, 1990a). The cortical new bone formation index was only 0.21% at 12 weeks and reached only 0.74% at nine months (Fig. 4). These measurements were significantly lower compared to autografts.

"Callus encasement" of the allograft remained confined to 2 to 6 mm of host–allograft junctions. No "callus encasement" occurred in the central 2 cm portion of all allografts at 4, 6, 8 12, and 16 weeks. Even at six and nine months, no "callus encasement" occurred around the central 2 cm portion of the allograft. The "callus encasement index" was 0% for all specimens (Fig. 5). This was in sharp contrast to autografts where "callus encasement" appeared from two weeks onwards.

Microangiographically, whilst some vessels could be seen to penetrate the allograft in the region of the host–allograft junctions, very few vessels could be seen to penetrate the cortical allograft in the central 2 cm portion even at nine months (Figs. 18 and 19). The revascularisation index remained very low at 0.06 mm/sq mm even at nine months (Fig. 7) — significantly lower compared to revascularisation occurring in autograft segments.

In contrast to the active repair processes occurring with non-vascularised autografts (Nather *et al.*, 1990b), very little reparative activity occurred in cortical allografts (Nather, 1990). Less than 2% of the allograft showed resorption and new bone formation. No "callus encasement" was seen with allograft segments. Deep-frozen, large, cortical allografts remained biologically inert for a long period of time in the adult cat.

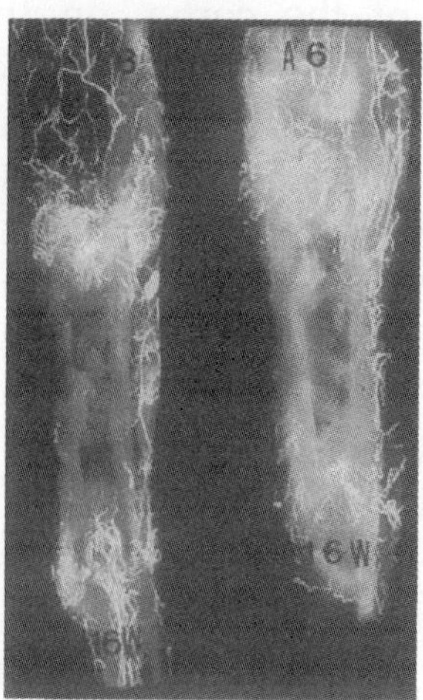

Fig. 18. Microangiogram of allograft at 16 weeks (A6). Only some vessels could be seen to enter the allograft in the region of the host–allograft junctions. In the central portion of the allograft, no vessel was seen to enter the bone.

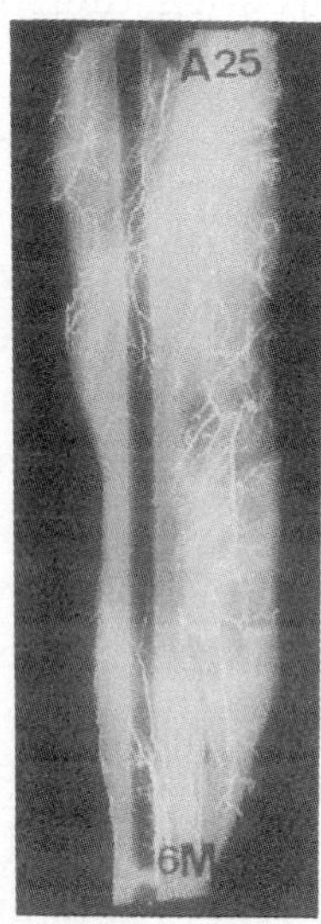

Fig. 19. Microangiogram of allograft at six months (A25). Hardly any vessels were seen to penetrate the cortex of the allograft. Only some vessels were seen at the host–allograft junctions.

9. Clinical Significance

The fact that deep-frozen allografts do not undergo significant resorption–apposition meant that allografts do not undergo much weakening with time after transplantation, a phenomenon occurring with non-vascularised autografts which initially become weak until more new bone formation occurs (Enneking *et al.*, 1975; Nather *et al.*, 1990d).

Allografts therefore act as "spacers" and remain relatively inert though union at the host–allograft junctions occurred without much difficulty. Union at host–allograft junctions occurred much later — 12 weeks (Nather, 1990a), compared to union at host–autograft junctions in adult cats — 8 weeks (Nather, 1990b).

10. Conclusions

Allografts are biologically inert. They do not exhibit osteogenesis or osteoinduction. At best they act as "osteoconductors", providing scaffolds for host cells to repopulate their physical structure. Whilst the extent of osteoconduction that occurs with cortical allografts is small and very limited, osteoconduction occurs more readily and to a larger extent with cancellous or cortico-cancellous allografts.

Since allografts have little osteogenic potential, large cortical allografts are best used in combination with autografts as "allograft–autograft composites" (Nather, 1999) or in combination with vascularised fibula transplants to augment the biological healing of such large cortical allografts (Capanna *et al.*, 1993).

11. Acknowledgements

The author would like to thank the National University of Singapore for the research grant RP 880334 "Use of allografts for bridging large bone defects" awarded to conduct this study. He would also like to thank Mr. S.C. Yong for all technical assistance provided, Mr. S.L. Tow and Mr. S.S. Moorthy for the excellent photographs taken and Dr. Wang LiHui and Mrs. D.P. Vathani for the secretarial assistance provided.

12. References

CAPANNA, R., BUFFALINI, C. and CAMPANACCI, M. (1993). A new technique for reconstruction of large metaphyseal bone defects — A combined graft (allograft shell plus vascularised fibula). *Orthop. Traumatol.* **2**, 159–177.

CONRAD, E.U. *et al.* (1995). Transmission of hepatitis C by tissue transplantation. *J. Bone Joint Surg. [Am]* **77A**, 214–224.

DELL, P.C., BURCHARDT, H. and GLOWCZEWSKIE, F.P. Jr. (1985). A roentgenographic, biomechanical, and histological evaluation of vascularized and non-vascularized segmental fibular canine autografts. *J. Bone Joint Surg. [Am]* **67A**, 105–112.

DZIEDZIC GOCLAWSKA, A., OSTROWSKI, K., STACHOWICKZ, W., MICHALIK, J. and GRZESIK, W. (1991). Effect of radiation sterilization on osteoinductive properties and the rate of remodeling of bone implants preserved by lyophilization and deep freezing. *Clin. Orthop.* **272**, 30–37.

ENNEKING, W.F., BURCHARDT, H., PUHL, J.J. and PIOTROWSKI, G. (1975). Physical and biological aspects of repair in dog cortical-bone transplants. *J. Bone Joint Surg. [Am]* **57A**, 237–252.

ENNEKING, W.F., EADY, J.L. and BURCHARDT, H. (1980). Autogenous cortical bone grafts in the reconstruction of segmental skeletal defects. *J. Bone Joint Surg. [Am]* **62A**, 1039–1058.

FIDELER, B.M., VANGSNESS, C.T., MOORE, T., LI, Z. and RASHEED, S. (1994). Effects of gamma irradiation on human immunodeficiency virus. *J. Bone Joint. Surg.* **76A**, 1032–1035.

MANKIN, H.J., GEBHARDT, M.C., JENNINGS, L.C., SPRINGFIELD, D.S. and TOMFORD, W.W. (1996). Long term results of allograft replacement in the management of bone tumours. *Clin. Orthop.* **324**, 86–97.

MONTGOMERY, D.M., ARONSON, D.D., LEE, C.L. and LA MONT, R.L. (1990). Posterior spinal fusion: Allograft versus autograft bone. *J. Spin. Dis.* **3**, 370–373.

NATARAJAN, M.V. (1998). Challenges and achievements in orthopaedic oncology. Proceedings 43rd Annual Conference of Indian Orthopaedic Association, 16–20 December 1998, Jabalpur, India.

NATHER A. (1990a). Healing of large diaphyseal allograft transplants. An experimental study. In: *Proceedings of The International Society for Fracture Repair*, Second Meeting, E.Y.S. Chao ed., Mayo Clinic, 6–8 September, p. 90.

NATHER, A., BALASUBAMANIAM, P. and BOSE, K. (1990b). Healing of non-vascularised diaphyseal bone transplants. An experimental study. *J. Bone Joint Surg. [Br]* **72B**, 830–834.

NATHER, A., BALASUBRAMANIAM, P. and BOSE, K. (1990c). Bone morphometry of revascularisation of a large avascular segment of bone. A microangiographic study. In: *Bone Morphometry*, H.E. Takahashi ed., Nishimura, Smith-Gordon, Tokyo, London, pp. 92–95.

NATHER A., GOH, J.C.H. and LEE, J.J. (1990d) Biomechanical strength of non-vascularised and vascularised diaphyseal bone transplants. An experimental study. *J. Bone Joint Surg. [Br]* **72B**, 1031–1035.

NATHER, A. (1999). Use of allografts in spinal surgery. *Ann. Transpl.* **4**, 7–10.

OSTRUP, L.T. and FREDERICKSON, J.M. (1974). Distant transfer of a free, living bone graft by microvascular anastomases. An experimental study. *Plast. Reconstr. Surg.* **54**, 274–285.

PHO, R.W.H. (1981). Malignant giant cell tumour of the distal end of the radius treated by a free vascularised fibular transplant. *J. Bone Joint Surg. [Am]* **63A**, 877–884.

SIM, F.H., BEAUCHAMP, C.P. and CHAO, E.Y.S. (1987). Reconstruction of musculoskeletal defects about the knee for tumour. *Clin. Orthop.* **221**, 188–201.

WEILAND, A.J. and DANIEL, R.K. (1979). Microvascular anastomoses of bone grafts in the treatment of massive defects in bone. *J. Bone Joint Surg. [Am]* **61A**, 98–104.

YAMAMURO, T. (1990). Replacement of the vertebrae with bioactive glass-ceramic prostheses. In: *Proceedings of 13th Singapore Orthopaedic Association Meeting in Conjunction with the 2nd Asia Pacific Association of Surgical Tissue Banking Meeting*, Nather ed., Singapore, 2–5 August, p. 60.

Advances in Tissue Banking Vol. 5

25 THE BIOLOGY OF MASSIVE BONE ALLOGRAFTS: UNDERSTANDING ALLOGRAFT BIOLOGY AND ADAPTING IT TOWARDS SUCCESSFUL CLINICAL APPLICATION

SHEKHAR M. KUMTA[*], LOUIS T.C. CHOW[†],
JAMES GRIFFITH[‡], LINDA L.-K. FU[§] and P.C. LEUNG[*]

[*]Department of Orthopaedics & Traumatology
[†]Department of Anatomical & Cellular Pathology
[‡]Department of Diagnostic Radiology & Organ Imaging
and [§]Musculoskeletal Tissue Bank
at Sir Y.K. Pao Centre for Cancer
The Chinese University of Hong Kong
Prince of Wales Hospital, Shatin, NT, Hong Kong, SAR

1. Introduction

Massive diaphyseal allografts are being increasingly used for reconstruction of skeletal defects following tumour resection (Springfield, 1997). Unlike prostheses, which require customisation to fit the defect (Schindler *et al.*, 1997), allografts may be tailored intraoperatively to match the size and extent of the bone resection. The biological incorporation of allografts is a slow and incomplete process (Enneking *et al.*, 1975; Enneking and Mindel, 1991). The understanding of this phenomenon is instrumental to the successful clinical application and utilisation of massive allografts.

2. Biological Aspects of Graft Healing & Incorporation

Deep-frozen allografts are largely inert and most cells die during the freezing–thawing process (Enneking et al., 1975). The bone matrix remains weakly antigenic, and following implantation, a weak but definite inflammatory immune response is elicited from the host. Any form of cortical bone healing takes place through initial resorption of the grafted bone followed by replacement by bone and bone cells from the host (Nather et al., 1990). In the case of allografts, this process of creeping substitution (Bruchardt, 1983) takes place at the host–graft interphase. Resorption is best effected at the endosteal or intramedullary surface. The periosteal surface of bone resists resorption or remodelling because of a thin layer of unmineralised bone matrix that prevents osteoclastic bone resorption (Chambers and Fuller, 1985). Although creeping substitution is initiated at graft–host interphase, the initial inflammatory response prevents effective penetration of host vasculature into the graft medullary canal (Enneking and Mindel, 1991). Thus, trabecular resorption of bone is limited to a few millimetres of allograft bone at the host–bone junction. On the periosteal surface, new bone laid down by the periosteum of the host envelopes the allograft for a short extent, usually a few centimetres. This envelope of new bone is crucial to the successful amalgamation of the host bone interphase (Figs. 1a, 1b and 1c). Because of ineffective penetration by host cells, massive bone allografts remain largely necrotic, acellular and with empty lacunae (Aho et al., 1994; Enneking and Mindel, 1991). Unlike normal bone, these large masses of mineralised but now acellular matrix are incapable of responding to stress. Living cells within the lacunae of normal bone are not only capable of sensing the extent and the direction of deformation under loading, but respond to it by increasing the deposition or resorption of bone as required. This phenomenon of stress adaptation is called remodelling and is a fundamental property of living bone, classically known as Wolfe's law. Massive allografts, being acellular, are incapable of remodelling and are therefore susceptible to fatigue failure unless special precautions are taken.

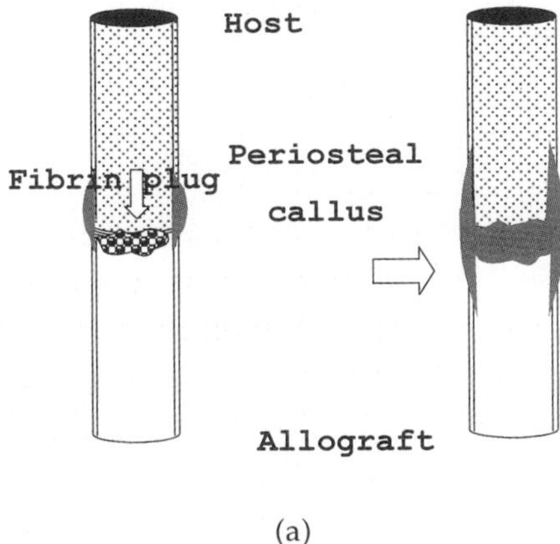

(a)

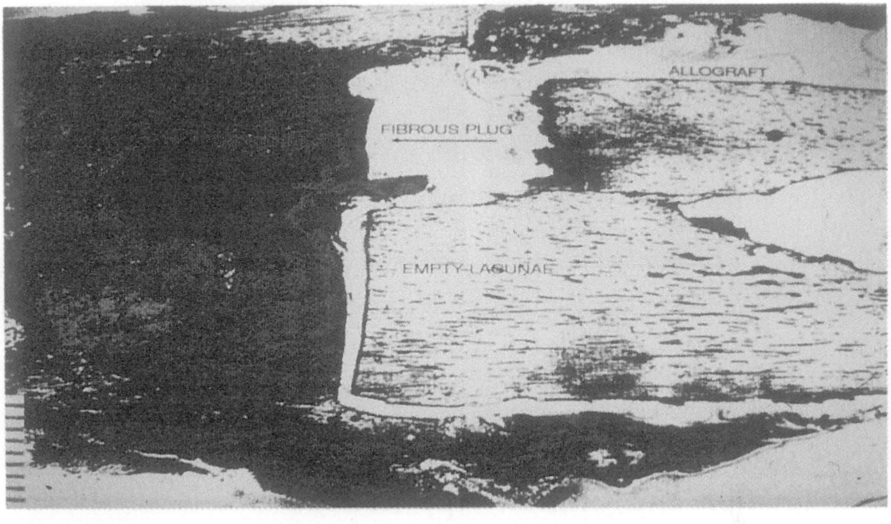

(b)

Fig. 1 (a) Diagrammatic representation of periosteal envelope emanating from the host bone and extending across the allograft. (b) Histological appearance of host–allograft junction retrieved following 12 months of implantation showing empty lacunae. An exuberant periosteal and endosteal host response is seen but with poor penetration into the allograft medullary canal, which has been blocked by a fibrous plug. (c) Enveloping callus emanating from the host bone as marked by arrows.

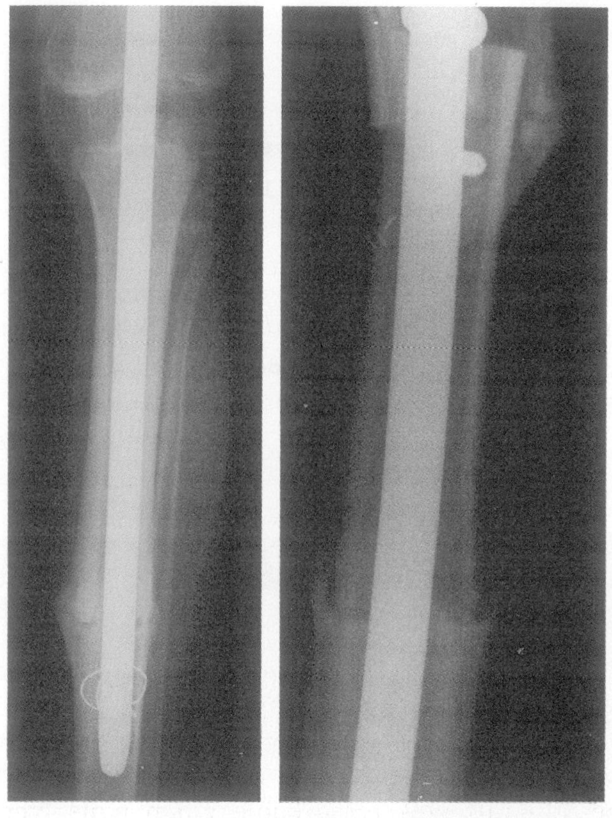

(c)

Fig. 1. (*Continued*)

3. Adaptation and Clinical Applications

Two major problems have been identified with the use of massive allografts

I. Difficulties with host–allograft union, and
II. Fatigue failure and allograft fracture.

Understanding the biology of massive allografts has enabled clinicians to overcome some of their problems through simple, effective and often innovative means, directed chiefly towards improving host–allograft interphase and preventing allograft fatigue failure.

3.1. Optimising the host–allograft interphase

3.1.1. Intramedullary nails preferred to surface plates

Studies on massive retrieved allografts have revealed that the initial junction between host and allograft is limited to a few millimetres and may be called a "spot-weld" (Enneking and Mindel, 1991). The role of the periosteum is therefore crucial as it provides a sound enveloping callus around the bone. It is hence necessary to preserve an envelope of periosteum and a layer of healthy soft tissue around the host bone junction to ensure the formation of an enveloping callus of bone.

Our previous studies have shown that surface implants interfere with this periosteal envelope (Kumta *et al.*, 1998). We scanned high-resolution radiographs of patients where allografts were stabilised with surface plates or intramedullary nails, and compared them using an image analysis program. Periosteal callus formation encasing the allograft was remarkable when nails were used and absent when surface plate was used (Fig 2). A higher incidence of junctional failure is therefore expected when plates are used for allograft stabilisation.

3.1.2. Increasing the surface contact area between host and allograft

Increasing the surface contact area may enhance the stability of the host bone interphase. A step-cut to approximate allograft with host bone results in a large surface contact area. Union across such a large surface is much stronger than that across conventional end-to-end apposition (Fig. 3). When a step-cut technique is used, stabilisation of the allograft must be secure or else displacement and failure may yet ensue. One may also increase the contact area

A Plate stabilization

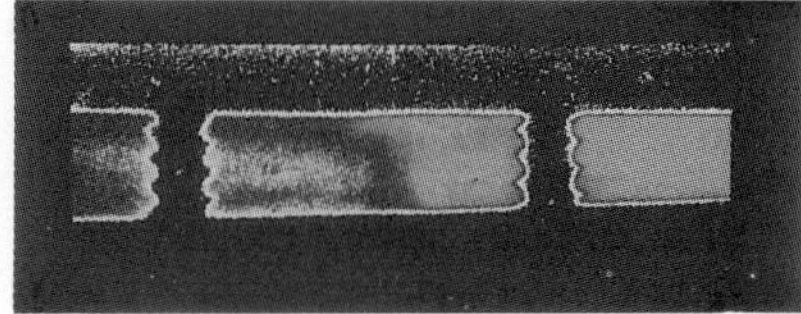

B Intramedullary Nail

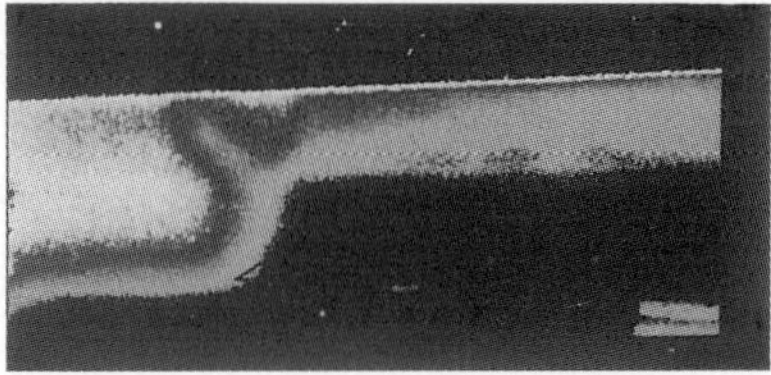

Fig. 2. High-resolution digitised images showing no callus under the plate (A). In contrast, callus is exuberant when intramedullary nail was used (B).

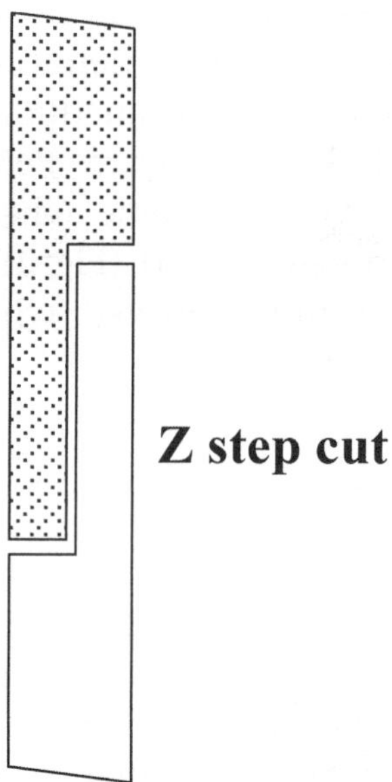

Fig. 3. Z step-cut increases allograft–host contact area and stability.

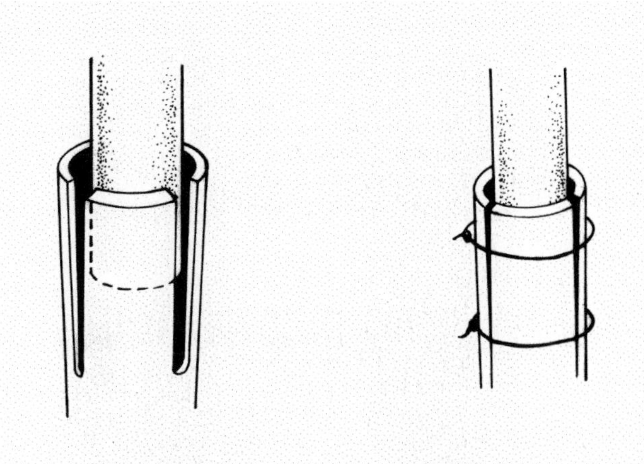

Fig. 4. Technique of telescoping allograft and host bone.

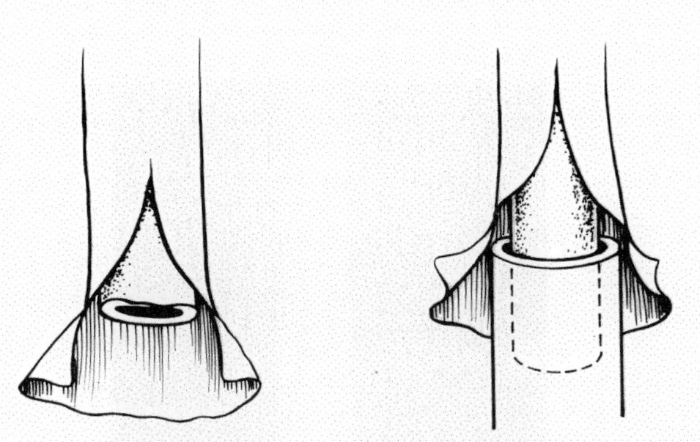

Fig. 5. Additional sleeve of periosteum used as to wrap around the allograft.

between graft and host bone by telescoping the host bone into the allograft (Fig. 4) (Kumta *et al.*, 1998). This is best applicable when there is a size discrepancy between host bone diameter and that of the allograft, as in children.

By telescoping the bone ends, junctional stability is enhanced and the available contact area is almost six times as that with conventional end-to-end apposition. One may retain an additional

                                                    S.M. Kumta et al.

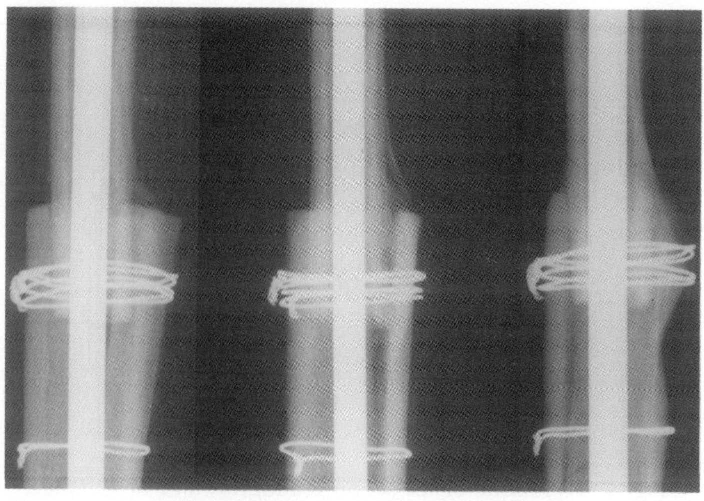

(a)

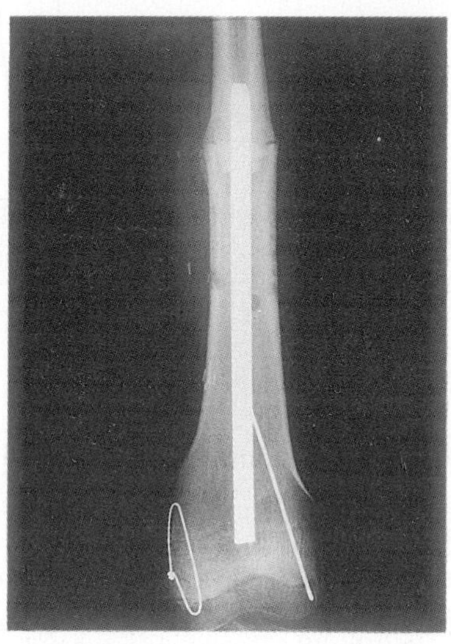

(b)

Fig. 6 (a) Telescoped junction showing progressive union through an enveloping callus. (b) Telescoped allograft with intramedullary nail and minimal internal stabilisation at the distal metaphyseal end.

sleeve of periosteum from the host bone and use it to envelop the allograft (Fig. 5). Excellent union was observed in our series with the use of this technique, with minimal additional internal stabilisation (Figs. 6a and 6b).

3.2. Protection against fatigue failure

3.2.1. Intramedullary nails versus plate

Although plates provide rigid fixation and were extensively used to stabilise fractures, their use for allograft stabilisation may not be ideal. Rigid metal plates may shield the underlying bone from stress and may result in stress fractures in the allograft just beyond the end of the plate (Fig. 7). Intramedullary nails, on the other hand,

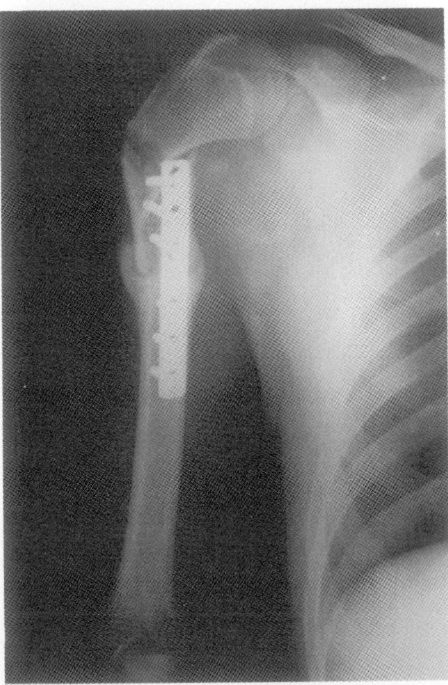

Fig. 7. Fatigue failure of allograft beyond the plate.

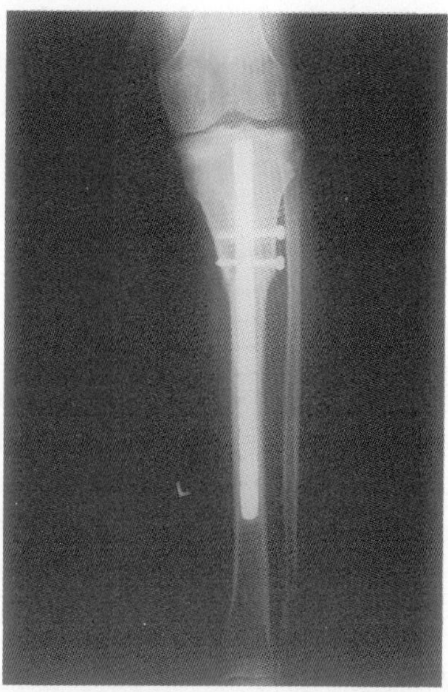

Fig. 8. Osteoarticular allograft tibia with excellent function at five years.

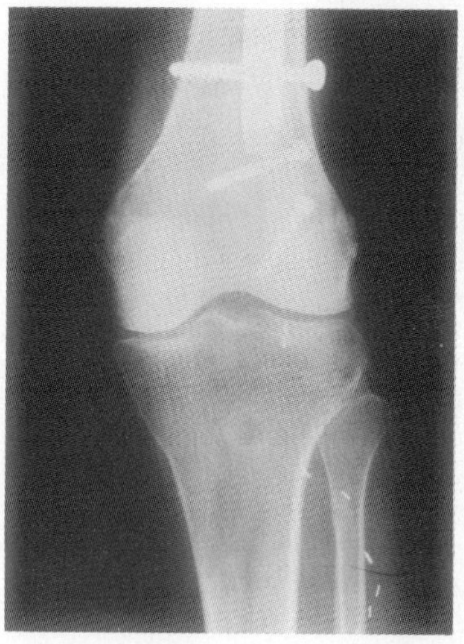

Fig. 9. Osteoarticular allograft replacement of the distal femur at five years following surgery and with excellent function.

allow an elastic and load-sharing means of stabilisation. Union of host–graft junction is not a problem as the soft tissue envelope is retained. The intramedullary nail shares load with the allograft and prevents fatigue failure under physiological and cyclical loading. Excellent functional results have been attained with the use of intramedullary nails allowing immediate weight-bearing and active mobilisation following allograft reconstruction (Figs. 8 and 9).

3.2.2. Enhanced remodelling potential of allografts

The essential problem in massive bone allografts is their inability to remodel under stress. In a study using an experimental rat model, Kumta *et al.* (1996) reported on the successful implantation of blood vessels into bone allografts. Rat allografts were implanted across a strong histocompatibility barrier. In one group, the femoral vascular bundle was implanted into the medullary cavity of deep-frozen allograft (Fig. 10a). A control group without vascular bundle implantation (Fig. 10b) was used for comparison. Following vascular

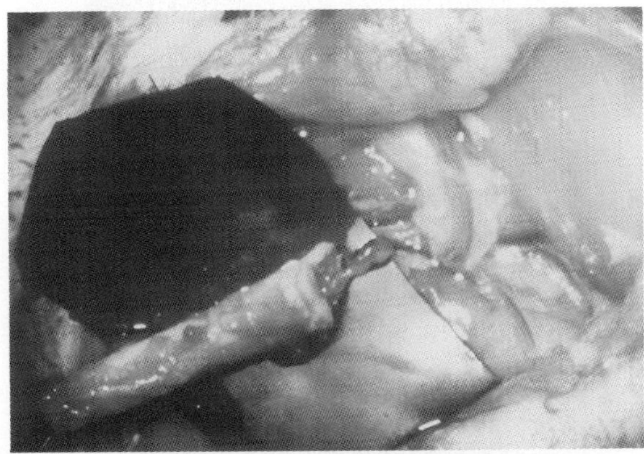

Fig. 10 (a) Vascular bundle implanted into femoral medullary canal of rat allograft. (b) Control without vascular implant. (c) Vascular proliferation within medullary canal and new bone formation spreading within the allograft (safranin stain; magnification 12×). (d) Lacunar repopulation and remodeling of bone with new bone formation (safranin-O stain; magnification 40×).

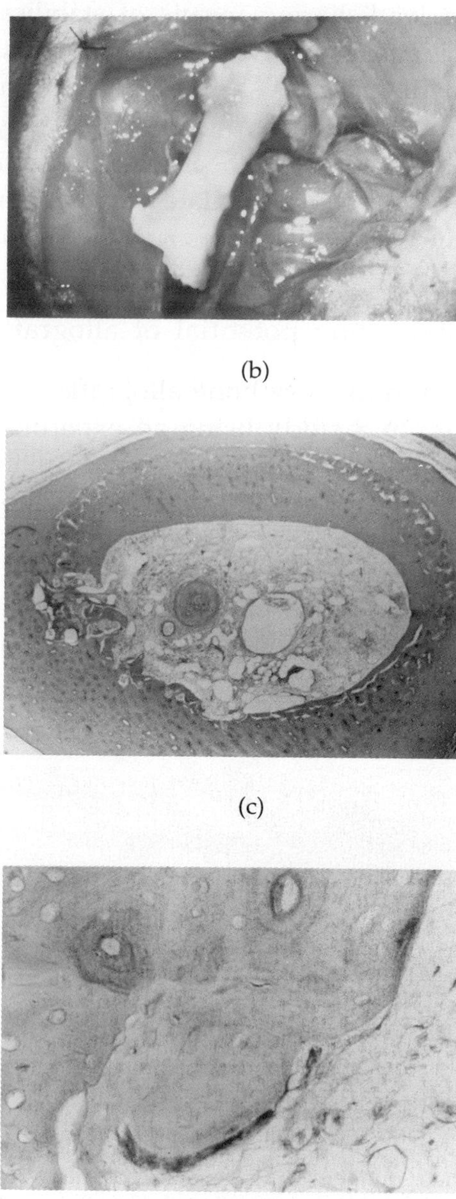

(b)

(c)

(d)

Fig. 10. (*Continued*)

bundle implantation, endosteal vascular proliferation, endosteal new bone formation and endosteal remodelling were observed in the allograft (Figs. 10c and 10d). By placing a vessel within the medullary canal, the immunological barrier towards neovascularisation seemed to be mechanically overcome. Lacunar repopulation of allografts was observed, while none of the control groups showed similar cellular repopulation. Using scanning electron microscopy, we observed a remarkable entry of leukocytes and red blood corpuscles within the lacunae of bone where vascular implantation was performed (Fig. 11).

Using a similar concept, Capanna *et al.* (1993) combined the use of vascular bone grafts with bone allografts, using an elegant reconstruction technique. By placing a vascularised bone graft (fibula) within the shell of an allograft, rapid hypertrophy and cellular repopulation of the graft were observed. The living bone and allograft fused to each other and were amalgamated as one within a short period (Fig. 12). Vascular bone grafts have excellent remodelling potential as they retain an intact blood supply. The vascularised bone graft quickly responds to stress and is capable

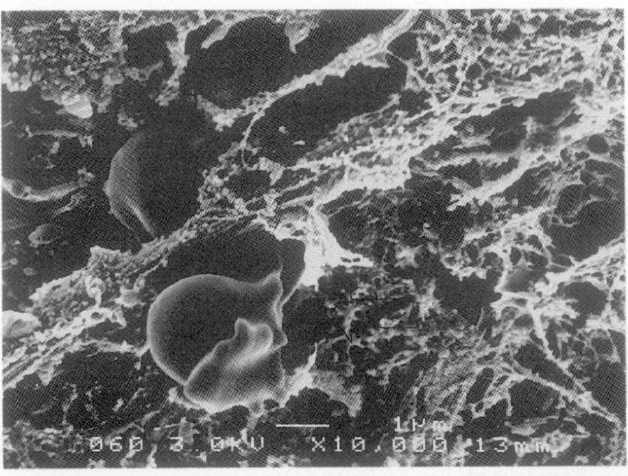

Fig. 11. Scanning EM photograph (magnification 10 000×) showing a blood corpuscle entering lacunae within the cortex.

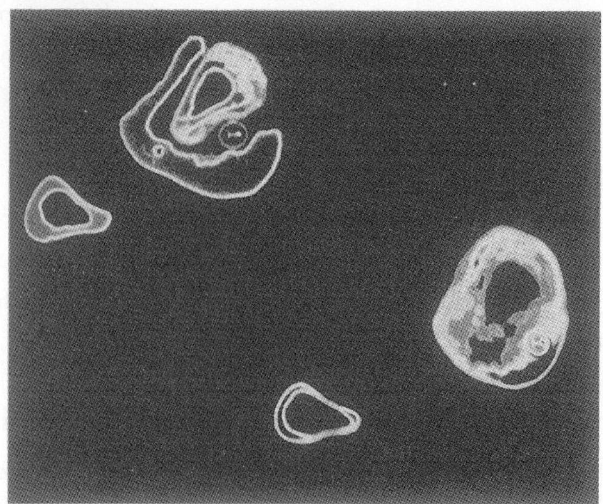

Fig. 12. Combined allograft vascular bone graft reconstruction. Vascularised bone graft within shell of allograft. Rapid incorporation and fusion within 12 months.

of remodelling, while its outer allograft shell provides a secure mechanical support. Not only does the vascularised graft hypertrophy under load-bearing, but it also induces new bone formation within the allograft as well as cellular repopulation of the otherwise inert allograft. We have studied hybrid reconstructions after retrieval either after death or amputation. The living bone induces early repopulation of the allograft and enables the otherwise inert allograft to remodel under loading. At the metaphyseal ends, where allograft bone is less dense (Figs. 13a and 13b), host cell populations quickly colonise the allograft and result in "formative remodelling". This process seems to bypass the obligatory requirement for cortical allografts to undergo resorption prior to host repopulation. Such a hybrid graft obviously has superior mechanical and biological properties, and heals much faster. The juxta-positioning of vascularised bone and allograft may produce a similar effect (Figs. 13b and 13c). The combination of living bone or vascular tissue enhances the biological potential of allografts and eliminates much of the disadvantages associated with allografts.

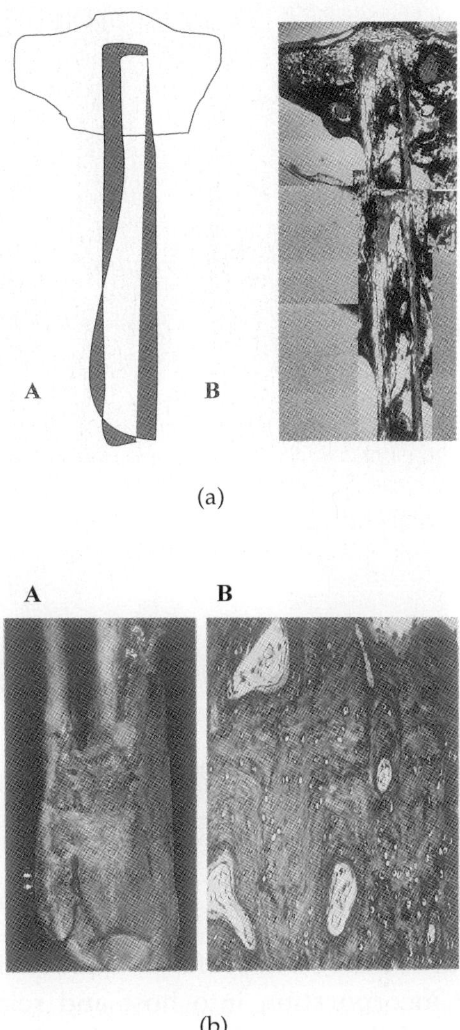

Fig. 13. (a) Schematic diagram (A) showing vascular fibula within allograft shell. Retrieved sections (B) showing hypertrophy and amalgamation of host bone with allograft. (b) Fusion of vascular fibula juxtaposed to allograft (A). Histological section shows extensive new bone formation around the original osteonal arrangement without resorption — so-called formative remodelling. (C) Vascular fibula juxtaposed with distal femoral allograft. Excellent healing of host–allograft junction, enhanced by contribution from the vascularised fibula. Patient has good extremity function nine years following surgery.

                                          S.M. Kumta et al.

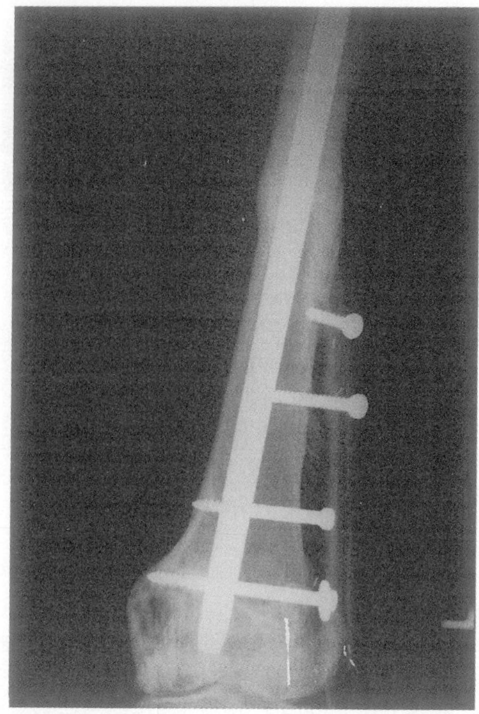

(c)

Fig. 13. (*Continued*)

The biology of massive allografts is characterised by their inert behaviour, slow incorporation into host and relative susceptibility to undergo fatigue failure. For the successful clinical applications of allografts, one must take into consideration these limitations. Secure host–allograft stabilisation, preserving a good biological soft tissue environment around the grafts, and enhancing their biological potential using vascularised tissue grafts are innovative means to ensure graft healing and prevent fatigue failure. Efforts are now underway to enhance cellular repopulation *in vitro* using stem cells from the recipient to colonise the allograft, prior to transplantation.

Pioneering work has been conducted by our department using cultured growth plate chondrocytes on a collagen matrix and a growth plate has been reconstructed *in vitro*. In the future, we expect such cellular manipulation to enable the host cell population to colonise various types of tissue grafts. As a result, such grafts will not remain inert. On the contrary, they will enhance the biological process of incorporation and eliminate problems of immune rejection.

4. Acknowledgement

We would like to thank Mr. Horace Ma for his secretarial support to the tissue bank and for preparing this manuscript.

5. References

AHO, A.J., EKFORS, T., DEAN, P.B., ARO, H.T., AHONEN, A. and NIKKANEN, V. (1994). Incorporation and clinical results of large allografts of the extremities and pelvis. *Clin. Orthop.* **307**, 200–213.

BRAUN, C. (1992). Autogenously vascularized bone grafts. Experimental model of a new bone-muscle composite graft. *Arch. Orthop. Trauma Surg.* **111**, 250–254.

BURCHARDT, H. (1983). The biology of bone graft repair. *Clin. Orthop.* **174**, 28.

CAPANNA, R., BUFFALINI, C. and CAMPANACCI, M. (1993). A new technique for reconstructions of large metadiaphyseal bone defects — A combined graft (allograft shell plus vascularized fibula). *Orthop. Traumatol.* **2**(3), 159–177.

CHAMBERS, T.J. and FULLER, K. (1985). Bone cells predispose bone surfaces to resorption by exposure of mineral to osteoclastic contact. *J. Cell Science* **76**, 155–165.

ENNEKING, W.F., BURCHARDT, H., PUHL, J.J. and PIOTROWSKI, G. (1975). Physiological and biological aspects of repair in dog cortical bone transplants. *J. Bone Joint Surg.* **57**, 237–251.

ENNEKING, W.F., EADY, J.L. and BURCHARDT, H. (1980). Autogenous cortical bone grafts in the reconstruction of segmental skeletal defects. *J. Bone Joint Surg.* **62A**, 1039.

ENNEKING, W.F. and MINDEL, E.R. (1991). Observations on massive retrieved bone allografts. *J. Bone Joint Surg.* **73**, 1123–1142.

KUMTA, S.M., YIP, K., ROY, N., LEE, S.K.M. and LEUNG, P.C. (1996). Revascularisation of bone allografts following vascular bundle implantation: An experimental study in rats. *Arch. Orthop. Trauma Surg.* **115**, 206–210.

KUMTA, S.M., LEUNG, P.C., GRIFFITH, J.F., ROEBUCK, D.J., CHOW, L.T.C. and LI, C.K. (1998). A technique for enhancing union of allograft to host bone. *J. Bone Joint Surg.* **80B**, 994–998.

NATHER, A., BALASUBRAMANIAM, P. and BOSE, K. (1990). Healing of non-vascularised diaphyseal bone transplants: An experimental study. *J. Bone Joint Surg. [Br]* **72B**, 830–834.

SCHINDLER, O.S., CANNON, S.R., BRIGGS, T.W. and BLUNN, G.W. (1997). Stanmore custom-made extendible distal femoral replacements. Clinical experience in children with primary malignant bone tumors. *J. Bone Joint Surg.* **79**, 927–937.

SPRINGFIELD, D.S. (1997). Allograft reconstructions. *Semin. Surg. Oncol.* **13**(1), 11–17.

26 EFFECT OF GROWTH FACTORS ON HEALING AND THE CLINICAL APPLICATIONS OF AUTOGENOUS PLATELET RICH PLASMA GEL TO ENHANCE BONE FORMATION

CHANG JOON YIM

Dankook University School of Dentistry
Infirmary Dental Hospital and Dankook University Hospital
Department of Oral & Maxillofacial Surgery
7-1 Sinbudong, Cheonan, 330-716
Republic of Korea

1. Introduction

A lot of clinicians and investigators tried to develop numerous bone grafting techniques to enhance and to confirm new bone formation of better quality. Autogenous platelet-rich plasma (PRP) is supposed to contain several growth factors which are able to promote hard tissue and soft tissue healing, such as platelet-derived growth factor (PDGF), transforming growth factor (TGF)-beta, insulin-like growth factor (IGF), etc. This paper reviews the effects of these growth factors in wound healing and bone healing, and discuss the clinical application of the autogenous PRP gel for mandibular or maxillary bone reconstruction with particulate bone grafts and dental implants.

2. Growth Factors in Wound Healing and Bone Healing

Growth factors can be defined as signalling peptides that act through specific cell surface receptors and paracrine or autocrine stimulation, or both, of cell proliferation and migration (Steenfos, 1994). Growth factors may enhance cell motility like classic endocrine hormone. About 30 growth factors have been identified, but not all are of importance in wound healing. Some of the most common growth factors supposed to play important roles in bone healing are described below.

The finding that growth factors play a part in wound healing opens important areas of research of clinical potential, which include acceleration of healing rates of normal soft tissue or chronic ulcerative lesions in medical field, and acceleration of healing of graft bone in and maxillofacial surgery.

Wound healing is a proliferative and complex cellular process similar to the growth of a cancer. The types of cells involved and the time sequence have been known for decades from histological studies of wound healing, but in the last decade, it has become clear that the cellular processes are initiated, controlled and terminated by growth factors, the discovery of which, to a large extend, results from studying the molecular biology of carcinogenesis. It is only since then that we have realised that growth factors play a part in physiological processes, such as wound healing. It has also been shown that growth factors may enhance cell motility, and it is likely that "classic" endocrine hormones participate with cytokines in the regulation of wound healing.

2.1. Mode of action

Growth factors are polypeptides. Because proteins do not normally cross cell membranes, polypeptide growth factors should bind to the receptors on the outer surface of the target cell for their action. The receptor is a protein that has an extracellular site for binding. A signal is transmitted into the intracellular site through the membrane and tyrosine kinase is activated. The signal reaches nuclear

DNA through little-known intracellular pathways, and there, transcription leads to suppression or induction of cell growth, such as production of the target protein, or cellular division and proliferation, or both. The effect of a growth factor relates both to its concentration and to receptor sensitivity. *In vitro* studies have shown that the effect is increased up to a certain concentration, but at higher concentrations, the effect is reversed.

The source of delivery of growth factors to a particular site may occur via one of the three pathways, such as endocrine, paracrine or autocrine delivery. Some growth factors such as IGF-1 and IGF-2 are delivered via the blood in an endocrine fashion. Certain other factors such as PDGF and FGF are synthesised by one cell and used by another cell after paracrine delivery. The other growth factors are produced and utilised by the same cell in a self-stimulatory autocrine fashion.

2.2. Wound healing phases

The wound healing process involves three phases — inflammation, proliferation and remodelling (Kanzler *et al.*, 1986; Lynch, 1991). It, however, is a continuous process in which the beginning of one phase and the end of another cannot be clearly defined, and there is considerable overlap between the phases.

Growth factors can be divided into three types, i.e. mitogen factors, chemo-attractant factors and transforming factors, according to their roles during wound repair. As mitogens, they signal cellular proliferation. Mitogens can be subdivided into competent factors and progression factors. The former factors stimulate cells to progress from the resting stage (G0) to a readiness state where cells replicate DNA and divide (G1). Once cells enter the G1 stage, the progession factors seem to be required to continue the cell cycle. As chemo-attractants, they stimulate cellular migration, which have either characteristics of chemotaxis which induces the target cell to move in a given direction, or chemokinesis which increases the rate of migration. As transforming factors, they alter the cell's phenotypic expression.

2.2.1. The inflammation (substrate) phase

Tissue injury activates biochemical amplification cascades that results in the local accumulation of platelets, neutrophils and monocytes in the wound space. Injury results in bleeding and the enzymatic activation of the clotting cascade, the complement cascade and the kinin cascade: activation of plasminogen, and the aggregation and activation of platelets. This activation of platelets results in the release of a number of substances, such as PDGFs and TGFs-beta, which stimulate the migration of macrophages, neutrophils and lymphocytes (Pierce *et al.*, 1989).

These immediate events are sometimes referred to as "the coagulation phase". Neutrophils and macrophages are the first cells to enter the injured tissue, and the main task of the neutrophils is to prevent bacterial infection. Macrophages seem to be the most important single type of cell in wound healing, as activated macrophages have various functions, including wound debridement and the release of growth factors.

The growth factors, in turn, stimulate a further influx of white cells and fibroblasts, as well as cells concerned with angiogenesis. Later, the lymphocytes enter the wound area, and they also secrete various growth factors and cytokines.

2.2.2. The proliferation (fibroplasia) phase

Stimulated by the released growth factors, fibroblasts, followed by endothelial cells, migrate into the wound to form granulation tissue, which is a connective tissue rich in blood vessels. The fibroblasts have a number of receptors for growth factors, and they secrete a number of molecules which lead to autocrine and paracrine stimulation of both fibroblasts and ingrowing capillaries. Simultaneously, the epithelial cells start to grow inwards from the wound edges to cover the wound. One of the most important molecules secreted by fibroblasts during this phase is collagen, which gives strength to the wound. During the proliferation phase, the wound acquires a high water content and concentration of the capillaries.

2.2.3. The remodelling (scarring) phase

Gradually, water and other compounds are lost from the wound. And the initially-produced collagen is gradually replaced by the more stable and interwoven type III collagen. The wound as a whole contracts because the amount of connective tissue and capillaries is reduced, and a scar is formed. The last phase may take up to several years, and deregulation may result in hypertrophic keloid scars. The role of growth factors in the formation of scar tissue is not fully understood, but it seems that TGF-beta is of importance.

2.3. Bone graft healing

Bone represents a highly regulated organ system for maintaining mineral homeostasis and structural integrity of the body. Bone metabolism is associated with cycles of active bone resorption and new bone formation. If bone grafts are transplanted to the hard tissue defects, they undergo cellular regeneration followed by remodelling. Axhausen divided such bone regeneration into two phases.

The first phase is one of cellular proliferation and production of osteoid in a random fashion. This bone lacks the arversian systems and lamellae of more mature bone. This phase I bone will undergo an obligatory resorption, which is then replaced by organised phase II bone. This physiology is common to all bone healing. The identical physiology is observed in the formation–replacement–remodelling–formation cycle of both internal and external fracture calluses and in normal skeletal remodelling.

In particulate bone graft transplantation, endosteal osteoblasts primarily, and mesenchymal fibroblasts secondarily, are responsible for bone formation. This initial phase of bone regeneration is directly proportional to the cellular density of the transplanted bone and will be the maximum amount of bone achievable by the graft system. There, PBCM grafts that transplant a greater quantity of osteoprogenitor cells have been found to produce superior bone ossicles in mandibular continuity defects over block-type grafts with fewer osteoprogenitor cells (Marx, 1994).

The second phase of bone is not derived from transplanted cells as is phase I bone. It is instead derived from host tissue cells that eventually replace phase I bone with mature, organised bone and establish an endosteum and a periosteum. As the osteoclasts resorb phase I bone, they are thought to secrete a coupling factor or release osteogenin from the mineral matrix of the resorbed bone, or both. This process occurs in normal everyday physiologic bone resorption. Such osteogenin release or coupling factor secretion couples bone resorption and new bone apposition through induction and mitogenesis of host connective tissue cells into functioning osteoblasts. Second-phase bone develops into a trabecular bone ossicle with more well-defined lamellae and a greater mineral density. The second-phase bone will only resorb and replace phase I bone in a 1:1 ratio at best. Such phase II resorption–remodelling occurs throughout the life of the particulate bone graft as it does in all other bone.

Clinically, phase II bone formation is enhanced by ensuring a cellular and vascular recipient bed. The vascularity is not only valuable for survival of the transplanted cells that produce the initial phase I bone but also for access of osteoclasts to initiate the phase II resorption–remodelling cycle. The cellularity must specifically consist of induced bone-forming cells, endosteum and periosteum. To this end, myocutaneous flaps or hyperbaric oxygen may enhance the vascular density and the specific type of cellular density necessary in the tissue bed; therefore, these entities have been used in bony reconstructions in irradiated or tissue-deficient patients.

2.4. Role of several growth factors

2.4.1. Platelet-derived growth factor (PDGF)

A glycoprotein, PDGF (MW 28–35 kDa) is a heterodimer protein containing A and B chains in humans, the latter exhibiting 90% sequence homology with the V-sis oncogene product. PDGF was first described in the alpha granules of platelets. It is also synthesised and secreted by other cells, such as macrophages and endothelium. It seems to be the first growth factor present in a wound, and it initiates connective tissue healing, including bone regeneration and repair. It is released from the platelet alpha granule, macrophages/monocytes and endothelial cells, as well as from normal osteoblasts and osteosarcoma cells. PDGF is present in small amount in bone and receptors for PDGF have been found on osteoblast-like cells. PDGF is a potent mitogen for mesenchymal cells, increasing proliferation and differentiation of cultured chicken and murine-cultured osteoblasts, but increasing calcium release from cultured murine calvarium in a prostaglandin-dependent manner (Joseph-Silverstein, 1987). The role of PDGF on bone formation and resorption in humans is currently unclear.

In lesser quantities, AA and BB homodimers exist in human beings with the same activity. The reason for the three distinct dimeric forms remains unclear, but differential binding by various receptor cells, such as endothelium, fibroblasts, macrophages and marrow stem cells, has been suggested. PDGF is known to emerge from degranulating platelets at the time of injury. Its mechanism is to activate cell membrane receptors on target cells, which in turn are thought to develop high-energy phosphate bonds in internal cyto-plasmic signal proteins. The bonds then activate the signal proteins to initiate a specific activity within the target cell. The most important specific activities of PDGF include mitogenesis (increase in the cell population of healing cells), angiogenesis (endothelial mitosis into functioning capillaries), and macrophage activation (debridement of the wound site and a second-phase source of growth factors for continued repair and bone regeneration). PDGF enhances healing

Table 1. Average amount of newly formed bone as a percentage of calvarial defect area.

	1 week	2 weeks	3 weeks
Control	6.85 ± 2.35[†]	7.80 ± 2.77[†]	23.36 ± 3.51
Experimental I	11.98 ± 3.34[ʃ]	10.59 ± 2.55[ʃ]	29.57 ± 8.69
Experimental II	31.46 ± 13.98[†ʃʃ]	32.88 ± 8.61[†ʃʃ]	32.55 ± 9.70

Significant difference between [†] and [‡], [ʃ] and [ʃʃ] in ANOVA ($p < 0.05$)

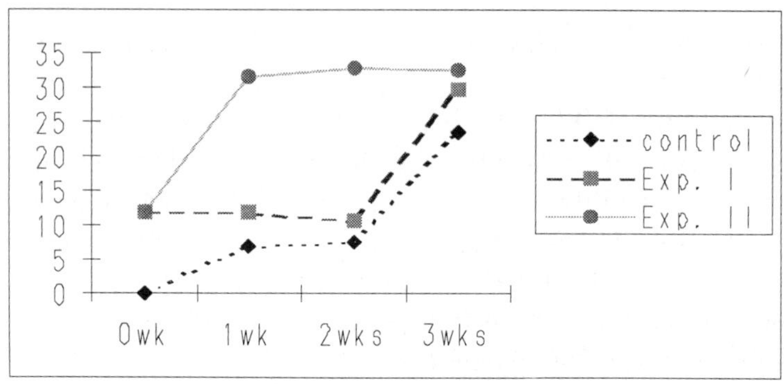

Fig. 1. The change in percentage of newly formed bone mass in the calvarial defect area.

rates of demineralised freeze-dried bone (DFDB) powders, healing rates of composite graft of DFDB powders and xenogenic bone minerals (Howes *et al.*, 1988; Hyun *et al.*, 2000; Kim and Yim, 2000).

PDGF-BB was added to the allogeneic DFDB transplanted into the calvarial defects of rats (Hyun *et al.*, 2000), which were divided into three groups, i.e. DFDB implant group, PDGF-added DFDB implant group and control group. The average percentage of newly formed bone mass in the calvarial defect area of the PDGF-added DFDB group was larger than that of the DFDB-only group (Table 1). The change of newly formed bone mass in the calvarial defect area showed as a curved linear graph (Fig. 1). PDGF-BB also promotes new bone formation in the bone defects filled with the bovine bone mineral (Kim and Yim, 2000).

There is approximately 0.06 ng of PDGF per million platelets, a fact that underscores this molecule's great potency. Stated in other terms, there is 6×10^{-17} g of PDGF, or about 1200 molecules of PDGF, in every individual platelet. Therefore, at least threefold or greater concentration of platelets, as was measured in PRP, can be expected to have a profound effect on wound healing enhancement and bone regeneration (Singh *et al.*, 1982; Bowen-Pope *et al.*, 1984; Marx *et al.*, 1998).

2.4.2. Transforming growth factor beta (TGF-beta)

TGF-beta (MW 25 kDa), refers to the superfamily of growth and differentiating factors of the bone morphogenetic protein (BMP) family which contains at least 13 described BMPs, is produced by osteoblasts and a variety of cells, including platelets (Joseph-Silverstein, 1987; Rifkin, 1989). It is present in abundance in the bone matrix, with bone representing its major storage site in the body. TGF-beta exhibits a complicated effect in bone. In the matrix, it is present in a latent form complexed with a 130 kDa binding protein, and it becomes released in an activated form following osteoclastic resorption of bone. The primary effect of TGF-beta is on bone formation, particularly in the early phase of osteoblast development. It increases chemotaxis of osteoblast precursors to the site of future matrix formation and increases cell proliferation. TGF-beta stimulates matrix protein synthesis by human osteoblasts and, when administered to rats, increases bone formation. TGF-beta, however, appears to inhibit differentiation of cultured rat calvarial osteoblasts, suggesting species differences.

The TGFs-beta referred to this contribution are TGF-beta1 and TGF-beta2 proteins, which are the more generic growth factors involved with general connective tissue repair and bone regeneration. TGF-beta1 and TGF-beta2 are proteins that have molecular weights of approximately 25 kDa. Like PDGF, they are synthesised and found in platelets and macrophages, as well as in some other cell types.

When released by platelet degranulation or actively secreted by macrophages, they act as paracrine growth factors (i.e. growth factors secreted by one cell exerting its effect on an adjacent second cell), affecting mainly fibroblasts, marrow stem cells and pre-osteoblasts. Each of these target cells, however, has the ability to synthesise and secrete its own TGF-beta proteins to act on adjacent cells in a paracrine fashion or act on itself as an autocrine growth factor. In the latter, it is secreted by a cell that acts on its own cell membrane.

TGFs-beta therefore represent a mechanism for sustaining a long-term healing and bone regeneration module and even evolve into a bone remodelling factor over time. The most important functions of TGF-beta1 and TGF-beta2 seem to be the chemotaxis and mitogenesis of osteoblast precursors. They also have the ability to stimulate osteoblast deposition of the collagen matrix of wound healing and of bone. In addition, TGFs-beta inhibit osteoclast formation and bone resorption, thus favouring bone formation over resorption by two different mechanisms.

TGF-beta directly inhibits both proliferation and differentiation of osteoclast precursor cells and inhibits the function of mature osteoclasts with reduction in TRAP and reactive oxygen radicals. TGF-beta released from the matrix during bone resorption could upregulate both calcitonin receptors in osteoclasts and PTH receptors in osteoblasts, thus inhibiting bone resorption. TGF-beta thus appears to exhibit a complex effect in many cells within bone, but has an overall effect of promoting bone formation and inhibiting osteoclastic resorption.

2.4.3. Insulin-like growth factors (IGFs)

These growth factors (MW 7.5 kDa) consist of two proteins, IGF-I (somatomedin C) and IGF-II (skeletal growth factor) which are secreted by osteoblasts. Both factors induce pre-osteoblast proliferation and differentiation, osteoblast collagen synthesis, and inhibit collagen breakdown. In human bone, the concentration of IGF-II is

50–100 fold greater than IGF-I whereas equivalent amounts of IGF-I are 4–7 times more active than IGF-II on bone formation. The biological effects of IGF are modulated by four specific binding proteins (IGF-BP 1–4). The role of these binding proteins are still under investigation. IGF-BPs appear to modulate the binding of IGF to cellular receptors and may either prolong the biological half-life of IGF or inhibit its biological activity. Like TGF-beta, IGF bound to a binding protein in the matrix may be released in an active form following osteoclastic resorption. Cultured osteoblasts *in vitro* release IGF-BP4 when PTH is added to the medium. In elderly women with fractures, while IGF-I levels in serum are normal, PTH and IGF-BP4 levels are increased, suggesting that increased PTH levels could indirectly cause a functional decrease in IGF-I activity. While osteoblasts express IGF type 1 (tyrosine kinase) and type 2 (mannose-6-phosphate) receptors, it is not clear which receptor(s) mediate the anabolic effect of IGF on bone.

Circulating IGF-I exerts a general effect on cell growth. Locally produced IGF-I, secreted by fibroblast and cells in bone and cartilage, is controlled by a variety of factors. The anabolic effect of PTH on bone is mediated by IGF-I which increases collagen synthesis. While 17-B-estradiol and GH increase transcription of IGF-I in human bone cells, there is no parallel increase in protein synthesis. Agents that increase cyclic AMP in bone, like PTH and PGE2, increase secretion of IGF-I. Corticosteroids reduce IGF-I synthesis and 1,25(OH)2D3 enhances binding of IGF-I to bone cells.

Human IGF-II exhibits 62% sequence homology with IGF-I, has higher affinity for the type II receptor and may exert its major effects through this receptor. Corticosteroids reduce the binding of IGF-II to osteoblasts. While IGF-I appears to be biologically more active than IGF-II, concentrations of the latter far exceed that of IGF-I in bone (Joseph-Silverstein, 1987; Rifkin, 1989).

2.4.4. Fibroblast growth factors (FGFs)

The matrix proteins, acidic and basic FGFs, are produced by osteo-blasts, bind heparin and are angiogenic factors, but their effects on bone *in vivo* are unknown. *In vitro*, they cause proliferation of osteoblast progenitor cells but inhibit differentiation, and do not appear to affect the osteoclast. Injected locally or parenterally into experimental animals, FGFs stimulate new bone formation and are secreted by some metastatic prostate cancer cells. However, their effects on bone may be indirect, mediated by such factors as TGF-beta (Baird, 1989; King, 1989).

3. Clinical Usage of PRP

Platelet-rich plasma is an autogenous source of platelet-derived growth factor, TGF-beta, and some other growth factors that are obtained by sequestering and concentrating platelets by gradient density centrifugation. This technique produces a concentration of human platelets of 338% and identifies platelet-derived growth factor and TGF-beta within them.

Platelets release PDGF, platelet-derived angiogenic factor (PDAF), TGF-beta and other growth factors from their alpha granules (Servold, 1991). The combination of these growth factors produces granulation tissue and stimulates cells to migrate into the wound space. Platelets could play a continuing role in growth factor production throughout repair (Knighton *et al.*, 1990).

In 1994, Tayapongsak *et al.* introduced the novel idea of adding autologous fibrin adhesive (AFA) to cancellous bone during mandibular continunity reconstructions. They identified earlier radiographic bone consolidation in 33 cases. They attributed this to enhanced osteoconduction afforded to osteocompetent cells in the graft by virtue of the fibrin network developed by AFA. They also reported the remarkable adhesive advantage of binding cancellous marrow particles during graft placement.

Since the early 1990s, Marx and his associates have been exploring the parallel but more specific sequestration and concentration of autogenous platelets in plasma and studying the growth factors contained within platelets in relation to their biologic enhancement of continuity bone grafts to the mandible.

They reported that platelet-rich plasma (PRP) indeed contains a concentration of growth factors and those growth factors, which were concentrated with a cell separator and added to the bone graft, produced an enhanced result in comparison with graft performed without its use. They emphasised that PDGF and TGF-beta are not the only growth factors that influence bone regeneration and neither are these the only growth factors contained in PRP, although it is an admittedly over-simplified model that focuses on the growth factors available to surgeons. According to their study, PRP increased platelet concentration when placed into grafts, showing the presence of at least three growth factors (PDGF, TGF-beta1 and TGF-beta2).

Using monoclonal antibody assessment, they have shown that cancellous cellular marrow grafts demonstrated cells that were capable of responding to these growth factors by bearing cell membrane receptors. They also showed the potential of PRP to increase the rate of bone formation in a graft and enhance the density of the bone formed at six months. The newly formed bone, with added platelet-rich plasma to grafts, evidenced a radiographic maturation rate 1.62 to 2.16 times to that of grafts without platelet-rich plasma. It also showed a greater bone density than that of the new bone grafted without platelet-rich plasma.

The author concentrates PRP from the patient's whole blood by platelet-pheresis or by double centrifugation method. One can use a platelet-pheresis machine for platelet concentration. The platelet concentrate (PC) was automatically separated from the patient's autogenous whole blood and the remaining portion of blood was returned to the patient. The double centrifugation method consists of a two-step centrifugation. The first step includes centrifuging the patient's whole blood at 2000 x*g* (gravity) for a duration of three minutes. The second step involves centrifuging the plasma and buffy coat separated from the first step at 5000 x*g* (gravity) for a duration of five minutes. The two-step centrifugation method is the modification of the PC sequestration standards of the American Association of Blood Banks. Usually, one obtains a 10% volume of

PRP from the whole blood processed and more than three-fold concentration rate from the original patients whole blood (1 cc PRP from 10 cc whole blood).

As mentioned earlier, the biochemistry of the recipient tissue and the graft itself is largely inherent. Other than soft tissue flaps and ensuring a healthy tissue bed, little else can be done and little else need to be done. However, at this point in time, early studies and experience with platelet-rich plasma (PRP) additions to the graft are promising, relating to early consolidation and graft mineralisation. The concept is that PRP forms a very specific form of the fibrin clot rich in platelets, which in turn release PDGF and other growth factors. This enhanced quantity of PDGF initiates the osteocompetent cell activity more completely than will otherwise inherently occur in the graft and clot. Additionally, the enhanced fibrin network created by PRP is thought to enhance osteoconduction throughout the graft, thus supporting graft consolidation. Furthermore, PDGF and TGF-beta, which are the family members of four major angiogenic growth factor families (Hom, 1992), stimulate angiogenesis during the early stage of wound healing.

Supplements of PDGF to demineralised bone matrix implants in older rats increased production of mRNA for collagen II, alkaline phosphatase activity and calcium content of the implant, whereas the other growth factors tested showed no such changes (Hows *et al.*, 1988). The results suggest that, under some conditions, bone induction is submaximal and can be increased by local supplement of rhPDGF-BB to allogeneic freeze-dried demineralised bone powders, which were transmitted into rat calvarial bone defects. PDGF-BB also enhances new bone formation with time, while the other groups without PDGF-BB were observed to produce slower and lesser bone formation (Hyun *et al.*, 2000).

In therapeutic applications, the administration of growth factors in combination may be more effective than the use of a single agent alone. This was suggested by the demonstration that the combination of PDGF and TGF-beta stimulated higher collagen deposition than TGF-beta alone in adriamycin-treated rats (Lawrence *et al.*, 1986; Lynch, 1987; 1989).

A volume of 6 cc of PRP can be gelated by adding 1 cc fo a mixture of 10% $CaCl_2$ and thrombin. Surgeons can add PRP gel to any type of particulate bone grafts, be it autogenous, allogeneic, or xenogenic grafts (Marx *et al.*, 1998; Yim, 1999; 2000).

Histologically, such grafts enter a long-term remodelling process. Normal skeletal graft cortex never becomes as thick as a normal jaw cortex and the graft itself retains a dense cancellous trabecular pattern. This dense cancellous trabecular pattern turns into quite an advantage when dental implants are placed as it promotes osseo-integration. It is an advantage when conventional dentures are placed as dense trabecular bone is very adaptable to a variety of functional stresses. Radiographically, the graft takes on the morphology and cortical outlines of a mandible or maxilla. The author successfully placed dental implant fixtures into newly-formed bone at the anterior maxillae three months after PRP has been added during autogenous grafting procedure.

The surgeon can use this knowledge of bone physiology to plan pre-prosthetic surgeries and schedule complete prosthetic rehabilitation. Essentially, the graft can begin full function at six weeks and earliest at four weeks if a rigid reconstruction plate is used. Subsequent pre-prosthetic procedures, such as skin graft vestibulo-plasties, have been performed. Together with vetibulo-plasties, osseo-integrated dental implants may be placed. Such implants osseo-integrate into bone grafts rapidly and may be activated at three months.

4. Summary

The surgeon can clinically apply autogenous PRP gel with the thorough knowledge of bone physiology to plan pre-prosthetic maxillo-mandibular bone reconstruction and schedule complete prosthetic rehabilitation. PRP is supposed to contain several growth factors which are able to promote the hard tissue and soft tissue healing, such as PDGF, TGF-beta, IGF, etc. Because they enhance the healing effects of soft tissue wound and bone, the autogenous

PRP gel can be applied for mandibular or maxillary reconstruction with particulate bone grafts and the dental implants may be surgically placed into the grafted bone.

A volume of 6 cc of PRP can be gelated by adding 1 cc mixture of 10% $CaCl_2$ and thrombin. Surgeons can add PRP gel any type of particulate bone grafts. The autogenous graft can begin full function at six weeks and earliest at four weeks if a rigid reconstruction plate is used. Such dental implants can osseo-integrate with the grafted bone rapidly and may be activated at three or four months. Subsequent pre-prosthetic procedures, such as skin graft vestibuloplasties, can be carried out. Dental implants may be placed at the time of maxillo-mandibular bone reconstruction or after their consolidation.

5. References

BOWEN-POPE, D.F., VOGEL, A. and ROSS, R. (1984). Production of platelet derived growth factor-like molecules reduced expression of platelet derived growth factor receptors accompany transformation by a wide spectrum of agents. *Proc. Natl. Acad. Sci. USA* **81**, 2396–2400.

HOWES, R., BOWNESS, J.M., GROTENDORST, G.R., MARTIN, G.R. and REDDI, A.H. (1988). Platelet-derived growth factor enhanced demineralized bone matrix-induced cartilage and bone formation. *Calcif. Tissue Int.* **42**, 34–38.

HOM, D.B. and MAISEL, R.H. (1992). Angiogenic growth factors: Their effects and potential in Soft tissue wound healing. *Ann. Otol. Rhinol. Laryngol.* **101**, 349–354.

HYUN, J.H., YIM, C.J., KIM, J.Y., KIM, J.K. and KIM, Y.K. (2000). The effect of PDGF on healing potential of the allogeneic demineralized freeze-dried bone transplanted in the calvarial defect of the rat. *Cell and Tissue Banking*, in press.

KANZLER, M.H., GORSULOWSKY, D.C. and SWANSON, N.A. (1986). Basic mechanism in the healing of cutaneous wound. *J. Dermatol. Surg. Oncol.* **12**, 1156–1164.

KIM, C.H. and YIM, C.J. (2000). Experimental study of PDGF's effect on healing response of the bovine xenograft mineral transplanted in the calvarial defect of the rat. *Proc. 4th Cong. Asian Assoc. Oral Maxillofac. Surg.*, Jeju, Korea.

KNIGHTON, D.R., FIEGEL, V.D. and DOUCETTE, M.M. (1990). Wound repair: The growth factor revolution. In: *Chronic Wound Care: A Clinical Source Book for Healthcare Professionals*, D. Krasner, ed., Health Management Publications, King of Prussin, PA.

LAWRENCE, W.T., SPORN, M.C., GORSCHBITH, C., NORTON, J.A. and GROTENDORST, G.R. (1986). The reversal of an Adriamycin induced healing impairment with chemoattractants and growth factors. *Ann. Surg.* **2**, 142–147.

LYNCH, S.E. (1991). Clinical and experimental approaches to dermal and epidermal repair: Normal and chronic wounds. In: *Interactions of Growth Factors in Tissue Repair*. Wiley-Liss Inc., New York, pp. 341–387.

LYNCH, S.E., COLVIN, R.B. and ANTONIADES, H.N. (1989). Growth factors in wound healing: single and synergistic effects on partial thickness porcine skin wounds. *J. Clin. Invest.* **84**, 640–646.

LYNCH, S.E., NIXON, J.C., COLVIN, R.B. and ANTONIADES, H.N. (1987). Role of platelet derived growth factor in wound healing: Synergistic effects with other growth factors. *Proc. Natl. Acad. Sci. USA* **84**, 7696–7700.

MARX, R.E. (1994). Clinical application of bone biology to mandibular and maxillary reconstruction. *Clin. Plast. Surg.* **21**, 377–392.

MARX, R.E., CARLSON, E.R., EICHSTAEDT, R.M., SCHIMMELE, S.R., STRAUSS, J.E. and GEORGEFF, K.R. (1998). Platelet-rich plasma, growth factor enhancement for bone grafts. *Oral Surg. Oral Med. Oral Pathol. Oral Radiol. Endod.* **85**, 638–646.

MOHAN, S. and BAYLINK, D.J. (1991). Bone growth factors. *Clin. Orthop. Rel. Res.* **263**, 30–43.

PIERCE, G.F., MUSTOE, T.A., LINGELBACH, J., MUSAKOWSKI, V.R., GRIFFIN, R.M. and DEUEL, T.F. (1989). Platelet derived growth factor and transforming growth factor-beta enhance tissue repair activities by unique mechanisms. *J. Cell Biol.* **109**, 429–440.

RAY, R.D. and HOLLOWAY, J.A. (1957). Bone implants. *J. Bone Joint Surg.* **39A**, 1119–1128.

REDDI, A.H. (1974). Bone matrix in the solid state: Geometric influence on differentiation of fibroblasts. In: *Advances in Biological and Medical Physics*, Vol. 15. J.H. Lawrence, J.W. Gofman and T.L. Hayes, eds., Academic Press, New York, pp. 1–18.

SERVOLD, S.A. (1991). Growth factor impact on wound healing. *Clin. in Pediatr. Med. Surg.* **8**, 937–953.

SINGH, J.P, CHAIKIN, M.A. and STILES, C.D. (1982). Phylogenetic analysis of platelet derived growth factor by radio-receptor assay. *J. Cell Biol.* **95**, 667–671.

STEENFOS, H.H. (1994). Growth factors and wound healing. *Scand. J. Plast. Reconstr. Hand Surg.* **28**, 95–105.

TAYAPONGSAK, P., O'BRIAN, D.A., MONTEIRO, C.B. and ARCEO-DIAZ, L.L. (1994). Autologous fibrin adhesive in mandibular reconstruction with particulate cancellous bone and marrow. *J. Oral Maxillofac. Surg.* **52**, 161–166.

YIM, C.J. (1999). Biology of demineralsed freeze-dried allogeneic bone powders and their clinical use. In: *Advances in Tissue Banking*, Vol. 3. G.O. Phillips, R, von Versen, D.M. Strong and A. Nather, eds., World Scientific, Singapore, pp. 87–111.

YIM, C.J. (2000). Mandibular reconstruction using bone allografts. In: *Advances in Tissue Banking*, Vol. 4. G.O. Phillips, R. von Versen, D.M. Strong and A. Nather, eds., World Scientific, Singapore, pp. 107–148.

Advances in Tissue Banking Vol. 5

27 BIOLOGY AND BIOMECHANICS OF ANTERIOR CRUCIATE LIGAMENT ALLOGRAFT RECONSTRUCTION

P. THIAGARAJAN and M. YEGAPPAN

Division of Adult Reconstructive Surgery
Department of Orthopaedic Surgery
National University Hospital
Lower Kent Ridge Road
Singapore 119074

1. Introduction

Various options for donor graft are available to reconstruct a torn anterior cruciate ligament (ACL). Several factors, however, need to be considered in graft selection for ACL reconstruction. These include initial graft tissue strength, graft fixation strength, morbidity related to tissue harvest and deficit, availability, associated problems and surgeon familiarity with a particular procedure. The surgeon must weigh the benefits and drawbacks of each graft before advising the patient on the appropriate selection of the graft material. There is little evidence to support the use of non-biologic grafts in the current literature.

There are essentially two types of biologic grafts available to the surgeon: autografts and allografts. Though the place of autograft reconstruction is well established, there are some concerns with the use of autografts for ACL reconstruction (Burks *et al.*, 1990; Ottero and Hutchenson, 1993; Shino *et al.*, 1993).

Patients with a pre-existing history of anterior knee pain and associated with severe chondral changes in the patella may not be ideal candidates for patellar tendon autograft. Previous surgery and trauma to the patellar or hamstring tendon may compromise the use of an autograft. The use of autograft is associated with some degree of morbidity and the patient may opt for an alternative graft. Particularly, in revision surgery or multiple ligament reconstructions, the availability of donor autografts may be limited. Hence, in such a situation an ACL reconstruction using an allograft tissue has been suggested (Shino *et al.*, 1984; Nikolaou *et al.*, 1986).

The available allograft tissues for ACL reconstruction include the patellar tendon, quadriceps tendon, hamstring tendons, the tendo-achilles, tibialis posterior tendon, flexor tendons of the foot and the hand, and also the fascia lata allografts. The potential for harvesting donor tissue for ACL reconstruction in a single donor is tremendous.

2. Allografts for ACL Reconstruction

Allograft tissue used for ACL reconstruction has advantages and disadvantages. The advantages include lack of donor site morbidity, availability of different types of allograft tissues for reconstruction and reduced operating time. Potential disadvantages that may be associated with allograft include potential disease transmission, long-term performance of the graft, possible delayed incorporation of the graft, immunological problems and availability.

Concerns with disease transmission, particularly viral diseases like human immunodeficiency virus (HIV) and hepatitis, is an important factor in the use of allograft tissue. Buck *et al.* (1989) calculated the risk of HIV disease transmission to be as high as 1 in 161 and as low as 1 in 1 667 600 if all of the currently available safeguards were employed (Buck *et al.*, 1989; 1990).

3. Preservation of Allograft Tissue

A concern for potential disease transmission has led to different processing methods for allograft tissue, some with profound undesirable effects in the human body. Ethylene oxide and gamma irradiation sterilisation had been advocated in the past to minimise bacterial and viral transmission. Ethylene-oxide-sterilised soft tissue allograft, however, has been associated with a high failure rate, and currently is no longer the preferred method of sterilisation due to its side effects (Jackson *et al.*, 1990; Roberts *et al.*, 1991).

In one study reported by Jackson *et al.* (1990), 6.4% of the 107 patients developed evidence of excessive inflammatory response in the form of lymphocyte and plasma cell infiltrates in the removed grafts. Prominent giant cell reaction, typical of a foreign body response was also observed. The authors also observed extensive widening of the femoral tunnel in one patient secondary to bone resorption.

The role of low-dose gamma irradiation remains controversial. It has been estimated that 36 kGy (3.6 Mrads) of radiation is required to inactivate the free HIV virus and possibly even a higher dosage for the cell-associated virus (Conway *et al.*, 1990). The effect of irradiation on the mechanical properties of soft tissue allograft is also of concern. Studies have shown that 30 kGy (3 Mrads) of irradiation can affect the mechanical properties substantially, hence caution must be advised against higher dosages (Gibbons *et al.*, 1991).

Deep-freezing is a widely accepted method of preserving allograft bone and soft tissue grafts. Experimental study in rats had revealed major histocompatibility antigens in the tendon cell components of allogenic tendons (Minami *et al.*, 1982). Treatment by freezing and thawing decreased the antigenicity more effectively than irradiation, glutaraldehyde or mitomycin C (Friedlaender, 1982; Minami *et al.*, 1982; Tomford *et al.*, 1983; Shino *et al.*, 1986; Jackson *et al.*, 1987; 1988).

A mechanical study on the properties of canine tendons revealed less changes in the tensile properties of tendons treated by irradiation followed by solvent preservation, than the reverse process, i.e. solvent preservation followed by irradiation (Maeda *et al.*, 1993).

The current trend seems to favour a deep-frozen allograft or a lyophilised graft without irradiation for a successful outcome of ACL reconstruction.

4. Animal Studies on ACL Reconstruction

In the literature, extensive studies have been performed to elucidate the course of events following anterior cruciate replacement, using both autografts and allografts in dogs, monkeys, rabbits, goats and sheep. Vascularity, immunology, biomechanical strength, remodelling and viability of the transplanted graft have been studied (Nikolaou *et al.*, 1986; Vasseur *et al.*, 1987; Shino *et al.*, 1988).

The allograft tissue used for the reconstruction of the ACL undergoes a complex remodelling process which has been traditionally divided into four phases: (i) avascular necrosis, (ii) revascularisation, (iii) cellular reproliferation, and (iv) remodelling (Clancy *et al.*, 1981; Arnoczky *et al.*, 1982). This process apparently takes approximately one year in a canine patellar tendon autograft reconstruction model (Arnoczky *et al.*, 1982). Vascular ingrowth begins at approximately two weeks and continues for a year (Malinin, 1993). The process of ligamentisation of the allograft occurs similarly to the autograft reconstructions, but at a slower pace. Studies have documented complete replacement of the allograft tissue with living normal tendon (Vasseur *et al.*, 1987).

Experimental ligament reconstruction in a canine model, using fresh-frozen patellar tendon allografts, revealed complete revascularisation of the transplanted graft by six months. The antero-distal portion of the graft was noted to be hypervascular, suggesting the importance of the infrapatellar fat pad as source of blood supply. A hypovascular area was noted in the mid-portion of the graft at 52 weeks. The graft was noted to be covered by a synovial membrane at three weeks following transplantation without any evidence of immunological reaction. Mesenchymal cell proliferation was evident by six weeks and the graft was completely covered by synovial membrane at 30 weeks. Histological findings similar to a normal ACL were evident at the end of one year following transplantation. The mechanical strength of the reconstructed grafts was insufficient at 30 and 52 weeks, though there was no significant difference between the allograft and autograft reconstructions.

Arnoczky *et al.* (1982) have shown that by four months, fresh-frozen allografts, in a dog model, were completely revascularised and at 12 months, the allograft tendon resembled a normal ACL histologically. Comparing autograft and allograft anterior cruciate ligament reconstructions at six months, in a goat model, Jackson *et al.* (1993) reported that autografts demonstrated a smaller increase in antero-posterior displacement. The values of maximum force to failure were two times greater in the autograft reconstructions and they also demonstrated a significant increase in cross-sectional area, an increase in density and the number of smaller diameter collagen fibrils compared to the allografts.

5. Biomechanics of Allograft Tissue Used for ACL Reconstruction

The structural and biomechanical properties of various autologous tissues used for ACL reconstruction had been investigated by Noyes *et al.* (1984). Studies have noted that it is preferable to implant grafts with greater stiffness and ultimate load than those of the native tissue to compensate for the decrease in these parameters in the early post-operative period.

The central 14 mm of the patellar tendon not only had a higher ultimate load of 2900 N, but also a higher stiffness of 685 N/mm than the ACL. If these data are extrapolated for a 10 mm strip of patellar tendon, then the ultimate load would be around 2070 N. The semitendinosus and gracilis tendons had ultimate loads which are lower than the ACL (1216 N and 838 N, respectively) but their stiffness was similar to the ACL (186 N/mm and 171 N/mm, respectively). From these data, one could conclude that at the time of implantation, both the central one-third of the patellar tendon and the semitendinosus and gracilis tendons used in conjunction, have suitable structural properties as ACL substitutes. The implanted graft must theoretically approximate these numbers, as animal studies have shown that following maturation, the graft regains only 80% of its initial strength (Clancy *et al.*, 1981).

Several studies had reported a significant decrease in the mechanical properties of freeze-dried allografts when compared with frozen allografts (Butler *et al.*, 1987; Jackson *et al.*, 1988). This discrepancy has been attributed to the time allowed for allograft reconstitution (Jackson et al., 1988). It has been noted that reconstitution of freeze-dried patellar tendon and fascia lata allograft for two hours resulted in significant reduction in ultimate strength as compared with freeze-dried allograft reconstituted for 24 hours.

Butler *et al.* (1987) found a significant reduction in the mechanical strength of patellar tendon and fascia lata after freeze-drying and ethylene oxide sterilisation. Paulos *et al.* (1987) showed a significant reduction in the tensile strength of human tendons after freeze-drying and 30 kGy (3 Mrads) of gamma irradiation. Gibbons *et al.* (1991) noted a dose-dependent effect of gamma irradiation on the mechanical properties of frozen goat bone–patellar-tendon–bone allografts. The allografts were not significantly affected by 20 kGy (2 Mrads) of gamma irradiation but weakened significantly after 30 kGy (3 Mrads) of irradiation. Gamma irradiation reduces the tensile strength of fresh-frozen patellar tendons minimally but impairs the tensile strength of freeze-dried ones significantly.

The effect of the initial mechanical properties of ACL substitutes cannot be evaluated following implantation in the humans. Hence, the results have to be extrapolated from animal studies.

6. Clinical Outcome of Allograft ACL Reconstruction

Noyes and Barber-Westin (1996) reported the long-term outcome of allograft reconstruction of the ACL in patients with an acute rupture of the ligament. Their conclusion was that there was no significant decrease in antero-posterior displacement of the knee, patellofemoral crepitus, pain or jumping score, or the over-all knee rating over a period of an average of 56 months following implantation. Based on this study, favourable results can be expected from the use of allograft tissue for reconstruction of the ACL.

Similar results from fresh-frozen allograft tissue have been reported by Shino *et al.* (1986). In another long-term study of human allograft ACL reconstruction, Shino *et al.* (1990) reported that 94% of patients had either good or excellent outcome at 57 months following reconstruction of the ACL. The Lachman and pivot shift tests were negative in over 90% of cases. A prospective study (Indelicato *et al.*, 1990) comparing the outcome of allograft reconstruction using freeze-dried and fresh-frozen tendon allografts showed no significant statistical difference in the two groups, though there was a trend towards improved functional and subjective outcomes in the fresh-frozen allografts. Indelicato *et al.* (1992) reported the successful use of fresh-frozen non-irradiated patellar tendon allografts in knees with chronically deficient ACL, with greater than 90% of patients having excellent and good functional outcomes. The authors concluded that allograft reconstructions have a similar outcome compared with autograft reconstructions.

Studies on arthroscopic and histological remodelling of transplanted allografts in humans have demonstrated no change in the macroscopic appearance of the ACL allografts from 11 months post-operatively onwards, and that the grafts reached histological maturity within the first 18 months (Shino *et al.*, 1988). Second-look arthroscopic evaluation of the reconstructed allograft ACL, using doppler flowmetry and histological evaluation in humans, had shown that at six months, the grafts exhibited a higher blood flow than the grafts which were reconstructed 12 to 89 months previously. Histological studies revealed that these ACL grafts remodelled with time, and that they reached stability and maturity at 18 months following implantation. These results confirmed the concept of age-dependent remodelling of allografts and their longevity in the human knee joint.

The process of ligamentisation of allograft tissue seems to be less uniform and the process takes much longer as compared to autograft tissue (Jackson et al., 1993). In another study (Shino *et al.*, 1995), at 12 months following anterior cruciate ligament reconstruction using allograft tendon in humans, the allografts were noted to comprise predominantly small diameter collagen fibrils (30 to 80 nm), which resulted in a unimodal pattern in the collagen fibril profile. The number of large diameter fibrils (90 to 140 nm) within the allogeneic tendon grafts had decreased. This predominance of small diameter collagen fibrils persisted in most specimens older than 12 months. They also noted that the anterior cruciate ligament allografts had collagen profiles that did not resemble normal tendon grafts or normal anterior cruciate ligaments, even several years after surgery. The loss of large diameter fibrils in the allografts six months or older, and their less tight-packing of collagen fibrils could be one potential explanation for the dramatic reduction of tensile strength of ACL allografts observed in previous experimental studies.

Outcome data on patients who had an allograft ACL reconstruction continue to provide a significant impetus to the understanding of the complex biological remodelling process, which sometimes fails. The consensus seem to favour a success rate for allograft reconstructions that is at least similar to the outcome of autograft reconstruction in carefully selected patients.

7. Conclusion

The evolution of allograft ACL reconstructions has been extensively studied in the literature. Studies on anatomy, biomechanics, biology and clinical data have increased our understanding of the behaviour and performance of allograft tissue, both in animal- and patient-based studies. There is ample evidence in the literature to support the use of allograft tissue for ACL reconstruction. However, the extensive use of allografts cannot be universally recommended for all patients due to the concern of potential disease transmission and biological failures. In clinical situations, when an autograft tissue is not available for reconstruction, allograft provides an ideal alternative. Allograft reconstructions are ideal in revision surgery. Selective use of allograft in athletes is recommended in view of the duration of biological incorporation.

Though the morbidity of allograft ACL reconstruction is much less than that of autograft reconstructions, the biological incorporation of allograft tissue is slower. Hence, the post-operative rehabilitation must be modified in order for the patient to obtain the maximum benefit of such a reconstruction. At present, deep-frozen allografts have the best outcome in the long term, and non-irradiated grafts seem to have an edge over irradiated grafts, irrespective of dosage.

With the advent of newer preservation techniques, primary sterile harvesting without the need for secondary sterilisation and the use of biological growth factors, the outcome of allograft ACL reconstruction can be expected to match that of autograft reconstruction.

8. References

ARNOCZKY, S.P., TARVIN, G.B. and MARSHALL, J.L. (1982). Anterior cruciate ligament replacement using patellar tendon. An evaluation of graft revascularization in the dog. *J. Bone Joint Surg. [Am]* **64A**, 217–224.

BUCK, B.E., MALININ, T.I. and BROWN, M.D. (1989). Bone transplantation and human immunodeficiency virus. An estimate of risk of acquired immunodeficiency syndrome (AIDS). *Clin. Orthop.* **240**, 129–136.

BUCK, B.E., RESNICK, L., SHAH, S.M. and MALININ, T.I. (1990). Human immunodeficiency virus cultured from bone. Implications for transplantation. *Clin. Orthop.* **251**, 249–253.

BURKS, R.T., HAUT, R.C. and LANCASTER, R.L. (1990). Biomechanical and histological observations of the dog patellar tendon after removal of its central one-third. *Am. J. Sports Med.* **18**(2), 146–153.

BUTLER, D.L., NOTES, F.R., WALZ, K.A. and GIBBONS, M.J. (1987). Biomechanics of human knee ligament allograft treatment. *Trans. Orthop. Res. Soc.* **12**, 128.

CLANCY, W.G. JR., NARECHANIA, R.G., ROSENBERG, T.D., GMEINER, J.G., WISNEFSKE, D.D. and LANGE, T.A. (1981). Anterior and posterior cruciate ligament reconstruction in rhesus monkey. *J. Bone Joint Surg. [Am]* **63A**, 1270–1284.

CONWAY, B., TOMFORD, W.W., HIRSCH, M.S., SCHOOLEY, R.T. and NAMKIN, H.J. (1990). Effect of gamma irradiation on HIV-1 in a bone allograft model. *Trans. Orthop. Res. Soc.* **15**, 225.

FRIEDLAENDER, G.E. (1982). Bone banking. *J. Bone Joint Surg. [Am]* **64A**, 307–311.

GIBBONS, M.J., BUTLER, D.L., GROOD, E.S., BYLSKI-AUSTROW, D.I., LEVY, M.S. and NOYES, F.R. (1991). Effects of gamma irradiation on the initial mechanical and material properties of goat bone-patellar tendon-bone allografts. *J. Orthop. Res.* **9**(2), 209–218.

INDELICATO, P.A., BITTAR, E.S., PREVOT, T.J., WOODS, G.A., BRANCH, T.P. and HUEGEL, M. (1990). Clinical comparison of freeze-dried and fresh frozen patellar tendon allografts for anterior cruciate ligament reconstruction of the knee. *Am. J. Sports Med.* **18**(4), 335–342.

INDELICATO, P.A., LINTON, R.C. and HUEGEL, M. (1992). The results of fresh-frozen patellar tendon allografts for chronic anterior cruciate ligament deficiency of the knee. *Am. J. Sports Med.* **20**(2), 118–121.

JACKSON, D.W., GROOD, E.S., ARNOCZKY, S.P., BUTLER, D.L. and SIMON, T.M. (1987). Cruciate reconstruction using freeze-dried anterior cruciate ligament allograft and a ligament augmentation device (LAD). An experimental study in a goat model. *Am. J. Sports Med.* **15**(6), 528–538.

JACKSON, D.W., GROOD, E.S., GOLDSTEIN, J.D., ROSEN, M.A., KURZWEIL, P.R., CUMMINGS, J.F. and SIMON, T.M. (1993). A comparison of patellar tendon autograft and allograft used for anterior cruciate ligament reconstruction in the goat model. *Am. J. Sports Med.* **21**(2), 176–185.

JACKSON, D.W., GROOD, E.S., WILCOX, P., BUTLER, D.L., SIMON, T.M. and HOLDEN, J.P. (1988). The effects of processing techniques on the mechanical properties of bone-anterior cruciate ligament-bone allografts. An experimental study in goats. *Am. J. Sports Med.* **16**(2), 101–105.

JACKSON, D.W., WINDLER, G.E. and SIMON, T.M. (1990). Intraarticular reaction associated with the use of freeze-dried, ethylene oxide-sterilized bone-patellar tendon-bone allografts in the reconstruction of the anterior cruciate ligament. *Am. J. Sports Med.* **18**(1), 1–10.

LAMBERT, K.L. (1983). Vascularized patellar tendon graft with rigid internal fixation for anterior cruciate ligament insufficiency. *Clin. Orthop.* **172**, 85–89.

MAEDA, A., INOUE, M., SHINO, K., NAKATA, K., NAKAMURA, H., TANAK, M., SEGUCHI, Y. and ONO, K. (1993). Effects of solvent preservation with or without gamma irradiation on the material properties of canine tendon allografts. *J. Orthop. Res.* **11**(2), 181–189.

MALININ, T. (1993). Allografts for the reconstruction of the cruciate ligaments of the knee: procurement, sterilization and storage. *Sports Med. Arthrosc. Rev.* **1**, 31–41.

MINAMI, A., ISHII, S., OGINO, T., OIKAWA, T. and KOBAYASHI, H. (1982). Effect of the immunological antigenicity of the allogenic tendons on tendon grafting. *Hand* **14**(2), 111–119.

NIKOLAOU, P.K., SEABER, A.V., GLISSON, R.R., RIBBECK, B.M. and BASSETT, F.H. (1986). Anterior cruciate ligament allograft transplantation. Long-term function, histology, revascularization, and operative technique. *Am. J. Sports Med.* **14**(5), 348–360.

NOYES, F.R. and BARBER-WESTIN, S.D. (1996). Reconstruction of the anterior cruciate ligament with human allograft. Comparison of early and later results. *J. Bone Joint Surg. [Am]* **78A**, 524–537.

NOYES, F.R., BUTLER, D.L., GROOD, E.S., ZERNICKE, R.F. and HEFZY, M.S. (1984). Biomechanical analysis of human ligament grafts used in knee-ligament repairs and reconstructions. *J. Bone Joint Surg. [Am]* **66A**, 344–352.

OTTERO, A.L. and HUTCHENSON, L. (1993). A comparison of double semitendinosus/gracilis and central third patellar tendon autografts in arthroscopic anterior cruciate ligament reconstruction. *J. Arthroscopy* **9**, 143–148.

PAULOS, L.E., FRANCE, E.P., ROSENBERG, T.D., DREZ, D.J., ABBOTT, P.J., STRAIGHT, C.B., HAMMON, D.J. and ODEN, R.R. (1987). Comparative material properties of allograft tissues for ligament replacement: Effects of type, age, sterilization and preservation. *Trans. Orthop. Res. Soc.* **12**, 129.

ROBERTS, T.S., DREZ, D. JR., MCCARTHY, W. and PAINE, R. (1991). Anterior cruciate ligament reconstruction using freeze-dried, ethylene oxide-sterilized bone-patellar tendon-bone allografts. Two year results in thirty-six patients. *Am. J. Sports Med.* **19**(1), 35–41.

SHINO, K., INOUE, M., HORIBE, S., HAMADA, M. and ONO, K. (1990). Reconstruction of the anterior cruciate ligament using allogenic tendon. Long-term followup. *Am. J. Sports Med.* **18**(5), 457–465.

SHINO, K., INOUE, M., HORIBE, S., NAGANO, J. and ONO, K. (1988). Maturation of allograft tendons transplanted into the knee. An arthroscopic and histological study. *J. Bone Joint Surg. [Br]* **70B**, 556–560.

SHINO, K., KAWASAKI, T., HIROSE, H., GOTOH, I., INOUE, M. and ONO, K. (1984). Replacement of the anterior cruciate ligament by an allogenic tendon graft. An experimental study in the dog. *J. Bone Joint Surg. [Br]* **66B**, 672–681.

SHINO, K., KIMURA, T., HIROSE, H., INOUE, M. and ONO, K. (1986). Reconstruction of the anterior cruciate ligament by allogenic tendon graft. An operation for chronic ligamentous insufficiency. *J. Bone Joint Surg.* **68**(5), 739–746.

SHINO, K., NAKATA, K., HORIBE, S., INOUE, M. and NAGAKAWA, S. (1993). Quantitative evaluation after arthroscopic anterior cruciate ligament reconstruction. Allograft versus autograft. *Am. J. Sports Med.* **21**(4), 609–616.

SHINO, K., OAKES, B.W., HORIBE, S., NAKATA, K. and NAKAMURA, N. (1995). Collagen fibril population in human anterior cruciate ligament allografts. Electron microscopic analysis. *Am. J. Sports Med.* **23**(2), 203–208.

TOMFORD, W.W., DOPPELT, S.H., MANKIN, H.J. and FRIEDLAENDER, G.E. (1983). Bone bank procedures. *Clin. Orthop.* **174**, 15–21.

VASSEUR, P.B., RODRIGO, J.J., STEVENSON, S., CLARK, G. and SHARKEY, N. (1987). Replacement of the anterior cruciate ligament with a bone-ligament — Bone anterior cruciate ligament allograft in dogs. *Clin. Orthop.* **219**, 268–277.

SECTION VII:

BIOMECHANICS OF ALLOGRAFTS

Advances in Tissue Banking Vol. 5

28 SOME PRINCIPLES OF BIOMECHANICS — STRUCTURAL AND MATERIAL PROPERTIES

BARRY P. PEREIRA

Department of Orthopaedic Surgery
National University Hospital
Lower Kent Ridge Road
Singapore 119074

1. Introduction

Biomechanics can be broadly defined as the study of the mechanics of living tissue. It examines the forces acting upon and within the structures, the behaviour and the function of biological systems, by applying and integrating mechanical engineering principles.

The main differences when comparing any engineering material to a biological tissue are that unlike the former, the latter is able to adapt and respond to its environment with self-repairing potentials and the ability to alter its properties and architecture. This makes the study of the mechanical properties of biological tissues dynamic and more challenging.

For allograft, several questions are often raised concerning its mechanical properties. The more important ones are related to the understanding of failure and fracture mechanisms — How strong is the allograft to be used? How would the allograft behave in response to the external loading? Can the allograft withstand the loading conditions when incorporated with the host? What are its limitations? When will it fail? Can the event of failure or fracture be predicted? Can the risk of failure be reduced? Some of these questions can be addressed if we have some basic understanding of the mechanical design of the material or tissue, and if we can measure its mechanical behaviour and limits when it is loaded.

2. Biomechanics of Tissue

When an external force or moment is applied to any tissue, the initial response of that tissue is to resist this applied load. The tissue begins to deform when the internal resistance against the applied load is overcome. Examples include pulling on a ligament and it stretches, or pressing onto a cartilage tissue and it depresses in. Deformation of the tissue would continue if the load continues to increase. A point would be reached when the tissue would finally fail. This failure could be a complete tear or crack across the tissue at one instant (more catastrophic in nature), or it could be gradual and progressive.

At the microstructural level, the deformation involves the displacement of constituent atoms and molecules that are resisted by the interatomic bonds that hold the material together. The stronger the bonds, the greater will be the resistance and the lesser the degree of deformation. This resistance would depend on (a) how many bonds there are within a given tissue (the structural property), and (b) what these bonds are made up of and how they are arranged and organised in relation to the applied external load (the material property). For a given tissue, the structural properties are essentially dependent on the shape and size, while the material properties describe the behaviour that is dependent on the material's composition and organisation of its constituents. The material property is often constant, regardless of its geometry. For collagenous tissue, some other factors affect the material properties. These include the mineral/collagen ratio, the collagen fibre orientation and the percentage of water content.

The advantages of determining the material property are (a) ranking or comparing the behaviour of various materials and tissues to loading, and (b) predicting their limitations and failure in a given loading environment.

2.1. Basic loading conditions

In understanding the basic structural and material properties, one must consider the folloring basic indirect loading conditions — axial loading, shear, bending and torsion, or combinations of these (Fig. 1). Axial loading includes loading an object in either tension or compression, where deformation of the material is in the direction of the applied load, perpendicular to the surface area on which the load is applied. Shear is when the load is applied parallel to and across a surface area resulting in deformation in the plane of the surface area and in the direction of the applied load.

Most tendons and ligaments function to resist and transmit forces in tension, while cartilage usually function to resist a combination

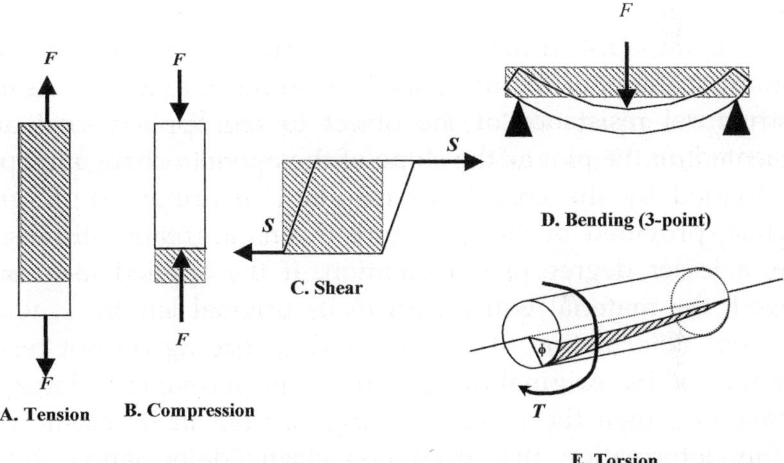

Fig. 1. Basic loading conditions. (A) Tension, (B) compression, (C) shear, (D) bending (3-point bending) and (E) torsion. The force applied to the object produces a certain amount of deformation. In the case of torsion, which is a twisting torque, this results in a rotation of the object about its long axis, where one cross-sectional end twists with respect to the other by an angle, ϕ.

of shear and compression. Bones, particularly long bones, experience a whole range of varied loading patterns. Apart from the more damaging direct loading patterns (e.g. tapping, penetration, crushing and impact loading), bones during various activities of daily living constantly undergo either tension, compression, shear, bending, torsion or combinations of all these.

3. Structural Behaviour — The Load-Displacement Curve

When a solid object of length, L, and uniform cross-sectional area, A, (width w and thickness t), is loaded in tension by a force, F, the object will deform (or stretch), increasing its length (Fig. 2A). The degree of deformation, x, can be recorded together with the amount of force applied to the object to produce this deformation. The plot between the applied force and resultant deformation is known as the force-deformation curve (Fig. 2B). This relationship can be described by the equation:

$$F = kx \tag{1}$$

where F is the applied load, x is the change in length, and k is the structural stiffness of the material. The structural stiffness describes the structural resistance of the object to the applied load and is represented on the plot as the slope of the curve (= change in applied load divided by the change in resultant deformation). A greater resistance provided by the structure means a greater stiffness and hence, a lesser degree of deformation. If the applied load is then removed, the material will return to its original length, L, with no permanent deformation. If loading and unloading do not result in a change in its original length (i.e. no permanent damage or deformation), then the object is being worked in its elastic region and the deformation that occurs is elastic deformation. Now, if the object is loaded beyond a critical load, where the bonds within the material cannot resist any further and break, some permanent deformation such as a micro-tear or crack will result. With a permanent deformation existing, the object is now working in the plastic region of the load-deformation curve. If the load is removed

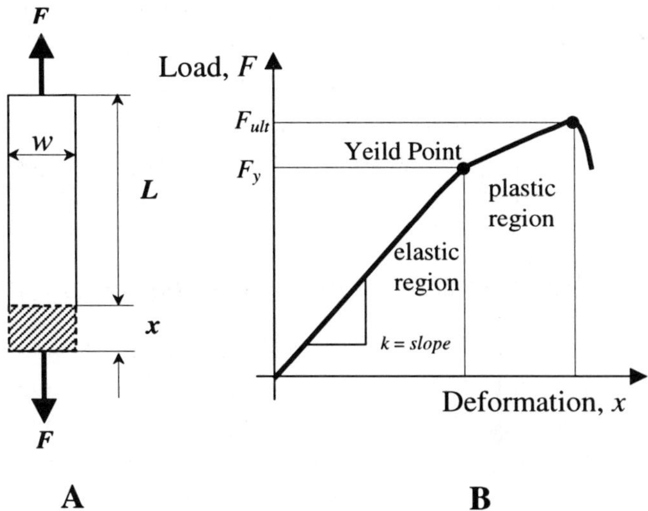

Fig. 2. Structural behaviour. (A) Specimen of length, L, width, w, and uniform thickness pulled in tension at a constant rate results in a deformation, x. (B) Plot of the load-deformation curve, k = slope of the curve (change in force divided by the change in the deformation) which defines the structural stiffness of the material, F_y = yield force, and F_{ult} = failure load.

this time, the object will not return to its original length. Plastic deformation would then have occurred. The object would still be functional thereafter when loaded, however, the elastic limits and stiffness may be altered as a consequence. An example would be a cortical screw that has been bent (a form of permanent deformation), yet able to function just as effectively, but perhaps with a weaker limit.

The point on the load-deformation plot, where increasing the load causes the change from elastic deformation to plastic deformation, is known as the yield point. The load recorded at this point is known as the yield load, F_y. The yield point divides the curve into an elastic region and a plastic region. If the material continues to be loaded after this yield point, with further deformation, a point will come when it will finally fail by snapping (or fracture). The load recorded when this happens is known as the ultimate (or failure) load, F_{ult}.

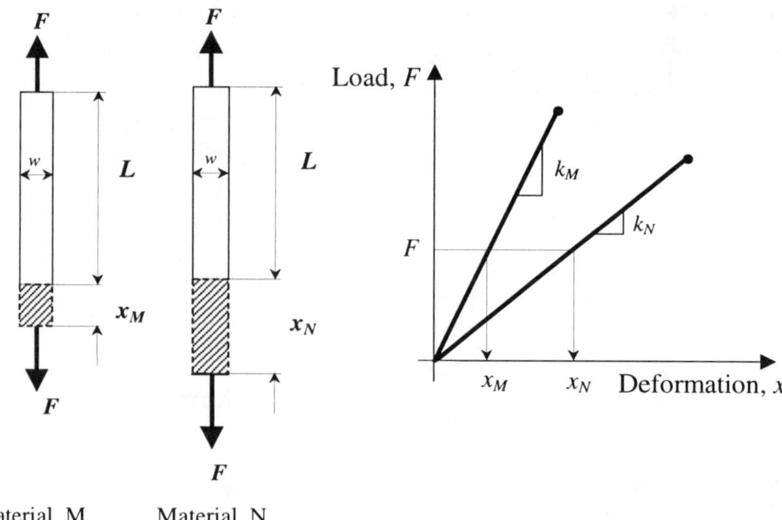

Fig. 3. Different materials, M and N, having the same initial length, L and cross-sectional area, A are pulled in tension by a force, F. (A) Material M is found to elongate by x_M and material N by x_N. (B) The load-deformation curve for both materials M and N show a difference in their slopes. The slope for material M is greater than material N. This would indicate that M is stiffer, and that M would deform less than N for the same given load.

With the load-displacment curve, different materials of the same length and cross-sectional area (width and thickness) can then be compared and ranked according to their structural stiffness (i.e. the slope of the curve) or their ultimate failure load. A material that is stiffer, i.e. having less deformation for the same load applied, would have a steeper load-deformation slope (Fig. 3) and a material with a higher ultimate load would be considered as stronger.

For a given material, the structural stiffness depends on the cross-sectional area and the length. This relationship for structural stiffness, k is given as

$$k \propto \frac{A}{L} \tag{2}$$

where A is the cross-sectional area of the object and L is the length of the object. Substituting this into Eq. (1), with some rearrangement, gives us the relationship for deformation x

$$x \propto \frac{F \cdot L}{A} \tag{3}$$

This relationship shows that the degree of deformation is directly proportional to the applied load, F, the original length of the material, L, and is inversely proportional to the cross-sectional area, A.

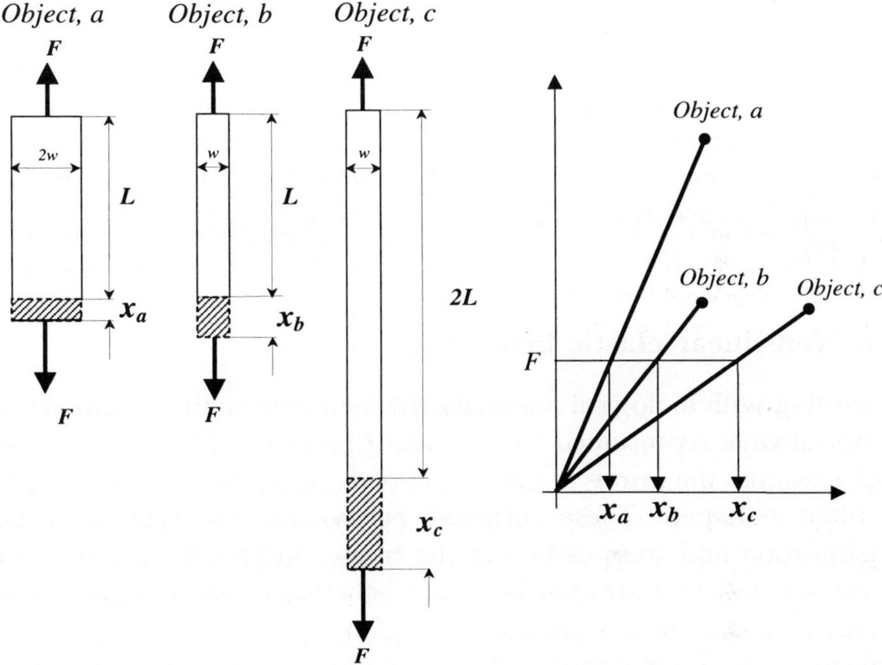

Fig. 4. Three objects a, b, c of the same material but of different lengths and cross-sectional areas. Objects b and c have the same cross-sectional area but object c is twice as long as b. Objects a and b have the same length but object a has twice the cross-section of b. The load-deformation curve shows that with longer specimens of the same material, the structural stiffness is reduced and hence more deformation results. On the other hand, with greater cross-sectional area, the material is stiffer and less deformation results.

For different materials, the above two equations would be given as

$$k = \frac{A}{L} \cdot E \tag{2a}$$

$$x = \frac{F \cdot L}{A} \cdot \frac{1}{E} \tag{3a}$$

where E is a material factor (or material property which will be subsequently defined as the elastic modulus of the material). The units for stiffness k are lb/in (pounds per inch) and N/mm (newtons per millimetre). (1 lb/in = 0.1752 N/mm; 0.001 N/mm = 1 N/m.)

Illustrating this with an example (Fig. 4) for a given applied load, F, an object that is comparatively longer will have a greater degree of deformation (referring to Eq. (3)) because its resistance (i.e. its structural stiffness) to the applied load is lower (Eq. (2)). Similarly, an object that has a larger cross-section would have less deformation (Eq. (3)) because the stiffness of that material would be greater (Eq. (2)).

3.1. Non-linear elastic behaviour

In dealing with biological materials, the load-deformation relationship is not always represented by a straight line (Fig. 5). For ligaments and tendons, the curve is often j-shaped, while for cortical bone it is often r-shaped. These different behaviours are typical of the organisation and composition of the tissue. Although they are non-linear (i.e. not in a straight line), the behaviours are still said to be elastic as the materials are able to regain their original length after unloading, without permanent deformation. Hence, these materials are often said to be non-linear elastic materials.

For ligaments and tendons, this non-linear behaviour can be explained by studying the arrangement of the collagen fibres and ground substance. At a relatively low applied load, the minimal resistance offered by the tissue is due to an initial uncrimping of the wave-like collagen fibres and the breaking of the loose bonds in the

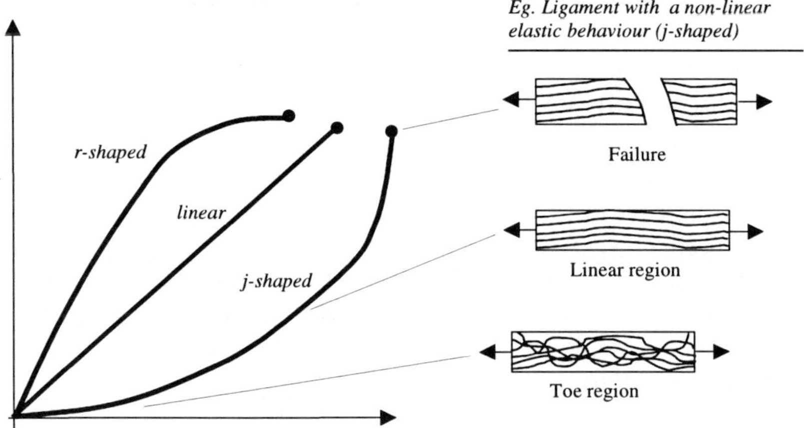

Fig. 5. Load-deformation curves of non-linear elastic materials.

ground substance that bind the collagen together. The tissue appears to stretch easily. When the fibres start to align to the increasing applied load, more fibres are recruited and aligned progressively, increasing the internal resistance of the material with increasing loads. This characterises the j-shaped curve from a low to a high stiffness with increasing loads. Cortical bone, on the other hand, is composed of collagen fibres that are bonded at their tips by very strong hydroxyapatite crystals. These minerals (crystals) give the cortical bone its strength and stiffness. Once these strong bonds are broken, the resistance to deformation and failure is then dependent on the collagen fibres itself. Hence, the noted change in its stiffness from a very steep slope to a gentler slope (r-shaped curve).

The work performed or the energy expended into deforming the object is equal to the applied load multiplied by the degree of deformation. Since the degree of deformation changes with the applied load, the total work done can be mathematically integrated from the load-displacement curve. This is represented by the area under the load-displacement curve for the given degree of displacement. The units used for work are ft-lb (foot-pound), N-mm (newton-millimetre) and J (joules). (1 ft-lb × 1.356 = 1 J; 1 J = 1 N-m = 1000 N-mm.)

3.2. Compression

In the case of compression, the analysis is similar to tension except that the deformation is a reduction or shortening in length (or height). Apart from bones, an obvious example of tissue that deforms in compression would be cartilage. The load-deformation curves will not be any different from those seen in tension. However, by convention, the compressive stresses are taken to be negative and the tensile stresses positive.

3.3. Poisson's ratio

So far, it has been assumed that for an object that is loaded axially, deformation only takes place along the direction of the applied load. In tension, the tissue lengthens and in compression, it shortens. However, in trying to retain its volume, a material that is axially loaded would also deform laterally to the applied load (Fig. 6). For example, if a thick rubber band is pulled in tension, it would not

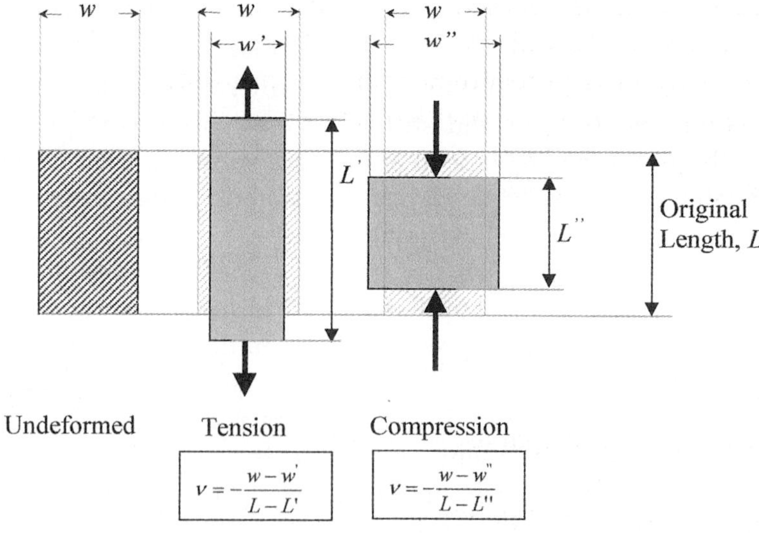

$$v = -\frac{w - w'}{L - L'}$$

$$v = -\frac{w - w''}{L - L''}$$

Fig. 6. Possion's ratio in uniaxially loaded specimen.

only increase in length, but would also be seen to have a reduction in its width as it tries to retain the volume of the material. Similarly, if you press your finger down on a soft sponge, it would not only depress downwards but would also bulge out sideways. For the case of uniaxial loading, this lateral deformation or strain is simply related to the amount of axial strain as the material is trying to maintain its volume. This relationship is described by the Poisson's ratio, υ, and given as

$$\upsilon = -\frac{\text{lateral strain}}{\text{axial strain}} \qquad (4)$$

This ratio differs for different materials and it gives a value as to how much lateral deformation that can occur when a material is loaded in a uniaxial direction.

4. Material Behaviour — Stress–Strain Curve

To remove the influence of shape and size on the mechanical property of an object, the force applied and the measured deformation should be normalised to its geometry. We will use the same example of an object of length, L, and cross-sectional area, A (Fig. 7A). When a force, F, is applied perpendicular to the cross-sectional area, A, the material tries to resist the applied force. The internal force intensity, or the resistance per unit of the cross-sectional area to the applied force is defined as stress (σ), which is simply given as

$$\text{Stress, } \sigma = \frac{F}{A} \qquad (5)$$

The units for stress are newtons/square metre (N/m^2) or pascal (Pa). [1 lb = 4.448 N; 1 pounds per square inch (psi) $\times$ 6.895 $\times 10^3$ = 1 N/m^2 = 1 Pa, 1 megapascal (MPa) = 1×10^6 Pa and 1 gigapascal (GPa) = 1×10^9 Pa].

The ratio of the elongation, x, to its original length, L, is defined as the strain, ε.

$$\text{Strain } \varepsilon = \frac{x}{L} \tag{6}$$

Note that strain does not have any units.

Thus, from the structural properties of load against displacement curve, which is dependent on the length and cross-sectional area, we can now have a normalised relationship which is independent of geometry from the stress-strain curve (Fig. 7B). Comparing the two plots, the yield load from the load-displacement curve now becomes the yield strength ($\sigma_y = F_y/A$) of the stress-strain curve; and the ultimate load becomes the ultimate strength ($\sigma_{ult} = F_{ult}/A$). The structural stiffness becomes the material stiffness, which is also

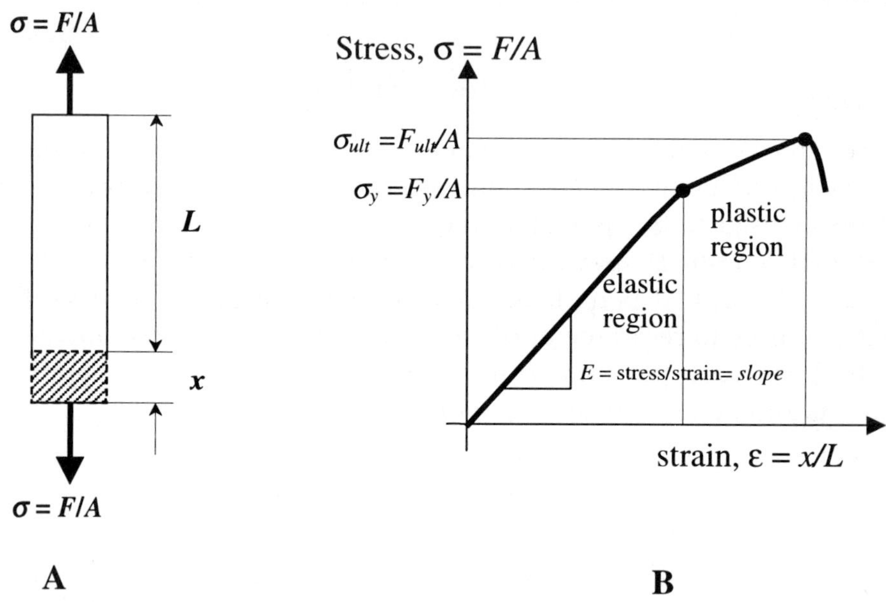

Fig. 7. Material behaviour. (A) Specimen of length, L, width, w and uniform thickness pulled in tension at a constant rate results in a deformation, x. (B) Plot of the stress-strain curve with the effect of geometry eliminated. The slope of the elastic region describes the elastic modulus of the material, E. σ = stress, ε = strain, σ_y = yield strength, σ_{ult} = ultimate strength.

known as the elastic modulus of the material, ($E = \sigma/\varepsilon$), and is the slope of the stress-strain curve in the elastic region only. This now allows us to compare and rank different materials regardless of shape and size.

The units used for the elastic modulus are lb/in^2 (pound per square inch), MPa or GPa, same as for normal stress, because strain is non-dimensional.

5. Elastic Strain Energy

When a material is loaded, a certain amount of energy is absorbed and stored due to the strain developed by the material. Within the elastic limits, this stored energy allows the material to recover to its original length after unloading. This energy is known as the elastic strain energy per unit volume, U, and can be represented by the area under the stress-strain curve (Fig. 8A).

This is a critical limit in determining the material's ability to resist fractures. The shape of the stress-strain curve (Fig. 8B) will give an indication of the type of facture that is expected of the material. If the slope of the curve is steep with a very small area under the curve, then failure would be abrupt with little plastic deformation. This type of material would be termed brittle (e.g. glass). Such materials will break, fracture or tear without absorbing much strain energy. If the area under the curve is large, with greater plastic deformation, then the material would be considered ductile, as there will be a greater degree of deformation before failure. These materials are able to absorb a lot of strain energy (as demonstrated by the large area under the stress-strain curve) and are considered tough. One way of observing the difference between the two types of material is that in a brittle fracture, the two fractured ends would normally be able to fit perfectly back together. In a ductile fracture, the two fracture ends would usually not be able to fit back perfectly, due to the plastic deformation that has occurred.

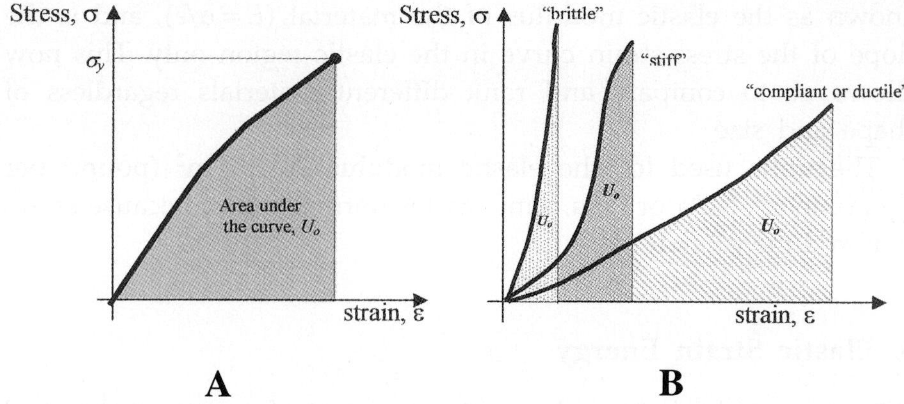

Fig. 8. (A) Fracture energy — area under the stress strain curve, Uo. (B) The area under the curve describes the material's toughness. The steep slope before fracture would suggest a brittle material with little plastic deformation, while a gradual slope with a large area under the curve would suggest a more compliant or ductile material. Ductile materials would fail with plastic deformation before complete failure occurs.

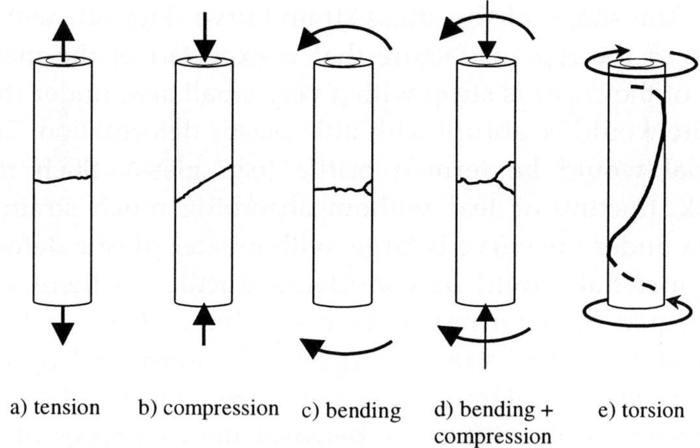

Fig. 9. Generalised mechanism of common long bone fractures. (a) In tension — tranverse fracture (e.g. some transverse patella fractures), (b) compression — oblique fracture (e.g. oblique fracture of the distal femur/humerus), (c) bending — transverse fractures with small butterfly fragment (e.g. transverse shaft fractures), (d) bending and axial compression — transverse fractures with large butterfly fragment, and (e) torsion — spiral fractures (e.g. spiral fractures of the tibia/humerus).

6. Long Bones

In the case of long bones, the loading profile may not simply be a case of tension, compression or shear. The other loading profiles include bending, torsion or combinations of all these patterns. Different loading directions would result in different types of fractures (Fig. 9).

7. Bending — Area Moment of Inertia

In determining the behaviour and response of an object to bending, several standard modes of bending are used. The more common ones are three-point bending, four-point bending and cantilevel bending (Fig. 10).

Taking the example of a cantilever beam (Fig. 11A) that is rigidly supported (or fixed) at one end, and applying a load perpendicular to the beam at its free end, the beam would tend to bend in the direction of the applied load. The maximum deflection would be at the point of the applied load (Fig. 11B). This results in the upper

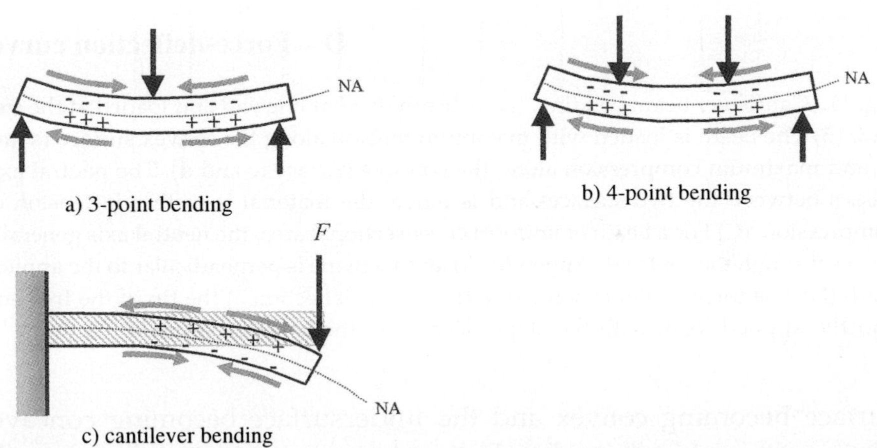

Fig. 10. Modes of bending. (A) 3-point bending, (B) 4-point bending and (C) cantilever beam bending. The concave side of the beam is in tension (+++) and the convex side in compression (−−−−).

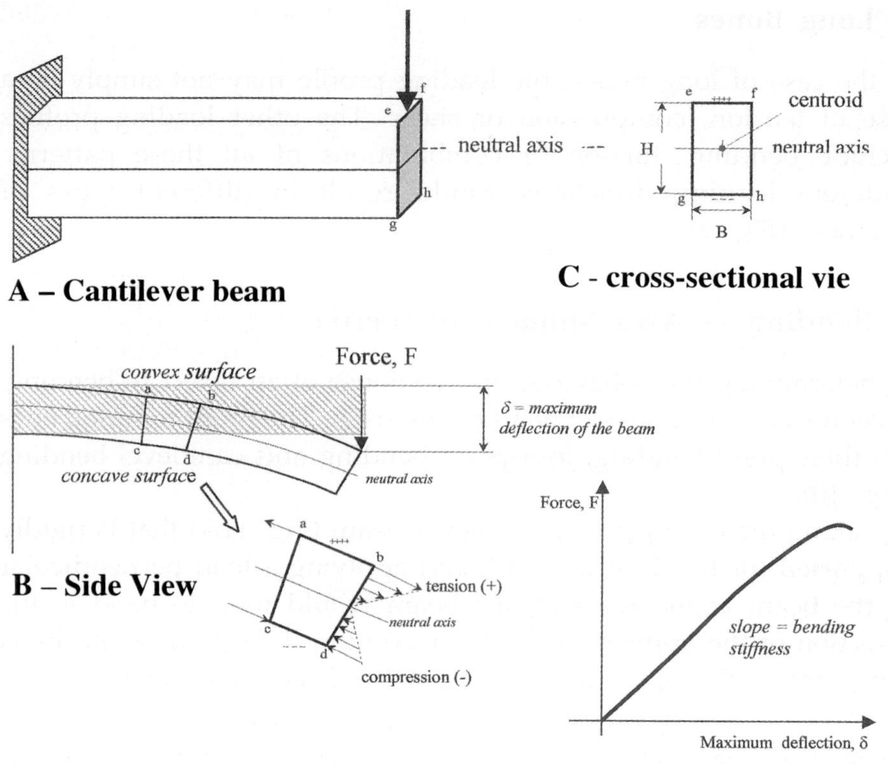

Fig. 11. Cantilever beam bending. (A) A beam fixed at one end and loaded at the free end. (B) The beam is loaded with maximum tension along the convex surface (a and b) and maximum compression along the concave surface (c and d). The neutral axis passes between the two surfaces and is where the material is neither in tension or compression. (C) For a beam of uniform cross-sectional area, the neutral axis generally passes through the centroid (Appendix A) and its plane is perpendicular to the applied load. (D) The force — deflection curve traces the deflection at the tip of the free end and the applied load, with the slope describing the bending stiffness.

surface becoming convex and the undersurface becoming concave. The upper surface is said to be in tension as it is stretched (tensile strain) downwards along with the applied load, while the lower concaved surface is in compression (compressive strain) as it is pushed inwards towards the rigidly supported end. The maximum strain occurs at these surfaces. At a level between the convex and concave surfaces, moving into the material, there would be a plane that would neither be in compression or tension (Fig. 11B), with no deformation occurring. This plane is known as the neutral axis (NA). For most cross-sections, the neutral axis would usually pass through the centroid of the beam's cross-section and would be perpendicular to the applied load (Fig. 11C).

The load-deformation diagram in this case is based on the applied load and the degree of deflection of the beam at the point of loading. This would be the maximum deflection, δ, for the case of a cantilever beam. The slope of the curve gives a representation of the bending stiffness or the flexural modulus (Fig. 11D).

An important geometric parameter that affects the stiffness of the material is the area moment of inertia. The area moment of inertia, I, is a mathematical representation of the distribution of area of a given cross-section about the neutral axis through the object. Specific formulae are derived for specific cross-sectional shapes (see Appendix A). The units used for I are in^4 (inches to the power of four) and mm^4 (millimetres to the power of four).

Generally, the greater the area moment of inertia, or in the physical sense, the greater the area that is distributed away from the neutral axis, the stiffer will be the material. We will consider two rectangular beams made from the same material, both with equal cross-sectional areas, but with different area moments of inertia because of the different heights and widths (Fig. 12). If a bending moment is applied to both beams, the one with the larger I would have a lesser degree of deflection, as it would be stiffer. A more generalised relationship for structural bending stiffness to its geometry, which simply defines the resistance of an object to an applied bending moment, would be:

$$\text{bending stiffness} \propto \frac{EI}{L^3} \tag{7}$$

where E is the elastic modulus, I is the area moment of inertia and L is the length of the beam. The relationship shows that the bending stiffness increases with I and E, and decreases with the L. The unit used for bending stiffness is N-mm (newton-millimetre).

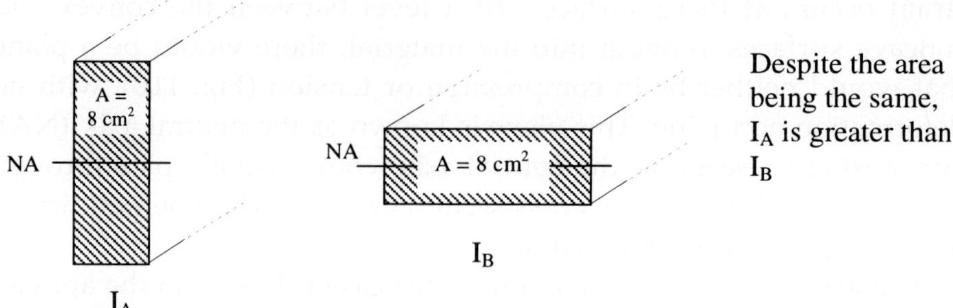

Fig. 12. The area moment of inertia of a beam affects the bending stiffness of the stucture. It describes the distribution of area about the neutral axis. The greater the area is distributed away from the neutral axis, the greater is the area moment of inertia. For a rectangular cross-section, it depends on the base and the third power of the height (Appendix A).

8. Torsion — Polar Moment of Inertia

Long bones are also subjected to twisting loads about their long axes. With an applied torque about the long axis of a long bone, the object, as before, will try to resist the external load. The resultant deformation is a twisting of the material about the axis of rotation (Fig. 13A). The degree of deformation is measured from the total angle of twist (angular deformation) of one end of the beam about the axis of rotation, with respect to the other end. The relationship of the angular deformation to its geometry, material properties and the applied torque is given as

$$\phi = \frac{T \cdot l}{G \cdot J} \tag{8}$$

where the angle of twist, ϕ, is in radians (2π radians $= 360°$), T is the applied torque (in Newton-metres), l is the length of the bar (in metres), G is the shear modulus (in N/m^2) and J is the polar moment of inertia.

The shear modulus, G, is a material property that describes the material resistance to shearing deformations and is analogous to the

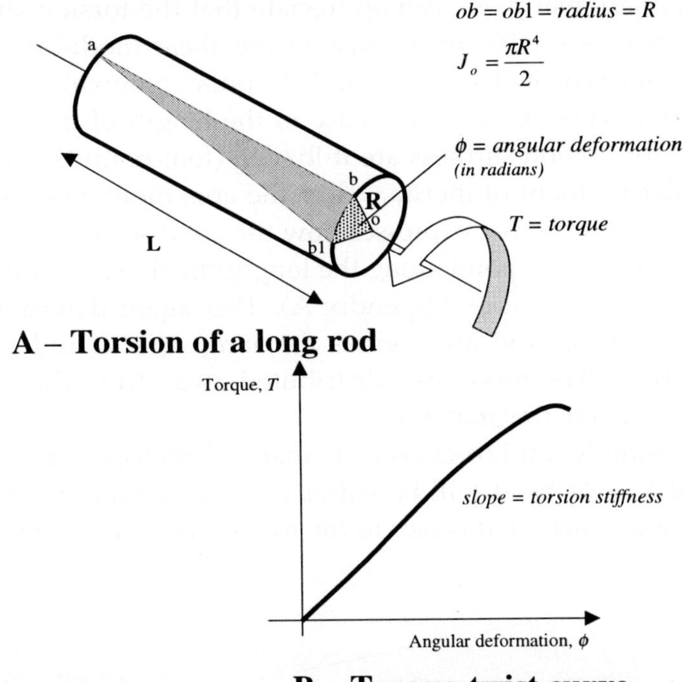

A – Torsion of a long rod

B – Torque-twist curve

Fig. 13. (A) A rod of radius, R, and length, L, in torsion would twist about the axis that the torque, T, is applied. The deformation is measured by the angular change of one end to the other (ob — ob1). (B) The torque-twist curves trace the angular deformation, ϕ, to the applied torque, T, with the slope describing the torsion stiffness of the rod.

elastic modulus, E. For most materials, the shear modulus is about ½ the elastic modulus (i.e. $G \approx$ ½ E).

From the torque-twist curve (Fig. 13B), the torsion stiffness can be determined from the slope of the plotted curve. The torsion stiffness describes the structural ability to resist deformation by twisting when a torque is applied. This is dependent on its geometry and the material properties and is given by the relationship,

$$\text{Torsion stiffness} = \frac{G \cdot J}{l} \tag{9}$$

From this relationship, we can appreciate that the torsion stiffness of an object increases with an increase in the shear modulus, *G*, of the material from which it is made and its polar moment of inertia, *J*. The stiffness decreases with increase in the length of the rod, *l*. The units used for torsion stiffness are ft-lb/deg (foot-pounds per degree).

The polar moment of inertia, *J*, like the area moment of inertia, is a mathematical term that expresses how the cross-section of a material is distributed about a point along the longitudinal axis that the torque is applied (Fig. 13B) (see Appendix A). This again determines how the distribution of the area about the long axis would resist the applied torque. The more area distributed away from the long axis, the stiffer will be the material.

As an example, an object with its material distributed away from the central axis of twist will be stiffer in torsion than an object with the same area distributed closer to the longitudinal axis (Fig. 14). The

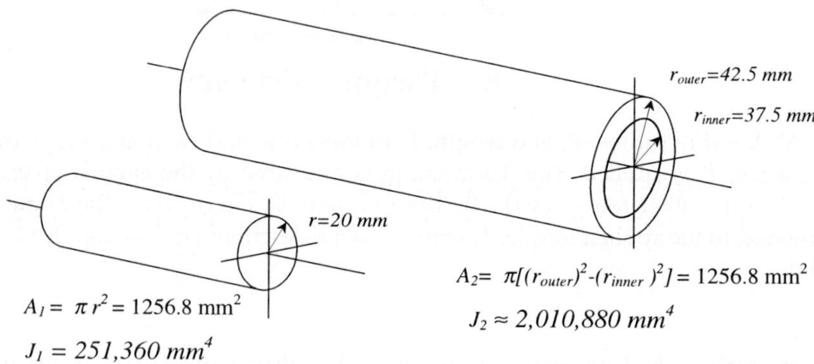

Between a solid rod and a hollow rod of equal cross-sectional area, the hollow rod has its area distributed further away (increase in outer radius by about 2 times) from the central longitudinal axis. This would give a greater torsion stiffness (by 8 times more) than the solid rod.

Fig. 14. The polar moment of inertia affects the structural resistance to torsion. The greater the polar moment of inertia, the greater the stiffness. We compare a solid rod and a hollow rod, both of equal cross-sectional area and length. The hollow rod would have a greater polar moment of inertia as more area is distributed away from the longitudinal axis. An increase in the outer diameter by two times results in a polar moment of inertia increase of eight times.

units used for polar moment of inertia, J, are in^4 (inches to the power of four) and mm^4 (millimetres to the power of four).

9. Viscoelastic Behaviour

So far, deformation of tissue was considered in a very static-loaded condition. This has also been independent of how fast the load is applied and how fast these materials respond to the load.

Tendons, ligaments and cartilage are materials that have a complex interaction between collagen, ground substance and water. The collagen would behave with a purely elastic response to the applied load as discussed previously. But to the ground substance and water, it would tend to resist the applied load in a way of retarding the strain on the collagen, similar to that of a damping system. This viscous behaviour will depend on the rate of the applied load and will also affect the rate at which the material deforms (the strain rate). This viscous behaviour is said to be rate-dependent, or time-dependent. An example is like trying to move your hand through water. The faster you try to move your hand through it, the greater would be the resistance (i.e. more viscous).

Materials that have both elastic and viscous elements are known as viscoelastic materials. Tissues are composite materials. Most of the times a simple understanding of the relationship of rate of loading (or strain rate) and stiffness is that, for viscoelastic materials, increasing the strain rate results in a stiffer response from the material. A slow loading rate on a viscoelastic material results in both the elastic and the viscous elements being deformed. The slow rate allows the viscous component to respond in tandem. For faster loading rates, the viscous element may not be able to respond just as fast, and hence, it creates a resistance. The outcome is a reduction of the degree of deformation, making the material appear stiffer. A greater discussion can be seen in the texts recommended at the end of this chapter.

9.1. Hysteresis in loading patterns

For a purely elastic material, the loading and unloading curves are

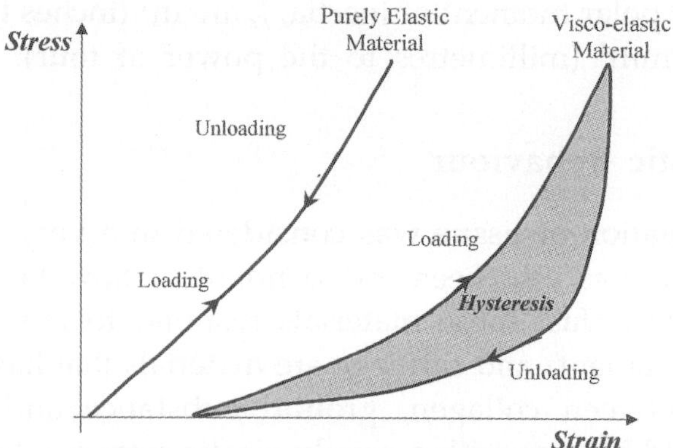

Fig. 15. The stress-strain curve for a non-linear viscoelastic material. Due to the presence of a viscous element that creates a resistance to loading, and is affected by the rate of loading, energy gone into working against this viscous resistance is lost when the material is unloaded. A hysteresis in the curve is observed when the energy recovered in unloading is less than the energy put in during loading. In a purely elastic material with no viscous component, the energy put into loading is equal to the strain energy recovered during unloading.

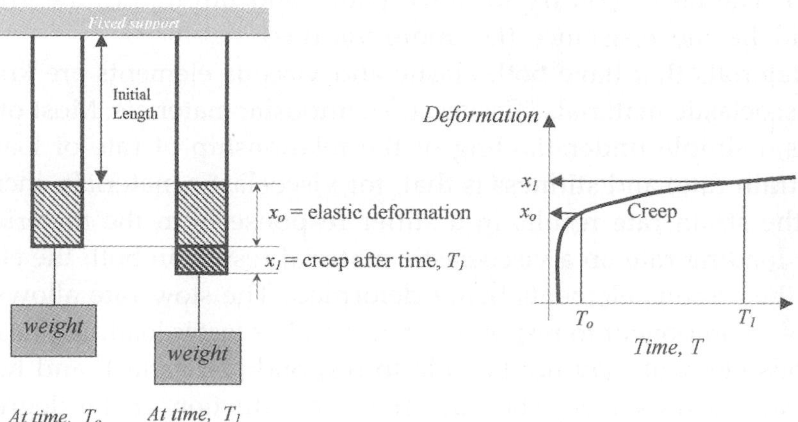

Fig. 16. Creep behaviour. A viscoelastic material that is initially loaded with a fixed load stretches by x_0. As initial load is resisted by a viscous element, some slow unloading of the material occurs. Since the load is fixed, the unloading amounts to additional stretching of the material until it finds a level where the viscous effect has been overcome. The rate at which the object is loaded has an effect on the amount of creep that occurs.

the same, as at most times, the energy loss is minimal (Fig. 17). The work put in to deform the material is fully recovered when the material unloads back to its original length. If we consider a viscoelastic material or structure, the loading and unloading patterns differ and result in a hysteresis loop (Fig. 15). This is because the work that goes into loading the viscous element is lost during the unloading. Hence, less energy is recovered. The amount of energy loss is also affected by the rate of loading, with more energy dissipated at higher loading rates. For collagenous tissues like tendon and ligaments, the energy lost (or dissipated) is fairly low (5–10%) making them very good elastic energy-storing elements in the limbs.

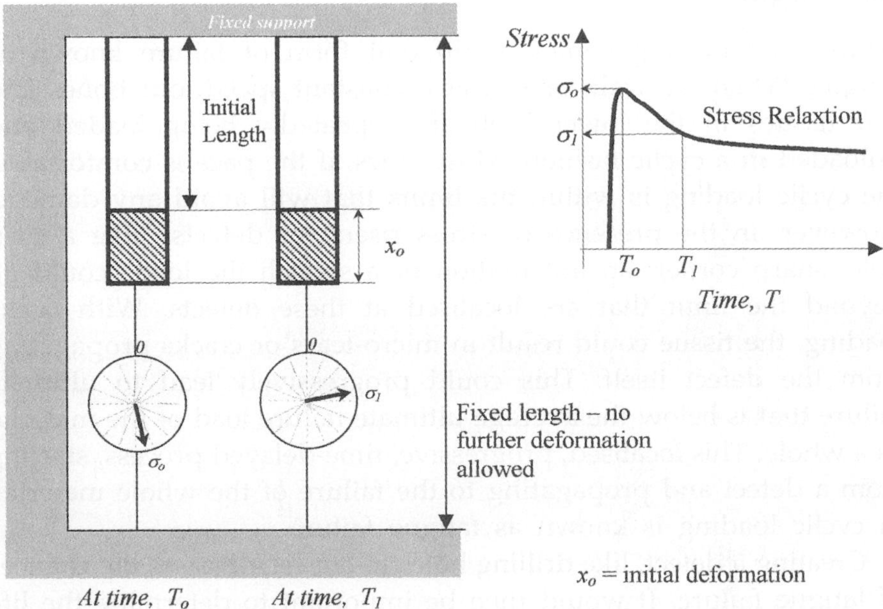

Fig. 17. Stress relaxation behaviour. A viscoelastic specimen that is initially stretched in tension by x_0 and then fixed in that position, would initially register a stress of σ_0. The initial work is resisted by an elastic and a viscous element. With time, a certain degree of unloading occurs, as the viscous element will have a time-delayed response and finally not contribute to any internal resistance, and as the length is fixed. This unloading is seen as a relaxation of the stress contributed by the elastic element only, resulting in a reduction in the stress to σ_1 as seen in the diagram.

Less stiff connective tissues like cartilage and skin, however, have considerable viscoelasticity with greater energy loss.

9.2. Creep and stress relaxation

Related to viscoelasticity are two physical behaviours — creep and stress relaxation. Creep is said to occur when a viscoelastic material that is subjected to a constant load continues to stretch over time (Fig. 16). Stress relaxation is a reduction in the internal resistance (stress) over time when a viscoelastic material is stretched and fixed in length without further deformation (Fig. 17).

10. Fatigue

With cyclic loading comes a different form of failure known as fatigue. When we walk or run at a constant speed, our bones and soft tissues in the lower limb are repeatedly being loaded and unloaded in a cyclic fashion. Most times, if the pace is comfortable, the cyclic loading is within the limits that will avoid any damage. However, in the presence of stress risers (or defects), like a scar, hole, sharp corner, an indentation or a scratch the loads could go beyond the limit that are localised at these defects. With cyclic loading, the tissue could result in micro-tears or cracks propagating from the defect itself. This could progressively lead to ultimate failure that is below the average ultimate failure load of the material as a whole. This localised, progressive, time-delayed process, starting from a defect and propagating to the failure of the whole material, in cyclic loading is known as fatigue failure.

Creating a defect, like drilling holes in bones, increases the chances of fatigue failure. It would then be important to determine the life span of the material in the presence of such defects. For this, experiments are usually carried out to test various samples of a material, each at different stress levels in cyclic loading (loading and unloading) until the material fails. The number of cycles to failure is then recorded for each of the stress levels, and both the stress level and the number of cycles to failure are plotted on a so-called S-N curve (stress versus number of cycles) (Fig. 18).

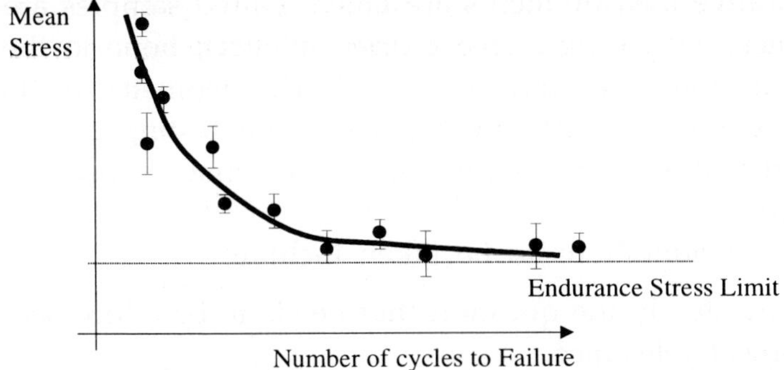

Fig. 18. The mean stress versus number of cycles to failure (S-N curve). The curve is plotted from several samples tested cyclically to various pre-determined stress levels and the number of cycles recorded when the specimen failed. An endurance limit is at a level of stress where the specimen can resist an infinite number of cycles without failure.

The S-N curve gives information about the number of cycles a aterial can withstand for a given stress level. A material would generally have a shorter cyclic life at higher stress. If the material works at a lower stress level, the number of cycles is greater, meaning a longer life span or fatigue life. Most materials have an endurance limit or fatigue limit, which is the stress level at which it can endure an infinite number of cycles without failure. This is seen on the S-N curve as its plateau. Typically, it would be better to allow the material to be loaded closer to the level of the endurance limit to increase the life of the material to cyclic loading. An introduction of a defect changes the endurance limit, thus changing the fatigue life.

11. Some Basic Guides to Conducting Experiments to Test Tissues for Their Mechanical Properties

When testing tissues or allografts for their structural and material properties it must be noted that trying to determine the non-uniform geometric properties, such as the cross-sectional area or the area moment of inertia, can be quite difficult. However, it can be simplified if comparative measurements are taken. Paired samples are usually taken when comparing a freeze-dried allograft bone to the normal bone in an animal or cadaver model. The geometry of the paired bones at identical points are the same. For testing of long bones, usually the straight mid-segment of the bone is used to ensure uniformity.

Other considerations to be taken include:

(i) State clearly the question that needs to be addressed and the clinical relevance.

(ii) Review the literature. Most of the time, the work has already been done and the answer available. Literature will also provide information on the parameters involved and the complexity of the problem.

(iii) Choose the appropriate model, e.g. animal, cadaver, bone, etc.

(iv) Carefully design your protocol to limit the variables and to focus on the particular question to be answered. This will include sample sizing, and most importantly the proper controls for the study.

(v) Ensure sufficient sample sizes for statistical significance and reproducibility.

(vi) Choose the appropriate mechanical test, e.g. tensile test for ligament and tendons, compression for cartilage and either torsion or bending for long bones.

(vii) It is essential to keep a proper log book and mantain detailed documentation of the whole study.

(viii) The key to answering question being researched comes from good analysis of the data, proper comparison with controls and previous data for confirmation and discussion with fellow research workers.

12. Conclusions

This chapter is only a brief introduction to the various terms used in biomechanics and those that are more closely related to biomechanics of allograft as a structure and a material. For further reading, the following books are recommended.

13. Recommended Books

MOW, V.C. and HAYES, W.C. (1997). *Basic Orthopaedic Biomechanics*, 2nd edn. Lippincott-Raven, New York, 453 pp.

NIGGS, B.M. and HERZOG, W. (1998). *Biomechanics of the Musculo-skeletal System*, 2nd edn. John Wiley and Sons, Chichester.

TENCER, A.F. and JOHNSON, K.D. (1974). *Biomechanics in Orthopedic Trauma: Bone Fracture and Fixation*, Martin Dunitz Ltd., London, 311 pp.

14. Appendix A — Useful Properties of Common Cross-Sections

A = area, I_o = area moment of inertia, J_o = polar moment of inertia. $\bar{y}$ = the distance of the centroid to the base of the cross-section.

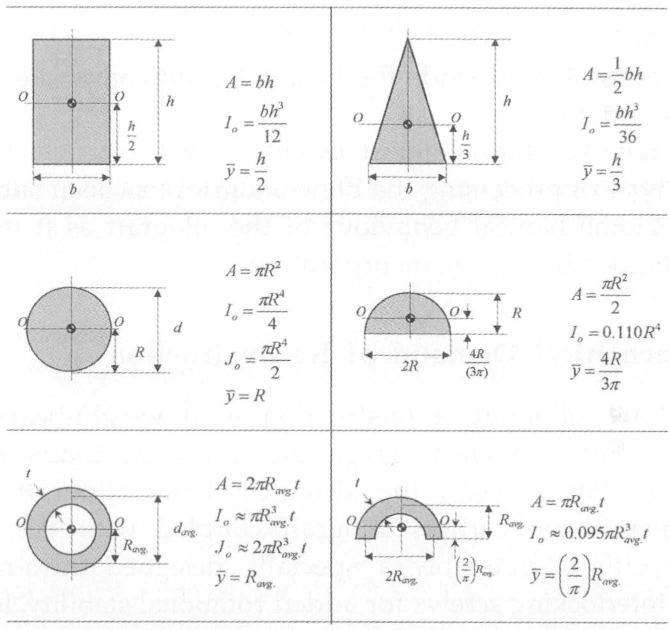

$$\text{Note} : R_{avg} = \frac{R_{outer} + R_{inner}}{2}$$

Advances in Tissue Banking Vol. 5
© 2001 by World Scientific Publishing Co. Pte. Ltd.

29 BIOMECHANICS OF BONE ALLOGRAFT TRANSPLANTATION

AZIZ NATHER

NUH Tissue Bank
National University Hospital
5 Lower Kent Ridge Road, Singapore 119074

From a biomechanical standpoint, the successful transplantation of bone allografts depends on four factors:

(i)   The physiological loads the host–allograft composite would be subjected to;

(ii) The type of bone allograft used;

(iii) The type of processing the bone allograft has been subjected to;

(iv) The biomechanical behaviour of the allograft as it unites and undergoes biological incorporation.

1. Biomechanical Demand of Reconstruction

Massive bone allograft reconstruction in a weight-bearing limb, e.g. lower limb, demands large physiological loads for early ambulation. For success, the strongest bone allograft must be used — deep-frozen cortical allograft coupled with the strongest internal fixation, preferably a specially designed intra-medullary nail with interlocking screws for added rotational stability. Resection-arthrosdesis for an osteogenic sarcoma involving the knee joint is best reconstructed using this method. Where the knee joint can be preserved and an osteoarticular allograft reconstruction is preferred, plating has to be done for internal fixation. For intercalary resection of tumour — cylindrical or hemi-cylindrical, plating must again be employed.

In other situations, where bone allografts are used to pack bone cavities as in giant cell tumour, aneurysmal bone cyst, simple bone cyst, fibrous dysplasia, enchondroma, chondroblastoma or to buttress depressed fractures as in depressed calcaneal fracture involving the subtalar joint, the biomechanical demand on the transplantation is much less. Weight-bearing is usually not needed for one to two months, though early mobilisation is required. No rigid internal fixation is necessary. Buttress plating is done for the lateral tibial condyle fracture and for calcaneal fracture to maintain the construct. For these purposes, morsellised bone allografts could be used either deep-frozen or lyophilised. Cortico-cancellous or cancellous bone allografts are usually employed.

2. Type of Bone Allograft Used

For reconstruction where the host–allograft composite is subjected to high physiological loads, especially for weight-bearing, the strongest type of bone allograft should be selected to withstan the loads. The strongest grafts are deep-frozen cortical long bones from deceased donors. Lyophilised cortical long bones should not be used. The choice of the strongest allograft is critical in determining the success or failure of the transplantation. Despite using deep-frozen cortical allograft in Mankin *et al.* (1983), series fracture of the allografts occurred in 15 out of 91 patients, an incidence of 16.5%.

In anterior spinal reconstruction following corpectomy for tumours and trauma of the spine, both deep-frozen as well as lyophilised cylindrical cortical allografts could be used. In the author's series (Nather, 1999) of 40 massive anterior spinal reconstructions using 25 deep-frozen and 9 lyophilised cortical allografts, no graft failure was seen. In all cases, strong instrumentation was used anteriorly. This showed that in the spine, for reconstruction of the anterior vertebral column following corpectomies, lyophilised cortical allografts were strong enough to withstand the physiological loads going through the reconstructed spine.

3. Effect of Different Methods of Processing on Biomechanical Strength of Bone Allograft

3.1. Deep-freezing

Sedlin (1965) showed that bones frozen at −20°C do not undergo any change in physical properties. Allograft bones are routinely preserved in electrical freezers at lower temperatures of −70°C to −80°C (enzymatic degradation being completely arrested at these lower temperatures) or cryopreserved in liquid nitrogen at −160°C to −180°C. Komender (1976) showed that bones deep-frozen at −78°C showed no change in bending, compression and torsion strength. Several authors showed that the torsional strength of bone remained unchanged at various temperatures from −20°C to 196°C (Komender, 1976; Pelkar *et al.*, 1983; 1984). Hamer *et al.* (1996) showed no change in bending strength when bones were frozen to −70°C.

3.2. Freeze-drying

Freeze-drying has been reported to cause a small increase of about 20% in the compression strength of the rehydrated bone (Pelkar *et al.*, 1984). In contrast, Komender (1976) also showed that lyophilisation increased the compression strength but rehydration of lyophilised bone restored the compression strength to normal. Triantafyllou *et al.*, (1975) showed that lyophilisation decreased the bending strength to 55–90% of controls. Pelkar *et al.* (1984) reported the observation of longitudinal microscopic and macroscopic cracks when the freeze-dried specimens were rehydrated. This could explain the reduction in strength with lyophilisation. On the other hand, Wolfinbarger *et al.* (1994) showed that there was no significant change of compression strength with deep-frozen, freeze-dried and rehydrated freeze-dried tricortical iliac crest wedges used for spinal fusion surgery.

Although freeze-drying generally weakens the bones, lyophilised grafts have been used successfully (Sneider and Bright, 1976; Spence *et al.*, 1976; Delloye 1999).

3.3. Radiation sterilisation

Several studies showed that the compression strength of bone allografts are not altered by radiation doses less than 30 kGy (Triantafyllou *et al.*, 1975; Komender, 1976; Bright *et al.*, 1983). Komender (1976) showed that 90% of torsion strength is maintained up to 30 kGy. In contrast, when the irradiation dosage was increased to 60 kGy, the specimens showed a reduction in bending, compression and torsion strength. The torsion strength was decreased to 65% by irradiation at a dose of 60 kGy and to 70% by a combination of irradiation at 30 kGy and freeze-drying. Triantafyllou *et al.* (1975) showed that the bending strength of bone was markedly reduced to 10–30% of controls by a combination of lyophilisation and radiation sterilisation at a dose of only 33 kGy.

In contrast, Hamer *et al.* (1996) showed that the bending strength of bone was reduced to 64% of control values after irradiation with 28 kGy and that the reduction in strength was also dose dependent. However, it is pertinent to note that the latest study by Zhang *et al.* (1994) showed that there was no statistical significant difference between irradiated and non-irradiated groups for both deep-frozen allografts and freeze-dried tricortical iliac crest allografts at a radiation dosage of 20–25 kGy. The authors recommended using 25 kGy for secondary sterilisation of human iliac crest wedges.

4. Biomechanical Healing of Allograft

In the healing of bone allograft, two factors are important in determining the ultimate strength of the construct:

- The fracture healing at the host–allograft junctions
- The biological incorporation of the allograft itself as shown by the parameters

— resorption activity
— new bone formation
— callus encasement index

(Dell *et al.*, 1985; Nather *et al.*, 1990)

4.1. Fracture healing of host–allograft junctions

Provided good apposition is achieved with a stable internal fixation, preferably by intra-medullary rodding, fracture healing of host allograft junction is usually achieved though it normally takes a longer time compared to the healing of host–autograft junctions (Nather, 1990; Nather and Goh, 2000). In the cat model, union was only achieved by 12 weeks with deep-frozen, cortical allografts compared to eight weeks with non-vascularised autografts.

4.2. Biological incorporation of allograft

Unlike non-vascularised autografts where significant biological incorporation occurred as quantitated by bone resorption index, new bone formation index and callus encasement index (Dell *et al.*, 1985; Nather *et al.*, 1990), deep-frozen cortical allografts remained biologically inert (Nather, 1990). There are little resorption activity, new bone formation and callus encasement.

5. Biomechanical Strength of Deep-Frozen, Non-Irradiated, Cortical Allografts

Nather and Goh (2000) studied the biomechanical strength of deep-frozen, non-irradiated, cortical bone allografts using the tibial diaphysis of the adult cat as the experimental model and compared it with the strength of vascularised and non-vascularised autografts (Nather *et al.*, 1990).

The large allograft (two-third of the tibial diaphysis) was procured from the right leg of a donor cat. During the procurement, the periosteum was removed and the graft collected under sterile conditions using the sterile double-jar technique for storage in the electrical freezer at −80°C. All allografts were stored for one month before they were transplanted into recipients (Fig. 1).

Internal fixation was done using an intramedullary rod. A total of (epiphyses shown to be closed on plain radiographs) were used, four for each observation period of 4, 6, 8, 12, 16, 28 and 36 weeks. At sacrifice, all specimens were fixed in 10% formalin together with the unoperated corresponding tibial segments (left) to act as controls (Fig. 2).

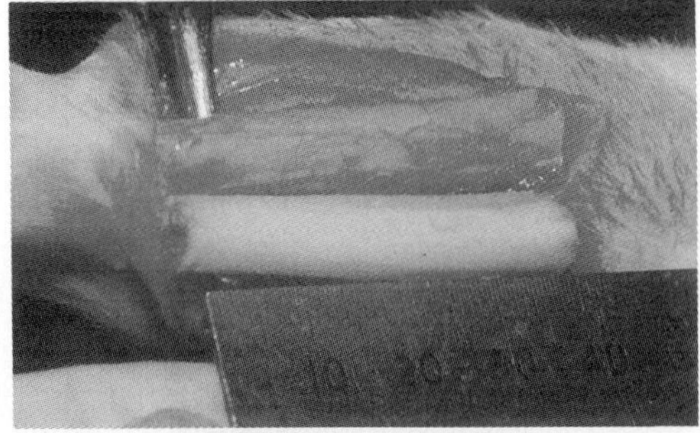

Fig. 1. Tibia in right leg of recipient cat osteotomised at both ends. Allograft (devoid) of periosteum placed beside it will be used to reconstruct this defect with intramedullary fixation.

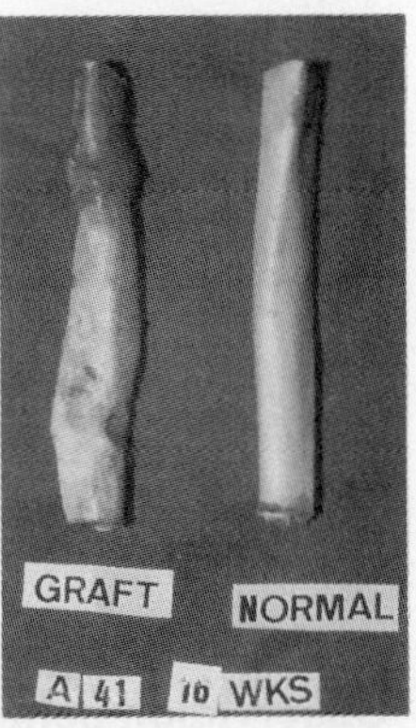

Fig. 2. At 16 weeks, the allograft shown on the left was thicker than the un-operated tibia on the right. Callus could be clearly seen at both host–graft junctions.

Each bone segment was embedded in rectangular jigs (moulds) of $3.2 \times 2.4 \times 3.2$ cm^3 using quick-setting dental cement, leaving the central 2-cm portion free for torsional testing.

Figure 3 shows the allograft mounted in rectangular jigs being loaded to failure with an external rotation torsional force. An oblique fracture is produced.

Figure 4 shows that deep-frozen, cortical, non-irradiated grafts did not achieve 100% torsional strength. The maximum torque

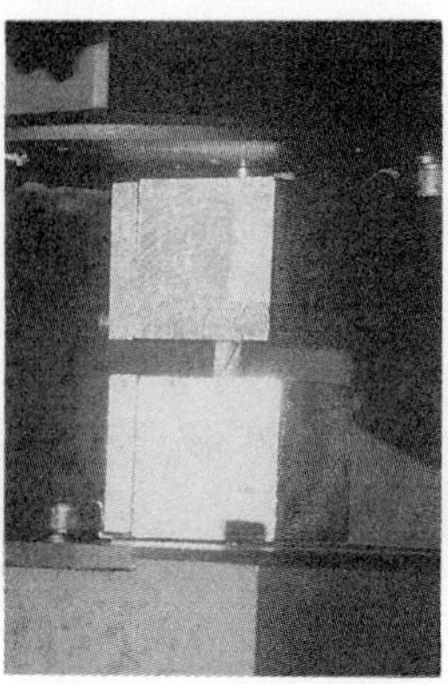

Fig. 3.   The allograft mounted in rectangular jigs being loaded to failure with an external rotation torsional force. An oblique fracture is produced.

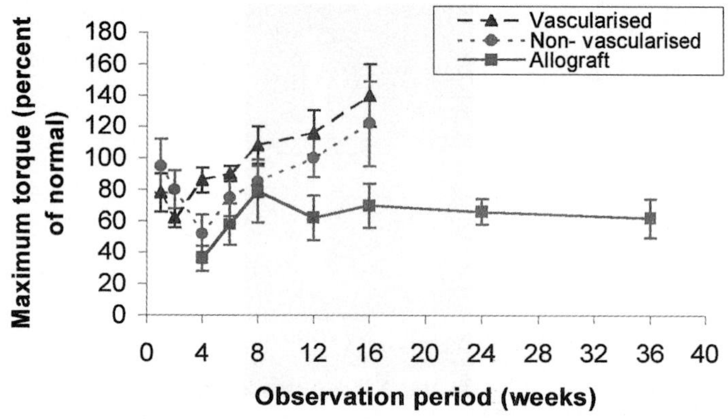

Fig. 4. Graph showing maximum torque of deep-frozen, cortical allografts, non-vascularised and vascularised autografts.

strength at nine months was only about 60% of the control value. In contrast, non-vascularised autografts attained 100% strength by 12 weeks. With vascularised autografts, 100% strength was achieved even earlier — eight weeks in the same experimental model (Nather *et al.*, 1990). Deep-frozen, cortical allografts were significantly weaker than non-vascularised and vascularised autografts at 4, 6, 12 and 16 weeks (p < 0.005).

As can be observed from Fig. 5 allografts showed higher values for torsional stiffness. The torsional stiffness achieved at six and nine months was about 80% of normal stiffness. In fracture healing, normal stiffness is achieved earlier than normal strength (Henry *et al.*, 1968; Davy and Connolly, 1982). With autografts in the adult cat, the same phenomenon was observed (Nather *et al.*, 1990). A 100% torsional stiffness was achieved by eight weeks in non-vascularised autografts.

The energy of absorption for allografts was also about 60% normal values from six weeks onwards and remained 60% even at nine months (Fig. 6). In contrast, 100% values were seen with non-vascularised and vascularised autografts by eight weeks in the adult cat.

Clinically, it must be recognised that deep-frozen, cortical allografts are significantly weaker than autografts. Therefore, for massive

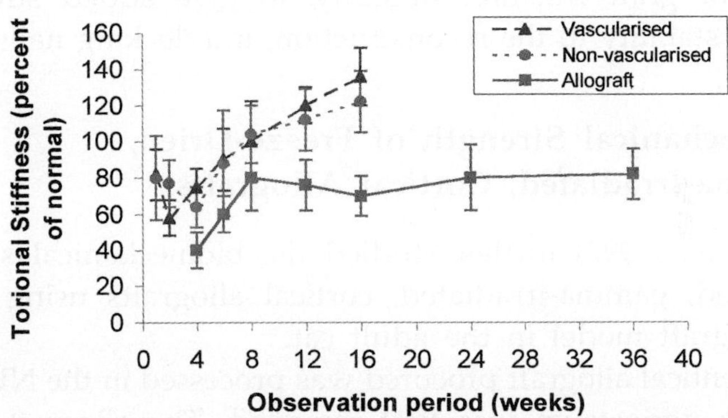

Fig. 5. Graph showing torsional stiffness of deep-frozen, cortical allograft, non-vascularised and vascularised autograft.

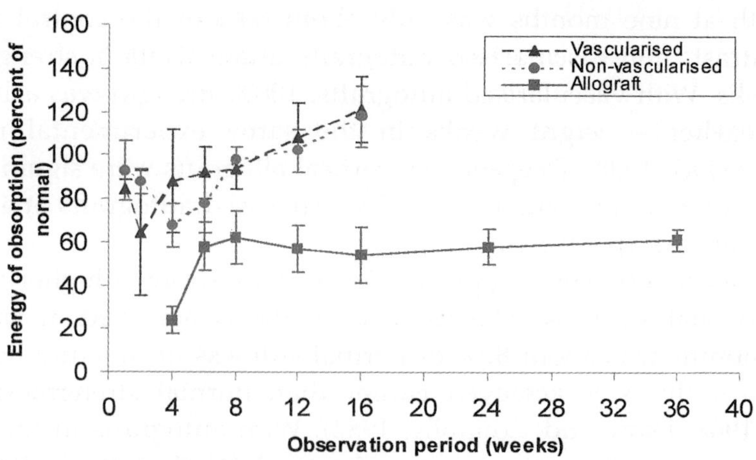

Fig. 6.   Graph showing energy of absorption of deep-frozen, cortical allografts, non-vascularised and vascularised autografts.

reconstruction of the extremities, to compensate for the intrinsic weakness of the allografts, strong, rigid, internal fixation must be employed. Specially designed intramedullary nails used for massive reconstruction of non-vascularised autografts (Enneking and Shirley, 1977) are preferred, to plates for internal fixation, especially in the lower limb, to allow for immediate weight-bearing and to reduce the rate of graft fracture. Recently, to give added strength and rotational stability to the reconstruction, interlocking nails are used.

6. Biomechanical Strength of Freeze-Dried, Gamma-Irradiated, Cortical Allografts

Nather *et al.* (1997) further studied the biomechanical strength of freeze-dried, gamma-irradiated, cortical allografts using the same tibial allograft model in the adult cat.

The identical allograft procured was processed in the NUH Tissue Bank. The periosteum was first removed. The allograft was then subjected to pasteurisation at 60°C for about three hours, and was then lyophilised till the water content was about 5%. The graft was then packed in double polyethylene bags in a laminar air-flow cabinet and was finally subjected to gamma irradiation in a gamma-chamber in the Physics Department, NUS, to a dose of 25 kGy.

Transplantation of these freeze-dried, gamma-irradiated allografts were performed in 28 cats, four for each observation period of 4, 6, 8, 12, 16, 28 and 36 weeks. The corresponding segment of the unoperated tibia (left) served as the control for each cat.

Torsional testing was performed using the same method, same equipment and jigs as were used for testing the torsional strength of deep-frozen, cortical allografts (Nather and Goh, 2000).

Figure 7 shows that the maximum torque of freeze-dried, irradiated, cortical allografts were significantly weaker than deep-frozen, cortical allografts. At nine months, the maximum torque was only 30% normal strength — half the strength of deep-frozen, cortical allografts.

Figure 8 compares the torsional stiffness of freeze-dried and deep-frozen, cortical allografts. No significant differences were noted except that at six months, the values for freeze-dried allografts were lower than those for deep-frozen allografts. At nine months, however, freeze-dried allografts achieved 60% torsional stiffness, similar to that of deep-frozen, cortical allografts.

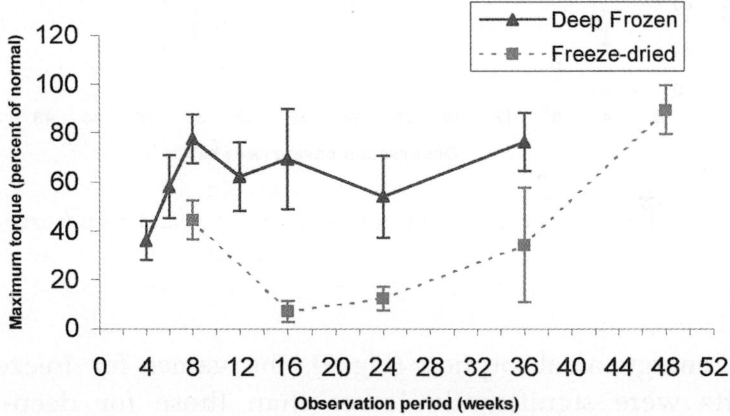

Fig. 7. Graph showing maximum torque of deep-frozen and freeze-dried cortical allografts.

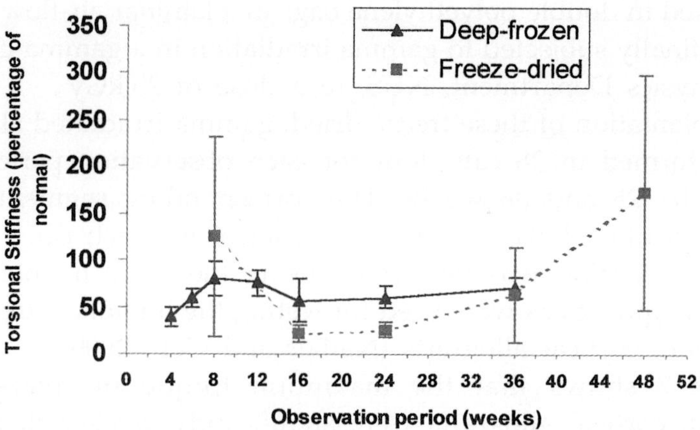

Fig. 8. Graph showing torsional stiffness of freeze-dried and deep-frozen, cortical allografts.

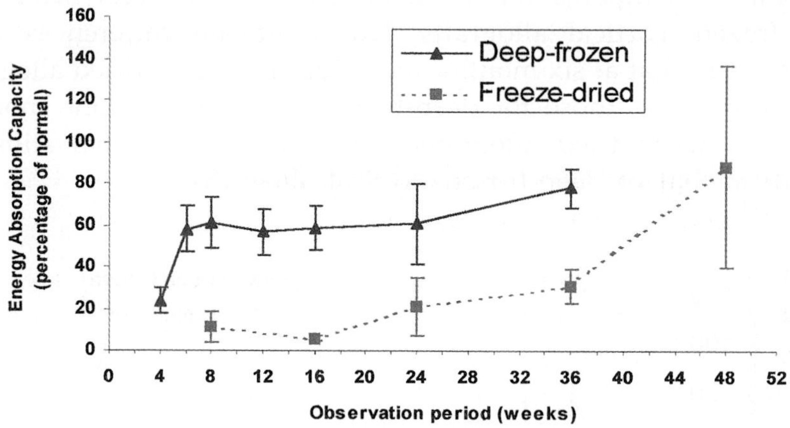

Fig. 9.   Graph showing energy of absorption of freeze-dried and deep-frozen, cortical allografts.

With energy of absorption (Fig. 9), the values for freeze-dried allografts were significantly lower than those for deep-frozen allografts at 8, 16, 24 and 36 weeks. At nine months, the values were less than half the values for deep-frozen allografts.

For clinical applications, it must be recognised that large, lyophilised, gamma-irradiated, cortical bone allografts are only half the strength of large, deep-frozen, cortical bone allografts. Therefore, they are not suitable for use in massive reconstruction of the extremities especially in the lower limbs where immediate weight-bearing is required. Even if strong, rigid intramedullary fixation is employed, the risk of graft fractures would be unacceptably high if lyophilised, irradiated allografts were used.

Lyophilised, gamma-irradiated allografts are useful as morsellised bone grafts for packing cavities in bones, such as simple bone cysts, aneurysmal bone cysts, fibrous dysplasia, benign tumours, and for packing depressed fractures, such as depressed lateral condyle fracture of the tibia ("bumper fracture") and depressed fracture of the calcaneum involving the subtalar joint. Such fractures are treated by elevating the fractures by packing with morsellised bone allografts and maintaining the construct by buttress plating. Lyophilised, gamma-irradiated, morsellised bone allografts are also useful packing cavities in the oral and maxillofacial regions.

7. Biomechanical Strength of Lyophilised Cortico-Cancellous Allografts

Nather *et al.* (1987) studied the compression strength of seventeen 12-mm lyophilised dowel grafts produced by the Bangkok Biomaterial Centre for Cloward's cervical fusion as compared with eight 12-mm deep-frozen dowel grafts from iliac crests of deceased donors in Singapore.

For standardisation, all dowel grafts were procured from a fixed reference point on the iliac wing 2 cm below and behind the anterior superior iliac spine.

The lyophilised grafts were tested after rehydration for one min (3), 5 min (7), 10 min (3) and 20 min (4).

The testing was done using the Shimadzu Universal Testing Machine Autograft DCS series with a compression test device of 500 kg force, between two rectangular moulds $4 \times 4 \times 2$ cm^3 with a central trough of 6 mm radius of curvature. The graft was tested to failure at a cross-head speed of 3 mm/min.

The results (Fig. 10) showed that with lyophilised grafts, the duration of rehydration was very important. At one and five min of rehydration, there was no difference in compression strength. However, after rehydration for 10 and 20 min, the strength was significantly reduced by 50%.

Deep-frozen cadaveric grafts were found to have the same compression strength as lyophilised grafts, provided the latter was not rehydrated for more than 5 min (Fig. 11).

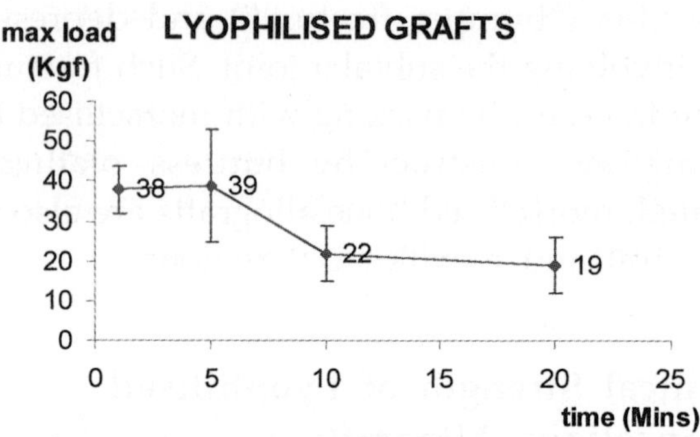

Fig. 10. Graph showing compression strength of lyophilised allografts after different periods of rehydration.

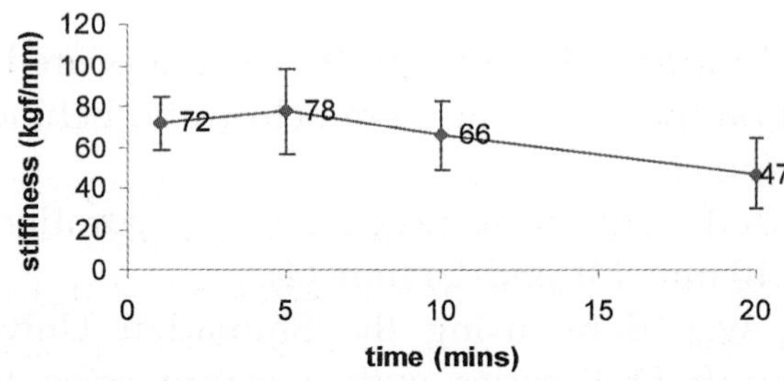

Fig. 11. Graph showing compression strength of deep-frozen and lyophilised grafts.

Clinically, one must recognise that lyophilised, cortico-cancellous allografts do become weakened with prolonged rehydration. When using such grafts, prolonged rehydration is not recommended. The lyophilised grafts could be transplanted without rehydration. Blood from the recipient bed gradually seeps into the graft and rehydrates it. There is therefore no need for prolonged rehydration with normal saline which will only weaken the graft unnecessarily.

8. Biomechanical Strength of Demineralised, Cortical Bone Allografts

With demineralised, cortical bone allografts, as would be expected after decalcification of bone, the biomechanical srength would be the weakest compared to lyophilised and deep-frozen cortical allografts. Itoman and Nakamura (1991) showed that in rats, using compression testing, deep-frozen, cortical allografts were stronger than lyophilised, cortical allografts, which in turn were stronger than demineralised, cortical allografts.

9. Summary

- Deep-frozen, cortical allografts are weaker than autografts
- Lyophilised, gamma-irradiated, cortical allografts are weaker than deep-frozen, cortical allografts
- Demineralised, cortical allografts are weaker than lyophilised, gamma-irradiated, cortical allografts.

10. Acknowledgments

The author would like to thank the National University of Singapore for the research grant RP 880334 "Use of allografts for bridging large bone defects" awarded to couduct this study. He would also like to thank Mr. S.C. Yong for all technical assistance provided, Mr. S.L. Tow and Mr. S.S. Moorthy for the excellent photographs taken, and Dr. Wang LiHui and Mrs. D.P. Vathani for the secretarial assistance provided.

11. References

BRIGHT, R. and BURCHARDT, H. (1983). The biomechanical properties of preserved bone grafts. In: *Bone Allografts: Biology, Banking and Clinical Applications*, G.E. Friedlaender, H.J. Mankin and K.W. Sell, eds., Little, Brown & Co., Boston, pp. 223–232.

DAVY, D.T. and CONNOLLY, J.F. (1982). The biomechanical behaviour of healing canine radii and ribs, *J. Biomech.* **15**, 235–247.

DELL, P.C., BURCHARDT, H. and GLOWCZEWSKIE, F.P. JR. (1985). A roentgenographic, biomechanical and histological evaluation of vascularised and non-vascularised segmental fibular canine autografts, *J. Bone Joint Surg.* **67A**, 105–112.

DELLOYE, C. (1999). The use of freeze-dried mineralised and demineralised bone. In: *Advances in Tissue Banking*, Vol. 3, G.O. Phillips, R. Von Versen, D.M. Strong and A. Nather, eds., World Scientific, Singapore, pp. 45–65.

ENNEKING, W.F. and SHIRLEY, P.D. (1977). Resection-arthrodesis for malignant and potentially malignant lesions about the knee using an intramedullary rod and local grafts, *J. Bone Joint Surg.* **59A**, 223–236.

FRIEDLAENDER, G.E. (1983). Guidelines for banking osteochondral allografts. In: *Osteochondral Allografts: Biology, Banking and Clinical Applications*, G.E. Friedlaender, H.J. Mankin and K.W. Sell, eds., Little, Brown and Co., Boston, pp. 177–180.

HAMER, A.J., STRACHAN, J.R., BLACK, M.M. *et al.* (1996). Biomechanical properties of cortical allograft bone using a new method of bone strength measurement. A comparison of fresh, fresh-frozen and irradiated bone, *J. Bone Joint Surg.* **78B**, 363–368.

HENRY, A.N., FREEMAN, M.A.R. and SWANSON, S.A.V. (1968). Studies on the mechanical properties of healing experimental fractures, *Proc. Roy. Soc. Med.* **61**, 902–906.

ITOMAN, M. and NAKAMURA, S. (1991). Experimental study on allogenec bone grafts, *Int. Orthop.* **15**, 161–165.

KOMENDER, A. (1976). Influence of preservation on some mechanical properties of human haversian bone, *Mater. Med. Pol.* **8**, 13–17.

MANKIN, H.J., DOPPELT, S.H., SULLIVAN, T.R. *et al.* (1982). Osteoarticular and intercalary allograft transplantation in the management of malignant tumours of bone, *Cancer* **50**, 613–630.

MANKIN, H.J., DOPPELT, J.H. and TOMFORD, W. (1983). Clinical experience with allograft implantation, *Clin. Orthop.* **174**, 69–86.

NATHER, A., GOH, J.C.H. and VAJARADUL, Y. (1987). Comparison of biomechanical strength of lyophilised versus fresh frozen cloward's cadaveric homografts, *Proc. 4th Int. Biomed. Engin. Symp.*, June, Singapore, pp. I-3-1–I-3-5.

NATHER, A., BALASUBRAMANIAM, P. and BOSE, K. (1990). Healing of non-vascularised diaphyseal bone transplants, *J. Bone Joint Surg.* **72B**, 830–834.

NATHER, A., GOH, J.C.H. and LEE, J.J. (1990). Biomechanical strength of non-vascularised and vascularised diaphyseal bone transplants, An experimental study, *J. Bone Joint Surg.* **72B**, 1031–1035.

NATHER, A. (1990). Healing of large diaphyseal allograft transplants. An experimental study, *Proc. Int. Soc. Fracture Repair*, September, Mayo Clinic, USA, p. 90.

NATHER, A., THAMBIAH, A., GOH, J.C.H. *et al.* (1997). Biomechanical strength of deep-frozen and lyophilised bone grafts, *Proc. 9th Int. Conf. Biomed. Engin.*, December, Singapore, pp. 93–96.

NATHER, A. (1999). Use of allografts in spinal surgery, *Ann. Transplant.* **4**, 7–10.

NATHER, A. and GOH, J.C.H. (2000). Biomechanical strength of large diaphyseal deep-frozen allografts. An experimental study, *Cell Tissue Int.* (in press).

PELKAR, R.R., FRIEDLAENDER, G.E. and MARKHAM, T.C. (1983). Biomechanical properties of bone allografts, *Clin. Orthop.* **174**, 54–57.

PELKAR, R.R., FRIEDLAENDER, G.E., MARKHAM, T.C. *et al.* (1984). Effects of freezing and freeze-drying on the biomechanical properties of rat bone, *J. Orthop. Res.* **1**, 405–411.

SEDLIN, E. (1965). A rheological model for cortical bone, *Acta Orthop. Scand.* **36**, (suppl 83): 1–77.

SCHNEIDER, J. and BRIGHT, R.W. (1976). Anterior cervical fusion using freeze-dried bone allografts, *Transplant. Proc.* **8**, (suppl 1): 73–76.

SPENCE, K., BRIGHT, R. and FITZGERALD, S. (1976). Solitary unicameral bone cyst: Treatment with freeze-dried crushed cortical bone allograft. A review of 144 cases, *J. Bone Joint Surg.* **58A**, 636–641.

TRIANTAFYLLOU, N., SOTIORPOULOS, E. and TRIANTAFYLLOU, J. (1975). The mechanical properties of lyophilised and irradiated bone grafts, *Acta Orthop. Belg.* **41**, 35–44.

WOLFINBARGER, L., ZHANG, Y., BAO-LING, T. *et al.* (1994). A comprehensive study of physical parameters, biomechanical properties and statistical correlations of iliac crest bone wedges used in spinal fusion surgery; II) Mechanical properties and correlation with physical parameters, *Spine* **19**(3), 284–295.

ZHANG, Y., HOMSKI, D., GATES, K. *et al.* (1994). A comprehensive study of physical parameters, biomechanical properties and statistical correlations of iliac crest bone wedges used in spinal fusion surgery: IV) Effect of gamma irradiation on mechanical and material properties, *Spine* **19**(3), 304–308.

SECTION VIII:

IMMUNOLOGY

Advances in Tissue Banking Vol. 5
© 2001 by World Scientific Publishing Co. Pte. Ltd.

30 BASIC PRINCIPLES OF TRANSPLANTATION IMMUNOLOGY

KAREN A. NELSON

Puget Sound Blood Center
921 Terry Avenue
Seattle, WA 98104
USA

1. Introduction

The immune system has evolved to protect us from pathogens via two types of responses. The *innate response* is the first line of defence and is not specific for the invader. This response is primarily mediated by phagocytic leukocytes: granulocytes and macrophages. The *adaptive immune response* is a specific response to the invader. It is mediated primarily by lymphocytes. An adaptive response is characterised by memory. The response to repeat exposures to the same invader is more vigorous than the first, and this memory is for life. Although the response to transplanted tissue contains elements of both types of immunity, this discussion will focus on the adaptive immune response. Space limits the ability to reference the primary sources for the concepts presented in this article. Recent editions of immunology texts are recommended sources of information not covered by the texts referenced.

2. Induction of the Immune Response by Presentation of Antigen

The adaptive immune response is set in motion by the interaction of lymphocytes with specialised cells which present antigen. Antigen-presenting cells (APCs) ingest foreign material and digest it internally. The resulting peptides are loaded into histocompatibility proteins (HLA) and displayed on the surface of the cell.

HLA molecules are heterodimers encoded by genes found on chromosome 6. The molecules are integral membrane proteins and share structural motifs with other members of the immunoglobulin supergene family. Each HLA molecule has a peptide-binding groove formed by a structure of alpha-helices and a beta-pleated sheet and also has a site which interacts with accessory molecules on T-lymphocytes. HLA molecules are inserted into the cell membrane and have a cytoplasmic tail (Fig. 1). The genes encoding for HLA class I and class II proteins exhibit a high level of polymorphism: there are literally hundreds of alleles for some loci. This amount of

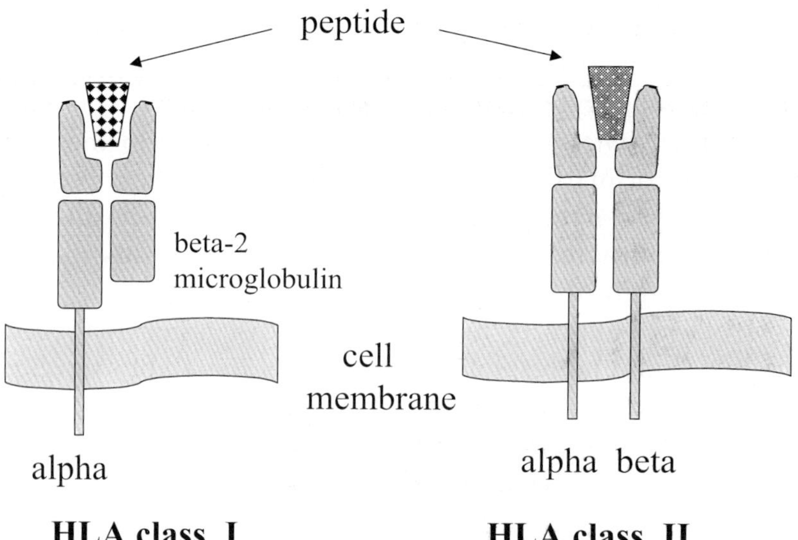

Fig. 1. HLA molecules are heterodimers inserted into the cell membrane.

polymorphism has arisen and has been maintained in order to allow presentation of peptides from any foreign invader that might prove dangerous to our survival. As expected, this polymorphism differs between peoples whose ancestors lived in different areas of the world and were exposed to different environmental pathogens. This is important when considering the chances of selecting HLA-matched donors and recipients for transplantation. Table 1 presents a recent tabulation of the number of alleles for each locus as published by the HLA Nomenclature Committee of the World Health Organisation (Bodmer *et al.*, 1999).

HLA class I antigens are expressed on the majority of nucleated cells in the body. They consist of a heavy chain carrying the HLA polymorphism associated with beta-2 microglobulin for cell surface expression. The peptides in the binding groove of HLA class I molecules are generated in the cytosol of the cell from internal proteins and loaded into the HLA molecules in the endoplasmic reticulum (ER). The structures that digest proteins into peptides, that transport peptides to the ER and that control entry into the ER are also encoded

Table 1. Extensive polymorphism of HLA genes.

Class I HLA Locus	Number of Expressed Alleles	Class II HLA Locus	Number of Expressed Alleles	MHC-Associated Locus	Number of Expressed Alleles
HLA-A*	118	HLA-DRA*	2	TAP1	6
HLA-B*	254	HLA-DRB1*	221	TAP2	4
HLA-C*	74	HLA-DRB3*	19	MICA	15
HLA-E*	5	HLA-DRB4*	7		
HLA-G*	13	HLA-DRB5*	12		
		HLA-DQA1*	19		
		HLA-DQB1*	39		
		HLA-DPA1*	15		
		HLA-DPB1*	83		

Adapted from Bodmer *et al.* (1999). Null alleles have been omitted from the tally.

in part in the complex of HLA genes. In virally infected cells, viral peptides are loaded into HLA class I molecules, identifying infected cells for destruction by T-lymphocytes. There are also tissue-specific differences in peptides presented by HLA class I proteins: recipients of kidney transplants have been shown to have T-cells responding to donor HLA–peptide complexes on renal cells that are not found on lymphocytes (Poindexter *et al.*, 1999).

HLA class II molecules also consist of two chains, both encoded by genes in the HLA complex. The three-dimensional structure of class II molecules is very close to that of class I molecules, the peptide-binding groove differs in being open on both ends to accommodate longer peptides. HLA class II molecules do not bind peptides in the ER. Their peptide-binding groove is blocked until transport to an endosomal vesicle containing digested peptides of extracellular proteins, as explained below.

HLA typing identifies the alleles of the HLA genes that were inherited by an individual from each parent. In transplantation, immune responses have been found to be different in class I and class II loci as follows:

Class I Loci   HLA A, HLA-B and HLA-C
Class II Loci   HLA-DR, HLA-DQ, and HLA-DP

Typing of all six loci is important for bone marrow or stem cell transplantation, in order to select a new immune system that will function well in the recipient. For organ or tissue transplantation, typing of HLA-A, HLA-B and HLA-DR is considered sufficient. These molecules are present at a higher density on the cell surface, and are thought to be the target of the majority of immune responses to donor antigens. However, responses to HLA-DP and to other class I antigens such as MICA, have recently been shown to be associated with graft loss. Most of the differences between alleles are substitutions of the amino acids that form the peptide-binding groove. Typing of these differences is difficult using the serological techniques that have been the gold standard for HLA typing. The majority of HLA typing is now performed using techniques which detect differences in DNA sequence corresponding to the amino acid substitutions (Nelson, 2001).

The processing and presentation of antigens from the environment outside of the cell are functions of dendritic cells, monocytes and macrophages, and B-lymphocytes. These cells have the ability to phagocytose cells or endocytose material bound to surface receptors: F_c or immunoglobulin. The material is enclosed in a series of endosomal vesicles of decreasing pH to which the cell adds digestive enzymes. The final vesicle in the series, which now contains peptides of the digested protein, coalesces with a vesicle from the Golgi containing HLA class II molecules. In this acidic compartment, the peptide-binding groove of the HLA molecule is opened, allowing binding of a peptide. Not all peptides fit, a peptide must have the appropriate amino acids at defined positions to fit into the binding pockets of the HLA molecule. The HLA molecule, now loaded with peptide, is transported to the surface of the cell and integrated into the membrane.

In transplantation, the HLA antigens of the donor are the target or antigen recognised by the T-lymphocytes. The T-lymphocyte receptor can recognise differences in sequence in the donor HLA antigens themselves and respond — a direct recognition of allo-antigen. Alternatively, the recipient's antigen-presenting cells ingest, digest and present peptides derived from donor tissue. When T-lymphocytes respond to the peptides, it is called an indirect recognition of alloantigen.

Indirect recognition is the main mode of sensitisation after tissue transplantation. Phagocytes are recruited to the surgery site as part of innate immunity. They ingest donor tissue in the process of repairing the injury and present the peptides to the recipient's T-lymphocytes.

Direct recognition is possible with transplants of fresh bone, cartilage, heart valves or corneas as these tissues may contain viable cells expressing HLA antigens and co-stimulatory molecules. Treatment of tissue to remove viable cells eliminates direct recognition of alloantigen. Processing tissues further to denature or remove donor HLA antigens also reduces chances for indirect recognition.

APCs also have other surface structures required for induction of an immune response. The "co-stimulatory" signal that these accessory molecules give to T-lymphocytes is essential for their proliferation and maturation. The molecules are identified by their cluster of differentiation or CD number. Co-stimulatory molecules include CD40, CD58, CD80 and CD86. The interaction of these molecules with their receptors on T-lymphocytes is a target for novel approaches to immunosuppression in transplant recipients. Monoclonal antibodies have been generated to bind to the molecules on the APCs and prevent delivery of the second signal to T-cells which are interacting with the MHC class II–peptide complex on that APC. The dendritic cell is emerging as the most potent APC due to its expression of high numbers of co-stimulatory molecules.

3. The Cellular Immune Response

T-lymphocytes have surface receptors (TCRs) which interact with the HLA proteins and their peptides; the presence of a foreign peptide triggers a response in a T-lymphocyte with the corresponding receptor. Most T-lymphocytes can only recognise foreign antigen when it is processed as peptides and presented by an HLA molecule. These T-cells use alpha and beta chains in their TCRs. Polymorphism is extensive, generated from germ-line genes by some of the same mechanisms that create different specificities for antibodies.

During development, T-cells traffic through the thymus where they are selected for the expression of TCRs that interact with self-HLA and peptides. In contrast, B-lymphocytes, with their surface receptors and immunoglobulin, can recognise peptides, proteins, lipids, nucleic acids, polysaccharides and chemical moieties. The TCR is made up of two chains and like HLA molecules shares motifs with other members of the immunoglobulin supergene family. On the cell surface, it is associated with the CD3 complex of proteins. If the binding of the TCR with the HLA–peptide structure is of sufficient affinity, a signal is transduced through the CD3 structure to give the first signal for T-cell activation. A small subset of T-cells use two different chains for their TCR, i.e. gamma and delta. This

TCR is also associated with CD3 but does not bind to HLA molecules and peptides. Some bind to lipoglycans produced by microbes. It is apparent that there is limited polymorphism as compared to the alpha-beta TCR.

The T-lymphocyte requires a second signal from the antigen-presenting cell to continue to respond. This second signal, called co-stimulation, is provided by the interaction of other receptors on the T-lymphocyte with structures on the antigen-presenting cell. The most potent co-stimulatory molecules on the antigen-presenting cell are CD80 and CD86. They interact with CD28 and CD152 on the T-lymphocyte. CD154 on the T cell interacts with CD40 on antigen-presenting cells. This interaction is also important for T-cell activation of B-lymphocytes. If the second signal is blocked, it halts the intra-cellular cascade of signals required for transcription of growth factors or cytokines required for further development of the T-cell and for development of other T-cells. The blocked T-cell is said to be anergic.

The T-lymphocyte plays a central, orchestrating role in both the cellular and humoral responses. There are different populations of T-lymphocytes with different functions. These populations can be distinguished by the expression of different CD antigens.

CD4 T-lymphocytes are the first to recognise foreign antigen. Their TCRs interact with HLA class II and peptides. The CD4 molecule becomes part of the CD3–TCR complex, binds to a site on the MHC class II molecule and helps stabilise the complex. CD4 T-cells make cytokines and growth factors that enable other antigen-presenting cells, CD8 T-lymphocytes and B-lymphocytes to respond. CD4 T-lymphocytes secrete cytokines that induce inflammatory responses. In the inflammatory response, elements of the innate immune system are activated. CD4 T-lymphocytes interact with B-lymphocytes to activate the humoral immune response. Growth factors and cytokines are discussed in the next section.

Mature, activated CD8 T-lymphocytes contain cytotoxic granules. They can kill infected cells or cells bearing donor HLA antigens. The TCR of CD8 T-cells interacts with HLA class I and peptides. The CD8 molecule becomes part of the CD3–TCR complex, binds to a site on the MHC class I molecule, and helps stabilise the complex.

The cellular immune response is marked by CD4 and CD8 lymphocytes trafficking into the transplant site. The activation of the cellular response most likely occurred in lymph nodes close to the transplant site or in the spleen. Donor cells may have migrated from the graft. Recipient dendritic cells or monocytes may have ingested material at the graft site and then migrated to lymph nodes or spleen. During activation, T-lymphocytes have undergone multiple rounds of cell division to increase the number of T-lymphocytes with TCRs specific for donor antigens. These T-lymphocytes have then matured to become cytokine producers or killer cells. Monocytes and other lymphocytes (called natural killer cells) also traffic into the transplant site due to recruitment by cytokines made by the T-lymphocytes.

4. The Humoral Immune Response

The humoral immune response is also activated in lymph nodes or spleen. Activation requires CD4 T-lymphocytes, antigen-presenting cells and B-lymphocytes. The B-lymphocyte has surface receptors for antigen: immunoglobulin or antibody. It requires signals or co-stimulation from the T-lymphocyte to become activated: to proliferate and mature into a plasma cell which makes antibody. The antibody molecule has a part called the variable region which binds to the antigen inducing the response, and a part called the constant region which can combine with other molecules or cells. The first antibody made in a response has an IgM constant region. If the response continues, interaction with other T-lymphocytes switches the antibody response to use an IgG constant region.

Antibody can interact with transplanted tissue in at least three ways. First, the variable region can bind to the HLA antigens on donor cells and the constant region can interact with plasma proteins called complement to destroy the donor cells. Second, antibody can bind to donor cells and mark them to be destroyed by lymphocytes and monocytes. Receptors on the lymphocytes or monocytes bind to the constant region of the antibody. Third, antibody can bind to donor cells and cause them to be "eaten" by phagocytes.

5. Immunological Memory

The induction or activation phase of the adaptive immune response lasts from one to seven days. During this time, the T-lymphocyte and B-lymphocyte populations are expanding by cell division and maturing into cells that make cytokines, killer granules or antibody. Towards the end of this period, lymphocytes appear at the site of transplant as described above, and the first antibody, IgM, appears in the blood.

Both T-lymphocytes and B-lymphocytes can mature into memory cells. After activation and proliferation, some lymphocytes become memory cells rather than effectors of the immune response. These memory lymphocytes reside in lymph nodes, spleen or bone marrow. If the same pathogen or donor HLA antigens are reintroduced, these cells rapidly respond by proliferating and maturing to provide effector T-lymphocytes and IgG antibody.

Recipients of tissue transplants may have been exposed to other people's HLA antigens as a result of blood transfusion, pregnancy or other transplants. If the HLA antigens expressed by the new donor are the same or similar to those in the previous exposure, there is a possibility of reactivating a memory immune response. Memory responses are more difficult to control than primary responses. Immuno-suppressive drugs used in organ transplantation target the early activation and proliferation phases of the immune response. These drugs are less effective in controlling a memory response.

6. Testing for Transplantation

Potential recipients of organ allografts are tested for humoral or cellular immunity to donor HLA antigens to avoid memory responses. The HLA class I and class II phenotypes are determined for the patient and donor. Other genetic polymorphisms may also be tested to determine the capacity of the recipient to mount an inflammatory response (Wilson *et al.*, 1997). Inherited differences in the intensity of production of TNF-alpha or TGF-beta cytokines may be important in predicting the recipient's ability to heal bone allografts due to their effects on osteoclasts (Fuller *et al.*, 2000; Roux and Orcel, 2000).

Testing for humoral immunity involves assays looking for IgG or IgM antibody which can bind to HLA molecules. These assays use lymphocytes from HLA-typed individuals or soluble HLA antigens immobilised on microbeads or ELISA trays. Techniques vary in sensitivity. The most sensitive techniques use fluorescence-activated flow cytometry for a quantitative measure of antibodies to HLA antigens. Testing with a panel of HLA antigens is performed during the time the patient is waiting for an allograft; the result is given as %PRA, meaning per cent panel-reactive antibody. It indicates the number of panel members to whom the patient has antibody and estimates the percentage of potential donors who would be ruled out for that patient due to prior exposure to HLA antigens of those donors. When a donor is identified, the antibody test is repeated using lymphocytes from the donor to ensure that the patient does not have immunological memory to that donor; this test is called the crossmatch. Figure 2 displays the results of a crossmatch of donor T-lymphocytes and serum with no antibody compared to serum with anti-donor antibody. The human IgG molecules binding to donor HLA antigens are detected by means of an anti-IgG reagent that is coupled to the flourochrome FITC (fluorescein isothiocyanate). The flow cytometer histogram displays the population of T-cells by the amount of FITC bound to their surface. The population of T-cells incubated with patient serum is compared to the population incubated with the negative control serum. This flow cytometry crossmatch is a very sensitive measure of anti-donor antibody.

After transplant, the appearance of antibody to donor antigens is highly correlated with incipient rejection. Assays to monitor patient sera for these antibodies alert clinicians to institute biopsy and anti-rejection protocols (Mckenna *et al.*, 2000). Recipients of large bone allografts who make antibody to their donor's class I HLA antigens also have poorer outcomes as compared to antibody-free recipients (Friedlaender *et al.*, 1999).

Measures of cellular immunity are used less frequently prior to transplant, but are used after transplant to identify patients who

Flow Cytometry Crossmatch

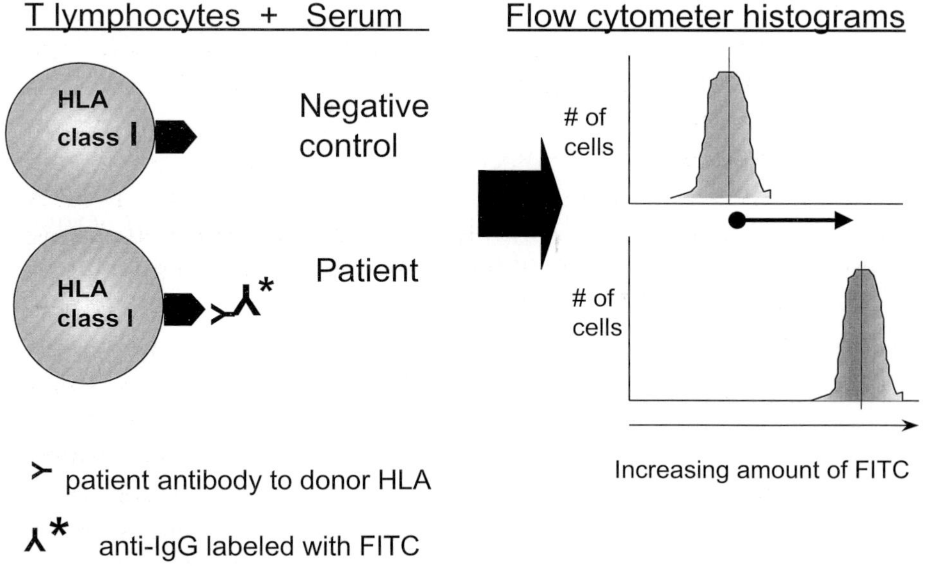

Fig. 2. Flow cytometry crossmatch.

have lost T-cells capable of responding to donor antigens and are candidates for protocols to reduce immunosuppressive medication. Recent advances include using fluorescence-activated cell analysis to identify phenotypes of T-cells responding to donor cells (Wells *et al.*, 1997) or using tetramers of HLA and peptides to identify T-cells with TCR specific for donor HLA (Mutis *et al.*, 1999).

7. Suggested Reading

ABBAS, A., LIGHTMAN, A.H. and POBER, J. (eds.) (2000). *Cellular and Molecular Immunology*, 4th edn., W.B. Saunders Co., Philadelphia.

JANEWAY, C., TRAVERS, P., WALPORT, M. and CAPRA, J.D. (eds.) (1999). *Immunobiology The Immune System in Health and Disease*, 4th edn., Garland Publishing, New York.

PARHAM, P. (ed.) (2000). *The Immune System*, Garland Publishisng, New York.

ROITT, I., BROSTOFF, J. and MALE, D. (eds.) (1998). *Immunology*, 5th edn., Mosby, London.

8. References

BODMER, J.G., MARSH, S.G.E., ALBERT, E.D., *et al.* (1999). Nomenclature for factors of the HLA system, 1998. *Tissue Antigens* **53**, 407–446.

POINDEXTER, N.J., STEWARD, N.S. and MOHANAKUMAR, T. (1999). Characterization of an HLA-A3 restricted human kidney specific T-cell clone, *Hum. Immunol.* **60**(10), 939–943.

NELSON, K. (2001). HLA typing. In: *Clinical Immunology* 2nd edn., R. Rich, T. Fleisher, B. Kotzin, W. Shearer and H. Schroeder, eds., Harcourt, London (in press).

WILSON, A.G., SYMONS, J.A., McDOWELL, T.L., *et al.* (1997). Effects of a polymorphism in the human tumor necrosis fiactor alpha promoter on transcriptional activation. *Proc. Nat. Acad. Sci. USA* **94**, 3195.

ROUX, S. and ORCEL, P. (2000). Bone loss: Factors that regulate osteoclast differentiation. An update. *Arthritis Res.* **2**, 451–456.

FULLER, K., LEAN, J.M., BAYLEY, K.E., *et al.* (2000). A role for TGF beta in osteoclast differentiation and survival. *J. Cell Sci.* **113**, 2445–2453.

McKENNA, R.M., TAKEMOTO, S.K. and TERASAKI, P.I. (2000). Anti-HLA antibodies after solid organ transplantation. *Transplantation* **69**, 31–326.

FRIEDLAENDER, G.E., STRONG, D.M., TOMFORD. W.W. and MANKIN, H.J. (1999). Long-term follow-up of patients with osteochondral allografts. A correlation between immunological responses and clinical outcomes. *Orthop. Clin. N. Am.* **30**, 583–590.

WELLS, A.D., GUDMUNDSDOTTIR, H. and TURKA, L.A. (1997). Following the fate of individual T-cells throughout activation and clonal expansion. Signals from T-cell receptor and CD28 differentially regulate the induction and duration of a proliferative response. *J. Clin. Invest.* **100**(12), 3173–3183.

MUTIS, T., GILLESPIE, G., SCHRAMA, E., FALKENBURG, J.H., MOSS, P. and GOULMY, E. (1999). Tetrameric, HLA class I-minor histocompatibility antigen peptide complexes demonstrate minor histocompatibility antigen-specific cytotoxic T-lymphocytes in patients with graft-versus-host disease. *Nat. Med.* **5**, 839–842.

SUBJECT INDEX

acetabulum   38, 52
achilles   360
ACL   494, 496, 497
ACL allografts   498
ACL reconstruction(s)   494, 495, 497–499
acromegaly   114
adaptive immune response   553
adductor magnus   27, 38
adhesion   150
AIDS   223, 227
allograft bone   424
allograft reconstruction(s)   496–498, 535
allograft transplantation   291, 438
allograft(s)   218, 290, 292, 294, 298, 300,
     301, 303, 356, 358–360, 363, 405, 407,
     412, 413, 422–424, 435–437, 443, 445,
     447, 449, 451, 455, 456, 458, 459, 461,
     463, 465, 467, 468, 470, 491–499, 507,
     531, 532, 534–538, 541–543, 545, 547,
     562
amnion   146, 147, 152, 153, 161, 163, 164,
     405, 414, 415
amnion grafts   409, 414
amniotic membrane(s)   150, 151, 162
angiogenesis   382, 384, 385, 390, 476,
     479
ankle   275
annulus fibrosus   47, 48
anterior   303
anterior cruciate ligament   491, 495
anterior cruciate ligament allografts   498

anterior cruciate ligament
     reconstruction   498
anterior cruciate replacement   494
anterior tibial artery   36
antibiotic(s)   191, 226, 301, 303
antibodies   175, 215, 223
anti-CMV   271
antigen(s)   74, 150, 192, 223, 224, 412,
     554–560, 562, 563
antigen-presenting cells (APCs)   554
anti-HCV   271
anti-HIV1   271
anti-HIV2   271
arm   282
aseptic   235, 236
autogenous transplantation   438
autograft reconstruction(s)   495, 498, 499
autograft(s)   407, 408, 411–414, 436, 437,
     440, 443, 448, 449, 451, 491, 492, 494,
     495, 498, 538, 541, 542, 547
axial loading   509
axilla   282

bacillus pumilus   353
bacteria   342
Bacteroides   187
basement membrane   129
biceps   32
bioburden   193, 200–204, 206–210,
     368
biomechanics   532

blastocyst 140–142

blood supply 63

blood vessels 97

B-lymphocytes 559

BMP(s) 420–428

bone allograft(s) 301, 435, 436, 456, 465, 467, 534, 535, 537, 545

bone autografts 434, 435

bone graft transplantation 477

bone graft(s) 296, 361, 424, 425, 435, 438, 467, 473, 488

bone graft(s) 473, 488

bone matrix 422

bone morphogenetic protein(s) 359, 361, 419, 428, 438, 481

bone(s) 73, 97, 98, 265, 270, 271, 273, 274, 284, 285, 294, 297, 298, 300, 301, 358, 360, 361, 363, 419–428, 434–436

bone–patellar-tendon–bone allografts 496

bovine spongiform encephalopathy (BSE) 183

brachial artery 20

brachial plexus 4

bremsstrahlung radiation 317

bullous keratopathy 150

burns 150

cadaveric 151

caesarean section 151

caesium-137 311

calcaneal tendons 303

calcaneo-fibular ligament 278

calcaneum 30, 275, 279, 545

calcaneum tendon(s) 280, 286

calcitonin 102

calvarium 58, 69

canaliculi 101

cancellous 44, 105

Candida albicans 187

carotid 68

carpal bones 8

carpal tunnel 16

cartilage 73, 112, 115, 119, 120, 122, 360, 361, 422, 436, 508

cauda equina 46

CD3 complex of proteins 558

chemical sterilisation 258

chondroblast(s) 114, 116, 120–122, 420

chondrocytes 109, 111, 115, 116, 119–122, 471

chorio-amnionitis 163

chorion 145–147

chorion frondosum 146

clavicle 3, 4

Clostridium perfrigens 187

Clostridium tetani 185

cobalt-60 311

coccyx 47, 51, 53

collagen fibrillogenesis 80

collagen I 424

collagen(s) 97, 74, 75, 78, 130, 147, 151, 152, 162, 359–363, 382, 384, 387, 392–395, 403, 404, 408, 414, 423, 425, 426, 471, 476, 477, 482, 483, 486, 498, 508, 514, 515, 527

compression 509, 516

compression fractures 44

Compton effect 315

conjunctival defects 150

coracoclavicular ligament 4

cornea 270, 274

cortex 487

cortical allograft(s) 441, 449, 451, 468, 536, 541, 542

cortical bone allografts 436

cortico-cancellous allografts   451, 547
Corynebacterium diphtheriae   185
cotyledons   145
creep   530
creeping substitiution   437
Creutzfeld-Jakob disease (CJD)   183, 225,
      352, 368
cruciate ligament   41
cubital fossa   6
culture   190, 201, 206, 209, 215, 220, 222,
      226, 267–270, 274, 285, 287, 289, 294,
      413, 427
curriculum   xix
   multimedia   xix
cytokine(s)   383, 385, 386, 393, 395, 404,
      405, 474, 476, 559–561
cytomegalovirus   216, 358

D_{10} 353, 355
D_{10} value   210
deceased donor(s)   265, 266, 274, 275,
      288, 535, 545
deep-frozen   465
deep-frozen allografts   451, 456, 499, 543
deep-frozen bones   303
deep-frozen cortical allograft   535, 538,
      547
deformation   509, 510
demineralised bone   426
dendritic cells   134
dermal cells   132
diaphysis   98, 111, 113
diploma course   xx
disinfection   193, 194
distance learning   xix
donor antigens   562
donor autografts   492
donor HLA   563
donor procurement   271

donor(s)   235, 265, 271, 273, 274, 292,
      294, 297, 301, 303, 304, 342, 356,
      358, 407–409, 412, 414, 425, 435,
      492, 538, 555–557, 559–563
dorsalis pedis artery   36
dose   328
dosimetry   336
double-jar   292
   sterile   292

ECM   93
elastic deformation   510
elastic strain energy   519
elastin   92, 130, 131
elbow   3
electromagnetic radiation   317
endochondral   99
endosteal   449
endosteal osteoblasts   477
endosteum   103, 109, 420, 478
Enterococcus faecalis   187
epidemic   178
epidermis   126
epidermopoiesis   137
epiphysis   98, 111, 113, 114
Epstein-Barr virus   213, 217
erector spinae   49
Escherichia coli   181, 187
extensor digitorum longus   33
external iliac artery   35
extracellular matrix   73, 74, 133, 384, 392

facet joints   49
facial nerve   65, 70
facial palsy   70
factors   475
fascia lata   280, 288, 286, 303, 304, 306,
      496
fascia lata allograft(s)   492, 496

femoral artery   35, 55
femoral head procurement   267
femoral head(s)   266–268, 275, 278, 286,
     292, 294
femoral nerve   38
femoral vein   55
femur   25, 38, 39, 41, 52, 98, 236, 266,
     275, 278, 286, 288, 427, 434, 435
fibroblast growth factors   483
fibroblast(s)   103, 114, 120, 122, 130, 132,
     133, 147, 152, 163, 164, 381, 383–387,
     389, 390, 392–395, 402–405, 409, 413,
     414, 476, 477, 479, 482, 483
fibrocartilage   121
fibronectin   131
fibula   28, 41, 278, 279, 434, 443
filopodia   101
fingers   3
foot   29, 241
foramina   44
force   510
force-deformation curve   510
forearm   3
fore limb   3
fracture(s)   114, 420, 422, 424–426, 443,
     458, 463, 535, 538, 540, 542, 545
freeze drying   358
freeze-dried allograft(s)   496, 544
freeze-dried bone   480
freeze-dried bone grafts   359
freeze-dried cortical bone allografts   436
fresh   152
fresh-frozen allograft   497
frozen   152
frozen allografts   496
fungi   183, 342

gamma   152, 311, 493

gamma irradiation   292, 436, 493, 496,
     543
gamma radiation   312–314, 316, 318, 331,
     370
gene therapy   426, 428
gene transfer   426, 427
glenoid fossa   59, 61
glenoid labrum   9
gloves   249
good manufacturing practices   333
good radiation practices   334
gown   249
graft bone   474
graft donor   423
graft failure   407
graft incorporation   438
graft(s)   151, 152, 297, 301, 303, 304, 358,
     362, 367, 406–411, 413–415, 422–425,
     438, 456, 461, 467, 468, 470, 477, 478,
     480, 484–488, 491–494, 496–498, 535,
     538, 540, 545–547, 556, 560
great saphenous vein   37
greater trochanter   25
growth   475
growth factors   419, 420, 428, 473–476,
     484, 559

α-herpesviruses   214
β-herpesviruses   214
γ-herpesviruses   214
Haemophilus influenzae   187
hallucis longus   33
hamstrings   32
Haversian canal(s)   105, 107
HbsAg   152, 271
HBV   213, 225
HCV   152, 213
head   150

heart 270
Helicobacter pylori 187
hemiarthroplasty 266
hemidesmosome 129
hepatitis 213, 214, 216, 354, 358, 367, 492
hepatitis A 179
hepatitis B 179, 188, 213, 223, 265
hepatitis B core IgG/IgM 152
hepatitis C 265
hip 240, 266, 435
hip bone 52
histocompatibility proteins (HLA) 554, 557
histogenesis 108, 120
HIV 222–225, 358, 359, 367, 492
HIV1 265
HIV-1 152
HIV-1 P24 antigen 152
HIV2 265
HLA antigens 560–562
HLA class I 555
HLA class II molecules 556
HLA typing 271
Hofbauer cells 147
HTLV-1 152
human immunodeficiency virus 367
humeral bone 284
humeral head 284
humerus 5, 98, 282, 284, 288
    head of 9
hyaluronan 88

IGF 487
iliac artery 54, 55
iliac bone 282
iliac crest(s) 51, 52, 275, 286, 287, 424, 425, 536, 537, 545
iliac vein 55
iliacus 30

immune system 553
implants 69
inferior dental artery 63
inferior dental nerve 62, 69
innate response 553
intercellular matrix 73, 97
intercondylar eminence 28
International Atomic Energy Agency (IAEA) xix
intervertebral discs 44, 47, 49
intramembranous 99
ionisation 366
irradiation 152, 312, 337, 354–356, 360, 362, 363, 366, 367, 370, 436, 493, 494, 496, 537
irradiation sterilisation 334, 493
ISO 11737-1 207
ISO documents 203

joint 425
joints of Lushka 45

keratinisation 137
keratinocyte(s) 127, 128, 380, 383–386, 390–392, 394, 395, 405, 408, 409, 413
kidney(s) 270, 274
Klebsiella 187
knee 38, 39, 266, 277
kyphotic 45

lacunae 101, 105, 109, 111
laminin 131
Langerhans 127
Langerhans cells 135
large 449
lesser trochanter 54
ligament(s) 48, 271, 273, 360, 508, 527, 529
ligamentum 28

ligamentum patellae 28
ligamentum teres 25
limb 240, 241, 271, 287, 534
lingual nerve 70
liver 270, 274
living donors 265, 266, 286
load 511
load-deformation curve 510
load-displacement curve 510
lordosis 46
lower limb(s) 239, 274, 275, 277, 289, 436, 530, 534, 545
lyophilisation 536, 537

major histocompatibility antigens 493
major histocompatibility complex 134, 412
mandible 59–62, 65, 69, 484, 487
marrow 298, 300
mast cells 133
mastication 64
matrix 103, 111, 113
maxilla 66, 68, 69
maxillary sinuses 65
maxillary tuberosity 69
maxillofacial 434
melanocytes 128
menisci 277
mental nerve 62
mesoblasts 146
metacarpal 8
metaphysis 98, 113
metatarsal 29
microangiography 445, 447
microbiology 175, 176
microorganisms 342
muscles 30, 49, 53, 64
Mycobacterium tuberculosis 181, 190

nasal cavity 65, 68
neck 150
nerve fibres 125
nerve root(s) 42, 43, 46
nerve(s) 69, 97, 409
nucleus pulposus 47, 48

obturator nerve 38
ocular surface disorders 150
olfactory nerve 70
ophthalmology 150
orbits 65
organ allograft(s) 561
organ transplantation 561
organogenesis 420
orofacial reconstruction 66
orthopaedic 434
ossification 108, 109, 111
ossification centre(s) 99, 108, 114
osteoarthritis 266
osteoblast collagen 482
osteoblast(s) 103, 108, 109, 111, 113, 361, 419–421, 479, 481–484
osteoclast(s) 101, 102, 111, 113, 478, 482, 562
osteoconduction 436, 437, 451
osteocytes 101, 105, 109, 443
osteocytic osteolysis 101
osteogenesis 363, 436, 438, 451
osteoid 100, 109, 361
osteoinduction 361, 436, 437, 451
osteoporosis 44
osteoprogenitor 100, 103, 109
otolaryngologic 150

pair production 316
palate 66
pandemic 178

papilla 132
papillary dermis 131
paracetic acid 194
parathormone 102
pasteurisation 194, 542
patella 26, 39, 359, 492
patella tendon(s) 275, 280, 286, 303
patella-tendon–tibial-tuberosity 277
pectoral girdle 3
pedicle 44
pelvic 150
pelvic girdles 42
pelvis 51, 56
perichondrium 116, 120, 122
periosteum 64, 103, 109, 114, 298, 420, 438, 440, 443, 449, 456, 459, 463, 478, 538, 542
peroneus tertius 33
phalanges 29
photoelectric effect 315
physical sterilisation 258
placenta 139, 141, 142, 144, 145, 151
plantar flexors 34
plastic bones 274
plastic deformation 511
platelet-derived growth factor(s) (PDGF) 383, 384, 387, 419, 473, 475, 476, 479, 484, 486, 487
platelet-rich plasma (PRP) 473, 481, 484–488
Poisson's ratio 516
polynucleosis 158
popliteal artery 35
popliteal fossa 38
posterior cruciate ligament 41
posterior crural muscles 33
posterior tibial artery 36
premolar 62

prions 183
processing 344, 356, 358, 557
procurement 235, 236, 266, 267, 270, 271, 273, 274, 275, 277, 289, 344, 436
profunda femoris 35
prostheses 435, 436, 455
proteoglycans 80
Pseudomonas 187
psoas major 30, 54
psoas minor 30
pubic tubercle 51
pubis 240
pubis symphysis 56

quadriceps femoris 27
quadriceps tendon 492
quality 3, 25, 42, 51, 58, 73, 97, 115, 123

radial nerve 5
radiation 210, 309–321, 325, 327–329, 333, 339, 346–356, 359–368, 537
radiation dose 314
radiation stability 328, 329, 331
radiation sterilisation 328, 331, 333, 334, 338, 340, 346, 358, 368, 537
radiation sterilisation of tissue grafts xix
radioactivity 313
radioisotopes 311
radius 6, 282, 284, 288
rami 55, 59
ramus 62, 69
reconstruct 491
reconstructed allograft ACL 497
reconstruction(s) 287, 306, 422, 425, 435, 436, 455, 465, 467, 468, 473, 478, 484, 487, 488, 491, 492, 494, 495, 497, 499, 534, 535, 542, 545
regeneration 114, 122

regional training centre   xix
rehydration   303, 546
rejection   150
resorption   438, 443, 449, 456, 477, 479,
      481, 482, 493, 538
reticular dermis   131
retromolar   69
revascularisation   409, 412, 439, 443, 449
ribs   46
RPR (TPHA)   271

sacral canal   46
sacral plexus   55
sacral promontory   46
sacro-iliac joints   56
sacrum   46, 49, 51, 53, 56
sagittal split osteotomy   69
salmonella typhi   191
scapula   4
scar   150
sciatic nerve   32
sebum   136
sensory nerves   61
serological tests   152, 226
sesamoid   27
sesmoid   98
shaft   98
Sharpey's fibres   103
shear   509
shoulder   3, 42, 282, 435
sigmoid notch   59
skin   123, 124, 136–138, 186, 189, 226,
      236, 239, 250, 360, 361, 380, 392,
      394, 395, 405–407, 409, 411, 414, 530
skin allograft(s)   409, 411, 412
skin autografts   409, 412
skin graft(s)   138, 407–409, 488
skin grafting   149

skin xenografts   405, 409, 414
skull   45, 58, 65
soft tissue allografts   292
speech   64
spinal canal   43
spinal cord   42, 43
spinal fusion   425
spine   42, 44, 45, 425
stenosis   423
steoblasts   100
sterile   201, 265, 267–269, 273, 274, 285,
      286, 383
sterilisation   193, 194, 200–202, 209, 210,
      225, 236, 253–261, 327, 328, 333, 339,
      346, 347, 356, 360, 367, 493, 496, 499,
      537
   radiation   209
sterility   235, 240, 241
sterility assurance level   338
sternoclavicular joint   4
Stevens-Johnsons disease   150
Still's disease   61
Streptococcus pneumoniae   187
Streptococcus pyogenes   187
stress relaxation   530
stress–strain curve   517
structural stiffness   512
subdermal plexus   132
subpapillary plexus   132
symphysis   49, 69
symphysis pubis   51, 52
synovial joint   44
syphilis   152, 265

tarsal   29
teeth   73
temporo-mandibular joint surgery   70
tendo-achilles   30, 279

tendon(s)   73, 98, 360, 527, 529
TGFβ   384
thigh   31
thumb   3
tibia   28, 39, 41, 98, 275, 278, 279, 286,
      288, 438, 443, 445, 543, 545
tibial fracture   424
tibial nerve   34
tibialis anterior   32, 275, 282, 286
tibialis posterior   34, 275, 282, 286, 303
tissue   408
tissue bank   xx
tissue bank operators   xix
tissue culture   152
tissue regeneration   74
T-lymphocyte(s)   134, 558
T-lymphotropic virus   358
TMJ   61
TMJ ankylosis   61
torsion   509
total hip replacement   266
total knee replacement   266
trabeculae   111
transforming growth factor (TGF)   383,
      419, 473, 476, 477
transforming growth factor beta
      (TGF-beta)   481–484, 486, 487
transplant(s)   217, 218, 298, 358, 411, 434,
      436, 478, 556, 557, 560–562

transplantation   213, 225, 358, 406,
      408–410, 412, 413, 436, 443, 445,
      451, 470, 494, 495, 534, 535, 555–557
trigelminal nerve   61
triple-wrap   292
   sterile   297
TT virus   213
tuberosity   66
tumour(s)   150, 422, 425, 455, 535, 545

ulcers   150
ulna   8, 282, 284, 288
ultimate   511
upper limb   274, 282, 284

varicella-zoster   215
vertebra(e)   42–49, 53
vertebral artery   45
villi   146
viruses   183, 342
Volkman's canals   107, 114

wrist   282

xenogenic grafts   487
xenograft(s)   405, 407, 413, 414, 436, 437

yield point   511